State-of-the-Art Environmental Chemicals Exposomics and Metabolomics

State-of-the-Art Environmental Chemicals Exposomics and Metabolomics

Minjian Chen

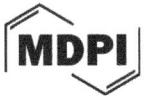

Basel • Beijing • Wuhan • Barcelona • Belgrade • Novi Sad • Cluj • Manchester

Minjian Chen
Department of Occupational Medicine
and Environmental Health
Nanjing Medical University
Nanjing
China

Editorial Office
MDPI AG
Grosspeteranlage 5
4052 Basel, Switzerland

This is a reprint of articles from the Special Issue published online in the open access journal *Toxics* (ISSN 2305-6304) (available at: www.mdpi.com/journal/toxics/special_issues/63NW1T7AB5).

For citation purposes, cite each article independently as indicated on the article page online and using the guide below:

Lastname, A.A.; Lastname, B.B. Article Title. *Journal Name* **Year**, *Volume Number*, Page Range.

ISBN 978-3-7258-2132-7 (Hbk)
ISBN 978-3-7258-2131-0 (PDF)
https://doi.org/10.3390/books978-3-7258-2131-0

© 2024 by the authors. Articles in this book are Open Access and distributed under the Creative Commons Attribution (CC BY) license. The book as a whole is distributed by MDPI under the terms and conditions of the Creative Commons Attribution-NonCommercial-NoDerivs (CC BY-NC-ND) license

Contents

About the Editor vii

Minjian Chen
Environmental Chemical Exposomics and Metabolomics in Toxicology: The Latest Updates
Reprinted from: *Toxics* **2024**, *12*, 647, doi:10.3390/toxics12090647 1

Xiao Ning, Yongli Ye, Jian Ji, Yanchun Hui, Jingyun Li and Po Chen et al.
Restricted-Access Media Column Switching Online Solid-Phase Extraction UHPLC–MS/MS for the Determination of Seven Type B Trichothecenes in Whole-Grain Preprocessed Foods and Human Exposure Risk Assessment
Reprinted from: *Toxics* **2024**, *12*, 336, doi:10.3390/toxics12050336 5

Xiao Ning, Lulu Wang, Jia-Sheng Wang, Jian Ji, Shaoming Jin and Jiadi Sun et al.
High-Coverage UHPLC-MS/MS Analysis of 67 Mycotoxins in Plasma for Male Infertility Exposure Studies
Reprinted from: *Toxics* **2024**, *12*, 395, doi:10.3390/toxics12060395 24

Chengzhi Liu, Shuang Chen, Jiangliang Chu, Yifan Yang, Beilei Yuan and Huazhong Zhang
Multi-Omics Analysis Reveals the Toxicity of Polyvinyl Chloride Microplastics toward BEAS-2B Cells
Reprinted from: *Toxics* **2024**, *12*, 399, doi:10.3390/toxics12060399 43

Jun Yao, Pengfei Zhou, Xin Zhang, Beilei Yuan, Yong Pan and Juncheng Jiang
The Cytotoxicity of Tungsten Ions Derived from Nanoparticles Correlates with Pulmonary Toxicity
Reprinted from: *Toxics* **2023**, *11*, 528, doi:10.3390/toxics11060528 57

Junyi Lv, Qing He, Zixiang Yan, Yuan Xie, Yao Wu and Anqi Li et al.
Inhibitory Impact of Prenatal Exposure to Nano-Polystyrene Particles on the MAP2K6/p38 MAPK Axis Inducing Embryonic Developmental Abnormalities in Mice
Reprinted from: *Toxics* **2024**, *12*, 370, doi:10.3390/toxics12050370 67

Haixin Li, Dandan Miao, Haiting Hu, Pingping Xue, Kun Zhou and Zhilei Mao
Titanium Dioxide Nanoparticles Induce Maternal Preeclampsia-like Syndrome and Adverse Birth Outcomes via Disrupting Placental Function in SD Rats
Reprinted from: *Toxics* **2024**, *12*, 367, doi:10.3390/toxics12050367 81

Zhaofeng Liang, Shikun Fang, Yue Zhang, Xinyi Zhang, Yumeng Xu and Hui Qian et al.
Cigarette Smoke-Induced Gastric Cancer Cell Exosomes Affected the Fate of Surrounding Normal Cells via the Circ0000670/Wnt/β-Catenin Axis
Reprinted from: *Toxics* **2023**, *11*, 465, doi:10.3390/toxics11050465 96

Bo Xu, Wei Gao, Ting Xu, Cuiping Liu, Dan Wu and Wei Tang
A UPLC Q-Exactive Orbitrap Mass Spectrometry-Based Metabolomic Study of Serum and Tumor Tissue in Patients with Papillary Thyroid Cancer
Reprinted from: *Toxics* **2022**, *11*, 44, doi:10.3390/toxics11010044 111

Kun Zhou, Miaomiao Tang, Wei Zhang, Yanling Chen, Yusheng Guan and Rui Huang et al.
Exposure to Molybdate Results in Metabolic Disorder: An Integrated Study of the Urine Elementome and Serum Metabolome in Mice
Reprinted from: *Toxics* **2024**, *12*, 288, doi:10.3390/toxics12040288 122

Huazhong Zhang, Jinsong Zhang, Jinquan Li, Zhengsheng Mao, Jian Qian and Cheng Zong et al.
Multi-Omics Analyses Reveal the Mechanisms of Early Stage Kidney Toxicity by Diquat
Reprinted from: *Toxics* **2023**, *11*, 184, doi:10.3390/toxics11020184 137

Jianjun Liu, Wenyu Kong, Yuchen Liu, Qiyao Ma, Qi Shao and Liwen Zeng et al.
Stage-Related Neurotoxicity of BPA in the Development of Zebrafish Embryos
Reprinted from: *Toxics* **2023**, *11*, 177, doi:10.3390/toxics11020177 149

Binxiong Wu, Yuntian Xu, Miaomiao Tang, Yingtong Jiang, Ting Zhang and Lei Huang et al.
A Metabolome and Microbiome Analysis of Acute Myeloid Leukemia: Insights into the Carnosine–Histidine Metabolic Pathway
Reprinted from: *Toxics* **2023**, *12*, 14, doi:10.3390/toxics12010014 166

Xinwei Xu, Lan Zhang, Yuyun He, Cong Qi and Fang Li
Progress in Research on the Role of the Thioredoxin System in Chemical Nerve Injury
Reprinted from: *Toxics* **2024**, *12*, 510, doi:10.3390/toxics12070510 182

About the Editor

Minjian Chen

Dr. Minjian Chen is a professor and doctoral supervisor at the Department of Occupational Medicine and Environmental Health at the School of Public Health, Nanjing Medical University. He is a member of the State Key Laboratory of Reproductive Medicine and Offspring Health of China and the Key Laboratory of Modern Toxicology of the Ministry of Education of China. He focuses on environmental exposomics, metabolomics, and reproductive and developmental health. He has taken the integration of exposomes and metabolomes as the key to discovering new reproductive and developmental toxicants and underlying mechanisms and established an efficient integrated analysis method of environmental chemical exposomes and metabolomes for the reproductive and developmental toxicological study; carried out extensive risk assessment based on the population study with a large sample size; screened out a series of reproductive and developmental toxicants; revealed the molecular mechanisms underlying reproductive and developmental toxicities; and contributed to the discipline of reproductive and developmental toxico-metabolomics. He has published 52 SCI papers in *EHP*, *Mol Cell*, and *Natl Sci Rev* as corresponding or first author (including co-authors); obtained 15 patents (all first); presided over three NSFC projects; won the Toxics 2022 Young Investigator Award and the Technical Innovation Award of Jiangsu Society of Toxicology (the first); and serves as an executive member of the Youth Committee of the Chinese Society of Toxicology (CST).

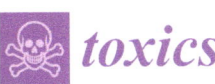

Editorial

Environmental Chemical Exposomics and Metabolomics in Toxicology: The Latest Updates

Minjian Chen [1,2]

1 State Key Laboratory of Reproductive Medicine and Offspring Health, Center for Global Health, School of Public Health, Nanjing Medical University, Nanjing 211166, China; minjianchen@njmu.edu.cn
2 Key Laboratory of Modern Toxicology of Ministry of Education, School of Public Health, Nanjing Medical University, Nanjing 211166, China

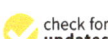

Citation: Chen, M. Environmental Chemical Exposomics and Metabolomics in Toxicology: The Latest Updates. *Toxics* **2024**, *12*, 647. https://doi.org/10.3390/toxics12090647

Received: 28 August 2024
Revised: 3 September 2024
Accepted: 3 September 2024
Published: 4 September 2024

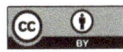

Copyright: © 2024 by the author. Licensee MDPI, Basel, Switzerland. This article is an open access article distributed under the terms and conditions of the Creative Commons Attribution (CC BY) license (https://creativecommons.org/licenses/by/4.0/).

1. Introduction

This Editorial introduces the Special Issue titled "State-of-the-Art Environmental Chemical Exposomics and Metabolomics". Due to the complexity and variability of human exposures, there is increasing interest in exploring the relationship between environmental exposures and human health from a more comprehensive perspective. This interest has spurred the development of the concept of chemical exposomes, which aims to thoroughly evaluate chemical exposures and their associated risks [1]. Metabolomics, which focuses on the high-throughput detection of endogenous chemicals, systematically identifies small molecule substrates, intermediates, and products of cellular metabolism, which are considered to be closest to the phenotype and provide important information for understanding physiological and pathological processes, making it highly significant in toxicology [2]. By integrating environmental chemical exposomics with metabolomics, researchers can gain valuable information for identifying key chemicals that lead to adverse outcomes and their toxic metabolic signatures, thereby clarifying the potentially harmful effects of these chemical exposures and the underlying mechanisms involved.

This Special Issue contains 13 articles—12 research papers and 1 review. The research papers focus on developing new methods for detecting specific chemical exposomes, exploring new aspects of exposome-related toxicity, applying metabolomics, and integrating metabolic information with exposomics and other omics across different biological layers in toxicology. The review article focuses on a neurotoxicity-related system linked to metabolism targeted by multiple chemicals. These articles advance our understanding of environmental chemical exposomes and metabolomics within toxicology.

2. An Overview of Published Articles

Detecting chemicals related to the exposome involves the development of new methods, which is both necessary and challenging. Mycotoxins, secondary metabolites produced by molds and fungi, are a major concern due to their potential contamination of agricultural products and various foods. These toxins pose risks to human health and livestock and are an integral part of the exposome. For external exposure, Ning et al. (contribution 1) introduced a novel, convenient, and sensitive quantitative method for detecting trace levels of seven type B trichothecene mycotoxins in preprocessed whole-grain foods. This method was applied to 160 food samples from China, revealing mycotoxin contamination in 70% of the samples, with whole-wheat dumpling wrappers exhibiting the highest contamination rate, posing a significant health threat. For internal exposure, Ning et al. (contribution 2) developed a highly sensitive and comprehensive analytical method for quantifying 67 mycotoxins in human plasma using mass spectrometry. This method identified 40 mycotoxins, including 24 emerging ones, in 184 plasma samples from both infertile and healthy males. Notably, infertile males had significantly higher levels of multiple mycotoxins, especially ochratoxins A and B and citrinin; this highlights the need for further research investigating the link between mycotoxins and male infertility.

This Special Issue presents four articles addressing novel exposures within the chemical exposome—two focus on nanomaterials, while the other two concentrate on micro/nanoplastics. These studies employed metabolomics and integrated information from other omics and biological layers, such as transcriptomics, to provide new insights into the pulmonary and reproductive toxicities associated with these materials. Liu et al. (contribution 3) examined the effects of polyvinyl chloride microplastics (PVC-MPs) on human lung cells, finding that PVC-MPs reduced BEAS-2B cell viability. Bioinformatics analysis, through analyzing the changes in the metabolome and transcriptome, showed that PVC-MPs disrupted lipid metabolic pathways including glycerophospholipid metabolism, glycerolipid metabolism, and sphingolipid metabolism, affecting 530 genes and 3768 metabolites. Yao et al. (contribution 4) reported the cytotoxicity of tungsten ions in BEAS-2B cells, including chromatin condensation and organelle damage; however, they noted that the ion chelator EDTA-2Na reduced these effects, suggesting potential therapeutic strategies. Lv et al. (contribution 5) investigated the embryotoxic effects of polystyrene nanoplastics (PS-NPs) in mice and human trophoblastic cells, finding that 30 nm PS-NPs caused abnormal embryonic development, a reduced placental weight, and altered the p38 MAPK pathway. PS-NPs also impaired HTR-8/SVneo cell vitality and migration. Li et al. (contribution 6) assessed the impact of titanium dioxide nanoparticles (TiO_2 NPs) on pregnant rats and their offspring. The authors found maternal preeclampsia-like symptoms, fetal growth restriction, and impaired trophoblastic cell invasion into the endometrium due to autophagy. Another significant component of the chemical exposome featured in this Special Issue is cigarette smoke. Exosomes are natural carriers secreted by cells to transport a diverse range of cargo, including numerous biological molecules such as proteins, nucleic acids, and metabolites, between different cells. Liang et al. (contribution 7) explored the effects of cigarette smoke, revealing that smoke extract enhanced stemness and epithelial-to-mesenchymal transition (EMT) in gastric cancer cells, finding that exosomal circ0000670 promoted gastric cancer development via the Wnt/β-catenin pathway.

Metabolomics and changes in endogenous metabolites provide insights that are close to pathological states. Therefore, focusing on metabolite information, their regulation, and effects is an effective way to study disease biomarkers, pathogenesis, and chemical toxicities. Xu et al. (contribution 8) reported the metabolomic characteristics of papillary thyroid cancer (PTC) by analyzing serum and tissue between patients with and without lymph node metastasis using UPLC-Q-Exactive mass spectrometry, offering new perspectives on diagnosing and treating PTC. This Special Issue includes studies on the toxicity mechanisms related to endogenous metabolites, integrating metabolome data with exposome, transcriptome, and microbiome information, focusing primarily on amino acid, lipid, and nucleotide acid metabolism. Zhou et al. (contribution 9) examined the metabolic toxicity of molybdate at human-relevant exposure levels using an integration of inductively coupled plasma–mass spectrometry (ICP-MS)-based elementomics (element part of exposomics) and UPLC-Q-Exactive mass spectrometry-based metabolomics. The research reported that molybdate disrupted amino acid and lipid metabolism, potentially through altered cadmium levels, supported by human evidence. Zhang et al. (contribution 10) investigated diquat (DQ)-induced kidney damage using multi-omics analysis including transcriptomic, proteomic, and metabolomic analyses in a mouse model. They identified 869 genes, 351 proteins, and 96 metabolites affected by DQ treatment and found that DQ-induced kidney damage involved the dysregulation of the PPAR pathway and elevated Hmgcs2 expression and 3-hydroxybutyric acid levels. Liu et al. (contribution 11) investigated the neurodevelopmental toxicity of bisphenol A (BPA) in zebrafish larvae during their early development. BPA exposure from the cleavage to the segmentation stages significantly impaired the larvae's spontaneous movement. Transcriptomic analysis revealed 131 differentially expressed genes, and further examination showed that guanine deaminase mRNA levels and enzyme activity were notably decreased in BPA-exposed larvae. Guanine deaminase, which catalyzes the conversion of metabolite guanine to xanthine, is essential for degrading guanine-containing nucleotides. The researchers restored guanine deaminase levels through microinjection, which improved locomotor activity, suggesting that guanine deaminase may be a key target for BPA toxicity. Wu et al. (contribution 12) investigated metabolome and gut microbiome changes associated with acute myeloid leukemia (AML) in humans and mice, finding that the Carnosine–Histidine metabolic pathway may be crucial in AML progression, with gut microbiota like *Peptococcaceae* and *Campylobacteraceae* potentially being involved. The antioxidant system components are integral to metabolic processes; thus, studying how chemicals impact these systems connects chemical exposure with metabolism and disease. In this Special Issue, Xu et al. (contribution 13) provide a comprehensive overview of current toxicology research. They report that exposure to various chemicals, including morphine, metals, and methylglyoxal, disrupts the homeostasis of the thioredoxin system—which comprises NADPH, oxidoreductase thioredoxin, and thioredoxin reductase—leading to neurological injury. Conversely, resveratrol and lysergic acid sulfide have been found to alleviate chemical-induced nerve damage. The authors also discuss the underlying mechanisms, offering a foundational reference for future studies on the complex relationship between the thioredoxin system and chemical-induced nerve injury.

3. Conclusions

Continuously improving chemical exposome evaluation methods, including developing detection methods for individual internal and external exposures to emerging pollutants, continuously improving metabolomics research in detection methods, research technologies and integration with other omics, and continuously conducting database construction and data mining of exposome and metabolome based on big data and artificial intelligence are research directions of environmental chemical exposomics and metabolomics that need to be carried out in depth. The articles in this Special Issue offer new perspectives on environmental chemical exposome and metabolome research in toxicology, including advancements in detection method development, toxicity, and metabolic mechanism exploration, which enhances our understanding in this field and serves as a foundation for future research and policy making.

Funding: This research was funded by the China National Key Research and Development (R&D) Plan (grant number: 2021YFC2700600), the Natural Science Foundation of China (grant numbers: 82273668 and 81872650), the Excellent Young Backbone Teachers of "Qinglan Project" of Colleges and Universities in Jiangsu Province, and the Priority Academic Program Development of Jiangsu Higher Education Institutions (PAPD).

Acknowledgments: The Guest Editor of the Special Issue of Toxics, "State-of-the-Art Environmental Chemical Exposomics and Metabolomics", in the "Exposome Analysis and Risk Assessment", would like to express his gratitude for all the contributions given to this valuable collection.

Conflicts of Interest: The author declares no conflicts of interest.

List of Contributions:

1. Ning, X.; Ye, Y.; Ji, J.; Hui, Y.; Li, J.; Chen, P.; Jin, S.; Liu, T.; Zhang, Y.; Cao, J.; et al. Restricted-Access Media Column Switching Online Solid-Phase Extraction UHPLC–MS/MS for the Determination of Seven Type B Trichothecenes in Whole-Grain Preprocessed Foods and Human Exposure Risk Assessment. *Toxics* **2024**, *12*, 336.
2. Ning, X.; Wang, L.; Wang, J.-S.; Ji, J.; Jin, S.; Sun, J.; Ye, Y.; Mei, S.; Zhang, Y.; Cao, J.; et al. High-Coverage UHPLC-MS/MS Analysis of 67 Mycotoxins in Plasma for Male Infertility Exposure Studies. *Toxics* **2024**, *12*, 395.
3. Liu, C.; Chen, S.; Chu, J.; Yang, Y.; Yuan, B.; Zhang, H. Multi-Omics Analysis Reveals the Toxicity of Polyvinyl Chloride Microplastics toward BEAS-2B Cells. *Toxics* **2024**, *12*, 399.
4. Yao, J.; Zhou, P.; Zhang, X.; Yuan, B.; Pan, Y.; Jiang, J. The Cytotoxicity of Tungsten Ions Derived from Nanoparticles Correlates with Pulmonary Toxicity. *Toxics* **2023**, *11*, 528.

5. Lv, J.; He, Q.; Yan, Z.; Xie, Y.; Wu, Y.; Li, A.; Zhang, Y.; Li, J.; Huang, Z. Inhibitory Impact of Prenatal Exposure to Nano-Polystyrene Particles on the MAP2K6/p38 MAPK Axis Inducing Embryonic Developmental Abnormalities in Mice. *Toxics* **2024**, *12*, 370.
6. Li, H.; Miao, D.; Hu, H.; Xue, P.; Zhou, K.; Mao, Z. Titanium Dioxide Nanoparticles Induce Maternal Preeclampsia-like Syndrome and Adverse Birth Outcomes via Disrupting Placental Function in SD Rats. *Toxics* **2024**, *12*, 367.
7. Liang, Z.; Fang, S.; Zhang, Y.; Zhang, X.; Xu, Y.; Qian, H.; Geng, H. Cigarette Smoke-Induced Gastric Cancer Cell Exosomes Affected the Fate of Surrounding Normal Cells via the Circ0000670/Wnt/β-Catenin Axis. *Toxics* **2023**, *11*, 465.
8. Xu, B.; Gao, W.; Xu, T.; Liu, C.; Wu, D.; Tang, W. A UPLC Q-Exactive Orbitrap Mass Spectrometry-Based Metabolomic Study of Serum and Tumor Tissue in Patients with Papillary Thyroid Cancer. *Toxics* **2023**, *11*, 44.
9. Zhou, K.; Tang, M.; Zhang, W.; Chen, Y.; Guan, Y.; Huang, R.; Duan, J.; Liu, Z.; Ji, X.; Jiang, Y.; et al. Exposure to Molybdate Results in Metabolic Disorder: An Integrated Study of the Urine Elementome and Serum Metabolome in Mice. *Toxics* **2024**, *12*, 288.
10. Zhang, H.; Zhang, J.; Li, J.; Mao, Z.; Qian, J.; Zong, C.; Sun, H.; Yuan, B. Multi-Omics Analyses Reveal the Mechanisms of Early Stage Kidney Toxicity by Diquat. *Toxics* **2023**, *11*, 184.
11. Liu, J.; Kong, W.; Liu, Y.; Ma, Q.; Shao, Q.; Zeng, L.; Chao, Y.; Song, X.; Zhang, J. Stage-Related Neurotoxicity of BPA in the Development of Zebrafish Embryos. *Toxics* **2023**, *11*, 177.
12. Wu, B.; Xu, Y.; Tang, M.; Jiang, Y.; Zhang, T.; Huang, L.; Wang, S.; Hu, Y.; Zhou, K.; Zhang, X.; et al. A Metabolome and Microbiome Analysis of Acute Myeloid Leukemia: Insights into the Carnosine–Histidine Metabolic Pathway. *Toxics* **2024**, *12*, 14.
13. Xu, X.; Zhang, L.; He, Y.; Qi, C.; Li, F. Progress in Research on the Role of the Thioredoxin System in Chemical Nerve Injury. *Toxics* **2024**, *12*, 510.

References

1. Vermeulen, R.; Schymanski, E.L.; Barabási, A.L.; Miller, G.W. The exposome and health: Where chemistry meets biology. *Science* **2020**, *367*, 392–396. [CrossRef] [PubMed]
2. Gonzalez-Covarrubias, V.; Martínez-Martínez, E.; del Bosque-Plata, L. The potential of metabolomics in biomedical applications. *Metabolites* **2022**, *12*, 194. [CrossRef] [PubMed]

Disclaimer/Publisher's Note: The statements, opinions and data contained in all publications are solely those of the individual author(s) and contributor(s) and not of MDPI and/or the editor(s). MDPI and/or the editor(s) disclaim responsibility for any injury to people or property resulting from any ideas, methods, instructions or products referred to in the content.

Article

Restricted-Access Media Column Switching Online Solid-Phase Extraction UHPLC–MS/MS for the Determination of Seven Type B Trichothecenes in Whole-Grain Preprocessed Foods and Human Exposure Risk Assessment

Xiao Ning [1,2], Yongli Ye [1], Jian Ji [1], Yanchun Hui [3], Jingyun Li [2], Po Chen [2], Shaoming Jin [2], Tongtong Liu [2], Yinzhi Zhang [1], Jin Cao [2,*] and Xiulan Sun [1,*]

1. School of Food Science and Technology, International Joint Laboratory on Food Safety, Synergetic Innovation Center of Food Safety and Quality Control, Jiangnan University, Wuxi 214122, China; nx200730079@163.com (X.N.); yyly0222@163.com (Y.Y.); jijian@jiangnan.edu.cn (J.J.); yinzhizhang@jiangnan.edu.cn (Y.Z.)
2. Key Laboratory of Food Quality and Safety for State Market Regulation, National Institute of Food and Drug Control, Beijing 100050, China; lijingyun@nifdc.org.cn (J.L.)
3. Sanyo Fine Trading Co., Ltd., Beijing 100176, China
* Correspondence: caojin@nifdc.org.cn (J.C.); sxlzzz@jiangnan.edu.cn (X.S.); Tel.: +86-010-6709-5070 (J.C.); +86-0510-8591-2330 (X.S.)

Abstract: With increasing health awareness and the accelerating pace of life, whole-grain prepared foods have gained popularity due to their health benefits and convenience. However, the potential risk of type B trichothecene toxins has also increased, and these mycotoxins in such foods are rarely regulated. In this study, a quantitative method combining a single-valve dual-column automatic online solid-phase extraction system with ultra-high-performance liquid chromatography–tandem mass spectrometry (UHPLC–MS/MS) was developed for the first time using restricted-access media columns. This method can simultaneously determine trace residues of seven type B trichothecenes within 15 min. The method is convenient, sensitive (limit of detection and quantification of 0.05–0.6 µg/kg and 0.15–2 µg/kg, respectively), accurate (recovery rates of 90.3%–106.6%, relative standard deviation < 4.3%), and robust (>1000 times). The established method was applied to 160 prepared food samples of eight categories sold in China. At least one toxin was detected in 70% of the samples. Whole-wheat dumpling wrappers had the highest contamination rate (95%) and the highest total content of type B trichothecenes in a single sample (2077.3 µg/kg). Exposure risk assessment indicated that the contamination of whole-grain prepared foods has been underestimated. The total health risk index of whole-wheat dumpling wrappers, which are susceptible to deoxynivalenol, reached 136.41%, posing a significant threat to human health. Effective measures urgently need to be taken to control this risk.

Keywords: trichothecene mycotoxin; UHPLC–MS/MS; prepared food; whole-wheat dumpling wrappers

1. Introduction

Whole-grain prepared foods have gained widespread popularity due to their numerous health benefits, convenience, and diversity. However, whole-grain foods are usually less processed, they are more susceptible to fungal contamination, particularly by type B trichothecene toxins, represented by deoxynivalenol (DON). In 2020, European Food Safety Authority (EFSA) and in 2021, World Health Organization (WHO) both highlighted concerns about the presence of DON in cereals, especially noting whole-grain foods as significant sources of DON exposure. These reports emphasize the need for monitoring and managing the risk of fungal contamination in these food products to ensure consumer safety [1,2]. Although some countries have implemented regulations for DON, other known co–contaminating modified and emerging toxins have received little attention. In recent years, some studies have reported the individual toxicity of these derivatives, such as DON glycosylated (deoxynivalenol 3-glucuronide, D3G) or acetylated (3-acetyldeoxynivalenol, (3AcDON) and 15-acetyldeoxynivalenol (15AcDON)) derivatives, as well as their synergistic toxic effects with emerging toxins such as nivalenol (NIV). To date, comprehensive information on the composition and concentration of mycotoxins in prepared foods is very limited, highlighting the urgency of comprehensive monitoring and adequate risk assessment of mycotoxin contamination in these foods.

Liquid chromatography–tandem mass spectrometry (LC–MS/MS) analysis is the most powerful alternative analytical method for mycotoxins with different physicochemical properties, enabling sensitive, fast, and reliable multi–target analysis in food matrices [3,4]. However, the complex food matrix makes it crucial to perform sample pretreatment steps to pre–concentrate the target compounds and reduce matrix effects. Solid–phase extraction (SPE) is a popular method for preparing complex samples [5]. Compared with traditional offline SPE, online SPE coupled with UHPLC–MS/MS contributes to the automation of the analytical process. To our knowledge, the currently reported SPE–LC–MS methods for simultaneous analysis of multiple trichothecenes are all offline modes, which are cumbersome, time–consuming, and labor–intensive, especially when dealing with a large number of samples [6]. Therefore, establishing an automated online SPE–UHPLC–MS/MS method will significantly improve the efficiency of analysis, reduce solvent consumption, and minimize environmental pollution. Unfortunately, due to the ease of SPE column clogging caused by macromolecules such as proteins in the samples, this robustness defect severely hinders the large-scale application of online automated mode to food samples [7]. Restricted access media (RAM) provides an effective approach to address this limitation. The chromatographic column packing simultaneously bonds hydrophilic groups with steric hindrance and hydrophobic groups for retention. Through two separation principles, it effectively prevents large molecules (such as proteins) from entering the adsorbent and causing analyte retention. To date, RAM chromatographic columns have not been applied to trace analysis of mycotoxins in food.

This study proposed an automated online SPE–UHPLC–MS/MS method using RAM columns for the simultaneous quantitative analysis of seven type B trichothecenes in wholegrain prepared foods. The method was validated in three sample matrices, including instant brown rice, oatmeal, and whole–wheat flour products, and the results met the acceptable criteria specified in European Commission Decision (EC) No. 2002/657/EC [8]. The proposed method is not only sensitive, accurate, and easy to operate but also successfully applied to analyze 160 actual samples collected from the Chinese market, covering eight different categories, including brown rice, whole-grain infant rice flour, oatmeal, instant oats, oatmeal cookies, whole–wheat bread, whole–wheat noodles, and whole–wheat dumpling wrappers. Finally, the exposure risk of these prepared foods susceptible to mycotoxin contamination was assessed by calculating the hazard quotient (HQ) and hazard index (HI). This is the first study on the analysis of trichothecenes and human exposure risk assessment in whole-grain–based prepared foods, providing a powerful tool and valuable reference for protecting consumers from the potential health risks of mycotoxin contamination.

2. Materials and Methods

2.1. Chemicals and Reagents

Acetonitrile (ACN), mass spectrometry grade, was purchased from Anple Laboratory Technologies Co., Ltd. (Shanghai, China); acetic acid (HAc), chromatographic grade, was provided by J&K Scientific Ltd., (Beijing, China); water was ultrapure water prepared by MilliQ. Seven standard solutions, each at a concentration of 100 μg/mL, were obtained from Romer Labs (Tulln, Austria), including DON, 3AcDON, 15AcDON, D3G, NIV, fusarenon-X (FusX), and de-epoxy-deoxynivalenol (DOM-1). Additionally, 180 whole-grain prepared food samples were purchased from the Chinese market. All chromatographic measurements were performed on a NASCA II UHPLC system (OSAKA SODA, Osaka, Japan), which consists of a NASCA II all-in-one machine (including a degasser, dual pumps, an autosampler, and a heating kit). Additionally, an external F3012 six–port valve, an F3202 degasser, and an F3301 dual pump form a two-dimensional liquid chromatography system connected to a QTRAP 5500 triple quadrupole-linear ion trap mass spectrometer (AB SCIEX, Toronto, SD, Canada). AB SCIEX Analyst chromatography software (1.5 version) was used for data acquisition and analysis. The pretreatment solid–phase extraction was carried out using a CAPCELL PAK MF C8 SG80 chromatographic column (5 μm, 150 mm × 2 mm, OSAKA SODA, Japan) with a pressure limit of 20 MPa. A CAPCELL PAK C18 MGII (2 μm, 100 mm × 2 mm) analytical column (OSAKA SODA, Japan) was used for chromatographic separation; a balance (METTLER TOLEDO, Greifensee, Switzerland); Fungilab ultrasonic device (FUNGILAB, Madrid, Spain); and Milli–Q UltrapUre Ion–Ex–TM ultrapure water system (MILLIPORE, St. Louis, MO, USA) were also used.

2.2. Preparation of Standard Solutions

The selection of concentrations for the mycotoxin standard solutions was based on their sensitivity to the instrument and their co-stability in the standard solutions. The mixed standard solution contained 2 μg/mL of 3AcDON, FusX, and NIV; 4 μg/mL of DON and DOM-1; 0.4 μg/mL of D3G; and 8 μg/mL of 15AcDON. All solutions were prepared in acetonitrile, stored in the dark at −20 °C, and diluted with the initial solvent for SPE–UHPLC–MS/MS analysis.

2.3. Online SPE–LC–MS/MS Method

2.3.1. Mass Spectrometry Conditions

The ion source was a Turbo–V electrospray ion source, operating in negative ion mode with a spray voltage of −2400 V, ion source temperature of 350 °C, spray gas (GAS1) at 25 psi, drying gas (GAS2) at 25 psi, and curtain gas at 40 psi. Multiple reaction monitoring (MRM) mode was used to monitor the analytes, with an entrance potential (EP) of −10 V, collision cell exits potential (CXP) of −15 V, and declustering potential (DP) of −100 V. The m/z values of the precursor and product ions for each substance, as well as the collision energy (CE) parameters in multiple reaction monitoring (MRM) mode, are shown in Table 1.

Table 1. Analytical parameters for the determination of 7 B type trichothecenes in ESI (−) using the UPLC–MS/MS method.

Analytes	Adduct	Retention Time (min)	m/z	Precursor Ion	Collision Energy (V)	Product Ion	Collision Energy (V)
DON	[M+CH$_3$COO]$^-$	7.43	355.1	295.1	−14	59.2	−50
D3G	[M+CH$_3$COO]$^-$	7.25	517.1	427.1	−30	457.1	−20
DOM	[M+CH$_3$COO]$^-$	8.34	339.1	249.1	−15	59.1	−50
FusX	[M+CH$_3$COO]$^-$	8.60	413.3	262.9	−22	59.1	−50
NIV	[M+CH$_3$COO]$^-$	6.40	371.1	281.1	−30	59.0	−46
3AcDON	[M+CH$_3$COO]$^-$	10.46	397.3	337.1	−13	307.2	−40
15AcDON	[M+CH$_3$COO]$^-$	10.33	397.3	59.0	−40	337.1	−9

2.3.2. Liquid Chromatography Analysis

The principle of the online SPE–LC–MS/MS method is shown in Figure 1a, and the gradient distribution of the two pumps and the corresponding positions of the six-port valve is shown in Table 2. At a low proportion of the organic phase, from 0 to 1.3 min, large molecular compounds such as proteins, fats, and starches that may be present in the sample are eluted, and the target substances are retained. At this time, the two-dimensional system balances the analytical column (column 2) through pump 2. From 1.3 to 11.1 min, after switching the six-port valve, pump 2 performs reverse flushing of column 1 and enters column 2, and the target substances enriched in column 1 enter pump 2 with the gradient conditions of the two–dimensional mobile phase to start the two-dimensional analysis process.

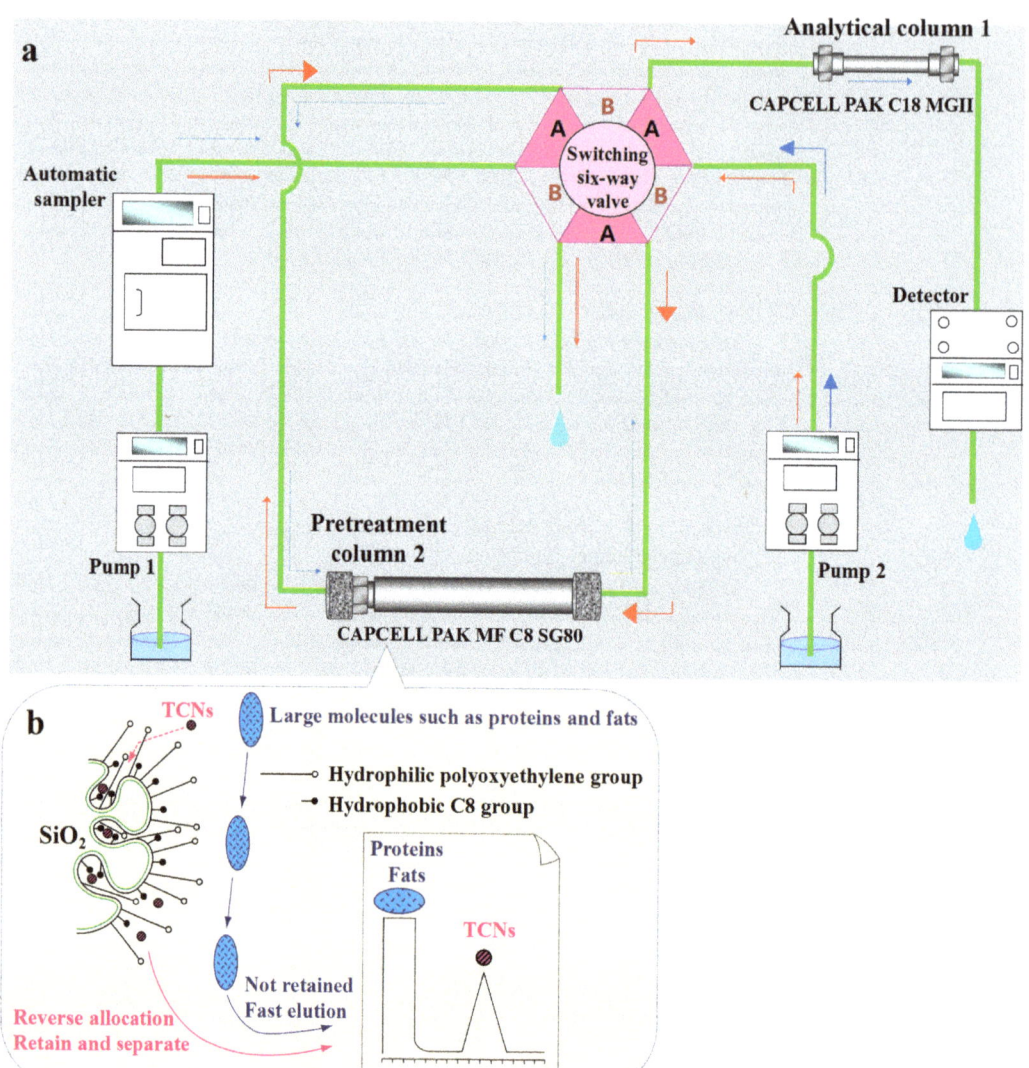

Figure 1. Schematic of the automated online SPE–HPLC system (**a**), and the extraction and clean–up principle of a RAM column (**b**).

Chromatographic columns: One-dimensional: CAPCELL PAK MF C8 SG80 (2 mm i.d. × 150 mm, particle size 5 μm) (OSAKA SODA, Japan); two-dimensional: CAPCELL PAK C18 MGII (2 mm i.d. × 100 mm, particle size 2 μm) (OSAKA SODA, Japan). The column temperature was 25 °C, and the injection volume was 10 μL.

Table 2. Linearity data, LOD, LOQ, and matrix effect (ME, %) for tested compounds by SPE–UPLC–MS/MS.

B-Type C-TCNs	Matrixs	Calibration Range (µg/kg)	Linear Equation	Correlation Coefficient (r)	LOD (µg/kg)	LOQ (µg/kg)	ME (%)
DON	Ready-to-eat brown rice	1–1000	y = 28,048x + 111,732	0.9991	0.4	1	−6.4
	Oatmeal		y = 27,171x + 137,284	0.9991	0.4	1	−10.6
	Whole wheat bread		y = 28,249x + 98,763	0.9998	0.3	0.9	−8.1
D3G	Ready-to-eat brown rice	0.2–200	y = 18,775x − 987	0.9996	0.06	0.2	−14.0
	Oatmeal		y = 17,106x − 1211	0.9993	0.05	0.15	−9.3
	Whole wheat bread		y = 17,614x − 373	0.9995	0.05	0.15	−10.0
3AcDON	Ready-to-eat brown rice	1–1000	y = 25,092x + 52,203	0.9992	0.2	0.8	−2.5
	Oatmeal		y = 24,956x + 34,251	0.9994	0.25	0.8	−6.6
	Whole wheat bread		y = 24,278x + 19,342	0.9994	0.3	1	−5.5
15AcDON	Ready-to-eat brown rice	2–2000	y = 12,969x + 10,982	0.9993	0.5	1.5	5.4
	Oatmeal		y = 13,311x + 41,537	0.9996	0.6	2	3.4
	Whole wheat bread		y = 12,510x + 38,762	0.9997	0.5	1.5	4.5
DOM-1	Ready-to-eat brown rice	1–1000	y = 22,102x + 12,324	0.9996	0.4	1	1.6
	Oatmeal		y = 24,397x + 10,981	0.9998	0.3	1	2.0
	Whole wheat bread		y = 22,274x + 8976	0.9993	0.4	1	2.6
FusX	Ready-to-eat brown rice	1–1000	y = 7115x + 3791	0.9998	0.2	0.8	−3.1
	Oatmeal		y = 6113x + 3429	0.9997	0.2	0.8	−6.2
	Whole wheat bread		y = 6202x + 2167	0.9995	0.3	1	−3.6
NIV	Ready-to-eat brown rice	1–1000	y = 10,810x + 8035	0.9994	0.3	1	−9.3
	Oatmeal		y = 9879x + 8035	1.0000	0.3	1	−12.8
	Whole wheat bread		y = 9976x + 8035	0.9994	0.3	1	−12.2

2.4. Samples and Sample Preparation

The method development and validation were conducted using three types of sample matrices: blank instant brown rice ($n = 6$), oatmeal ($n = 6$), and whole-wheat flour products ($n = 6$) collected from the Chinese retail market. All collected samples were ground into fine powder using a laboratory mill to achieve sufficient homogeneity and stored in sealed plastic bags in a dark environment at 4 °C until analysis.

After the method was validated to meet the acceptable criteria specified in European Commission Decision (EC) No. 2002/657/EC [8], it was applied to analyze 180 actual samples collected from the Chinese retail market, including brown rice, whole-grain infant rice flour, oatmeal, instant oats, oatmeal cookies, whole–wheat bread, whole–wheat noodles, and whole–wheat dumpling wrappers.

Extraction Procedure

Weigh 2.0 g of whole-grain prepared food. Add 10 mL of FA–ACN–water (1:84:14, v/v) mixture, vortex for 30 s, and extract by ultrasound for 10 min. After centrifugation (9000 r/min) for 5 min, pass the supernatant through a 0.22 µm filter membrane and set aside.

2.5. Method Validation

The optimized method was validated according to the existing procedures in [8,9]. The method can be used to analyze seven TCNs in nine types of samples, including cereal bars, oatmeal, whole-wheat bread, whole-wheat biscuits, whole-wheat steamed buns, whole-wheat noodles, instant rice, whole-wheat dumpling wrappers, and infant cereal rice flour. The performance characteristics evaluated include linearity, limit of detection (LOD), limit of quantification (LOQ), selectivity, matrix effect, recovery, repeatability, reproducibility, and robustness (details were described in the Supplementary File).

2.6. Risk Assessment

Given the severe toxicity of the target mycotoxins, it is crucial to assess their potential exposure risk to human health in whole-grain-based prepared foods by evaluating the contamination levels of the seven target mycotoxins and combining them with relevant food consumption data. The estimated daily intakes (EDIs) and hazard quotient (HQ) values of the mycotoxins were calculated using the following formulas:

$$\text{EDI} (\mu g/kg\, bw/day) = (C \times F)/bw$$

where, C is the average contamination concentration (μg/kg) of type B trichothecenes in whole-grain prepared food samples, and F is the average consumption (g/day) of whole-grain foods. As there are currently no authoritative statistics on the consumption data of whole-grain prepared foods in China, this study adopted the recommended daily intake value of whole grains for adults in the Chinese Dietary Guidelines, which is 100 g (the average of 50–150 g), as the food factor (F value) for estimating exposure [10]. bw is the human body weight (kg), and the default international average body weight for adults is 60 kg [11].

The EFSA has set tolerable daily intakes (TDIs) to assess the exposure risk of mycotoxins in food under controllable conditions. The TDI for DON is 1 μg/kg·day·bw, and the TDI for NIV is 0.7 μg/kg·day·bw [12,13]. Due to the limitations of toxicity studies on D3G, 3AcDON, 15AcDON, and FusX, there are currently no officially confirmed TDIs for these compounds. In 2017, EFSA conducted a comprehensive risk assessment of DON and its derivatives (including D3G, 3AcDON, and 15AcDON). The report supported the view of the Joint FAO/WHO Expert Committee on Food Additives, which states that the intake of 3AcDON and 15AcDON should be fully counted as DON equivalents, while 30% of the D3G intake should be counted as DON equivalents, and the TDI value of DON should be applied for risk assessment [14]. FusX may have similar toxic effects to NIV, and the TDI value of NIV can be used as a reference for risk assessment [15]. The hazard quotient (HQ) is usually introduced to represent the risk level of dietary intake of each toxin, which is calculated as the ratio of EDI to TDI, as shown in the following formula:

$$\text{HQ} (\%) = (\text{EDI}/\text{TDI}) \times 100$$

An HQ < 100% is considered an acceptable dietary exposure level for mycotoxins and does not pose a health threat to humans, while an HQ > 100% indicates that the dietary exposure level exceeds the permissible limit and poses a health threat and will therefore be considered a serious safety issue [16].

Furthermore, since the analyzed TCNs involve DON and NIV or their derivatives, and the interaction mechanisms between each toxin are not yet clear, the total risk can be estimated by directly combining the HQ values of each toxin and calculating the hazard index (HI, %) using the following formula:

$$\text{HI} (\%) = \sum \text{HQ}_i, \text{ where } i \in \{\text{DON, D3G, 3AcDON, 15AcDON, NIV, FUsX, DOM-1}\}$$

An HI > 100% for multiple mycotoxins indicates that dietary exposure may have a significant adverse effect on human health.

2.7. Data Analysis

When the mycotoxin levels detected in the samples were higher than the LOQ, the samples were considered positive, while samples with contamination levels lower than the LOQ were considered negative.

During the dietary risk assessment, mycotoxins that were not detected or below the LOQ were considered to be half of the LOD (LOD/2).

Statistical analysis was performed using SPSS software (version 22.0, IBM Corp., Armonk, New York, NY, USA) to calculate correlation coefficients (R2 ≥ 0.99). OriginPro software (2019b, OriginLab Inc., Northampton, MA, USA) was used to plot the spectra.

3. Results and Discussion

3.1. Selection of Sample Extraction

It is necessary to select a suitable extraction solvent for mycotoxins. Studies have shown that type B trichothecenes are highly soluble in organic solutions due to their lipophilic and hydrophobic properties [17]. The addition of a small amount of water promotes the wetting of the sample matrix and facilitates the penetration of organic solutions into the food. Furthermore, organic acids can disrupt the tight binding between the analytes and other food nutritional components (such as proteins and sugars), thereby promoting the extraction of mycotoxins [18]. Compared to methanol/water mixtures, the use of acetonitrile/water mixtures can effectively reduce the co-extraction of interfering substances from the samples and achieve satisfactory recoveries [19,20]. Therefore, this study compared the extraction effects of acetonitrile aqueous solutions containing 0.1%–1% formic acid. As shown in Figure 2, the mean recoveries of the seven mycotoxins extracted with six solutions were 39.7%, 48.2%, 58.3%, 70.9%, 79.3%, and 70.4%, respectively. Although none of the six solvents achieved ideal recoveries for all analytes after extraction without purification, it is worth noting that the analyte recoveries extracted with 1% formic acid–85% acetonitrile aqueous solution were tightly distributed in the box plot, with a median quartile (Q2) of 78.6% and a third quartile (Q3) of 80.3%, showing the relatively best extraction effect. Therefore, this solvent was chosen as the optimal extraction solvent for further purification and analysis.

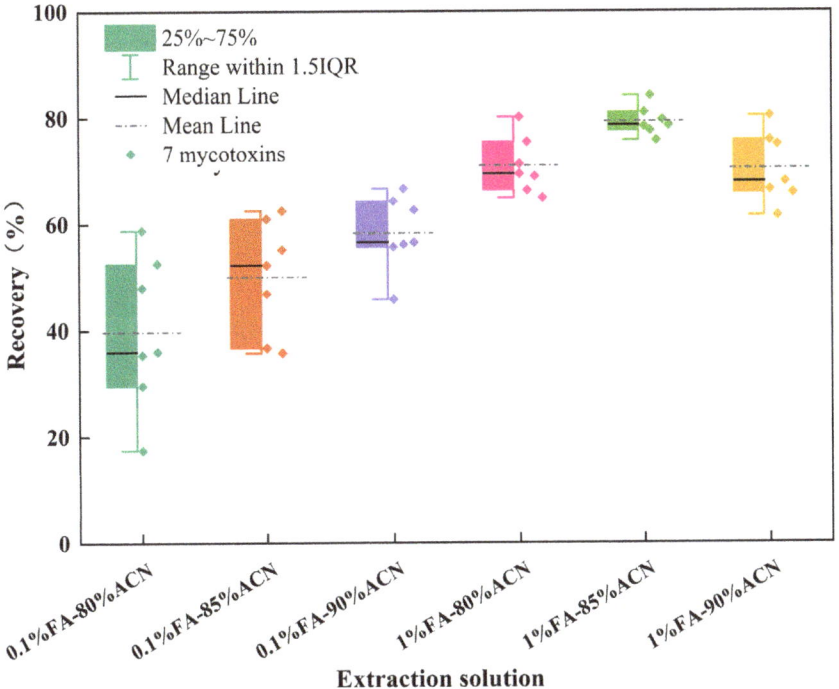

Figure 2. Average recoveries of 7 B-type trichothecenes extracted by 6 solutions.

3.2. Optimization of UPLC–MS/MS

Developing a suitable sample purification method is often considered the critical first step in the entire analytical chain, as it is the most time-consuming and error-prone step [21]. The RAM chromatographic column plays a key role in the online SPE analysis of complex food samples through two separation principles. As shown in Figure 1b, a uniform thin film coated with siloxane polymers is formed on the surface of high-purity silica gel. Simultaneously, hydrophilic groups with steric hindrance (polyoxyethylene) and hydrophobic groups (C8) for retention are bonded. Large matrix molecules such as proteins are affected by the steric hindrance of hydrophilic groups and the size exclusion effect caused by small pore size, and they are not retained but eluted directly at the dead time. In contrast, the target small molecule mycotoxins can interact with the hydrophobic groups to achieve retention and separation. In this study, we also attempted to use a CAPCELL PAK MF Ph–1 SG80 chromatographic column (4.6 mm × 150 mm, id, 5 μm, OSAKA SODA, Japan) with phenyl as the hydrophobic group for pretreatment. The retention capacity of the MF Ph–1 column was weaker than that of the C8 column, with NIV and D3G having retention times of 1.63 min, close to the dead time (1.2 min) at that point, which may cause loss during pretreatment valve switching and affect quantitative results. Therefore, it was abandoned.

To optimize the mass spectrometry method, a standard solution of a single compound was injected into the LC–MS/MS system. Analyses were performed in positive/negative ion mode, and the two highest-intensity ions observed for each analyte were used as Quantifier and Qualifier, respectively. When the mobile phase used 0.1% formic acid (FA) or 0.1% HAc as the aqueous phase, the corresponding precursor ions were $[M + H]^+$ or $[M+CH_3COO]^-$, respectively. Compared to positive ion mode, there was a trend of increased response intensity of analyte ions in negative ion mode, with increases ranging from 1.7-fold (D3G) to 6.0-fold (3AcDON). It can be seen that the $[M+CH_3COO]^-$ provided by HAc greatly enhanced the ionization of the analytes. When the HAc concentration was reduced from 0.1% to 0.01%, the signal intensity of 3AcDON and others increased by more than 1.8 times. Further reducing from 0.01% to 0.005%, all signal intensities continued to increase except for DON and FusX. However, the use of 0.005% HAc resulted in poor precision for all analytes, with the RSD range of peak areas for the tested mycotoxins (n = 3) between 11% and 32%. When the HAc concentration was 0.01%, the RSD was between 1% and 4%. Therefore, 0.01% HAc aqueous solution was selected as mobile phase (A), with ACN as mobile phase (B), and all compounds had good chromatographic peak shapes.

On this basis, the chromatographic separation conditions were further optimized to achieve satisfactory separation within a short analysis time. DON derivatives have similar structures and properties, especially the positional isomers 3AcDON and 15AcDON, which exhibit common precursor ions (m/z 397.3) and similar product ions. Therefore, baseline separation through gradient elution is necessary to achieve accurate quantification. In this study, key parameters were explored in terms of column type, flow rate, and gradient. As shown in Figure 3a, CAPCELL PAK C18 MGII is a moderately polar C18 column. At a flow rate of 0.25 mL/min, a mild gradient of 25–30% B was maintained for 5–8 min for elution, achieving baseline separation of 3AcDON and 15AcDON. Further research found that the CAPCELL CORE C18 column is a core-shell column with C18 as the bonded phase. The packing of core-shell columns has a solid core–porous surface structure, which, compared to fully porous packing, can achieve good retention and separation within a shorter analysis time, improving analytical efficiency. However, when using the CORE C18 column as the analytical column, the results are shown in Figure 3c. The analysis time was shorter than that of the MGII column, and the separation of 3AcDON and 15AcDON could not meet the analytical requirements, so it was abandoned. The ADME–HR column has a bonded phase of a sterically caged adamantyl group, a non-linear bonded phase. Due to the structural difference from the linear bonded phase, this column has ultra-high surface polarity while possessing certain surface hydrophobicity, making its retention effect on polar compounds and compounds containing polar groups superior to C18 columns, which is conducive to the separation of isomers. Therefore, we also tried using the ADME–HR column as the analytical column, but the results are shown in Figure 3b. Although the separation of 3AcDON and 15AcDON was better on this column, the peak shape was poor (peak too wide), so it was abandoned. Finally, the CAPCELL PAK C18 MGII was selected as the analytical column since after pretreatment with a front–end RAM column, quantitative analysis of seven compounds can be simultaneously performed within 11 min of a single injection. The extracted ion chromatogram is shown in Figure 3d.

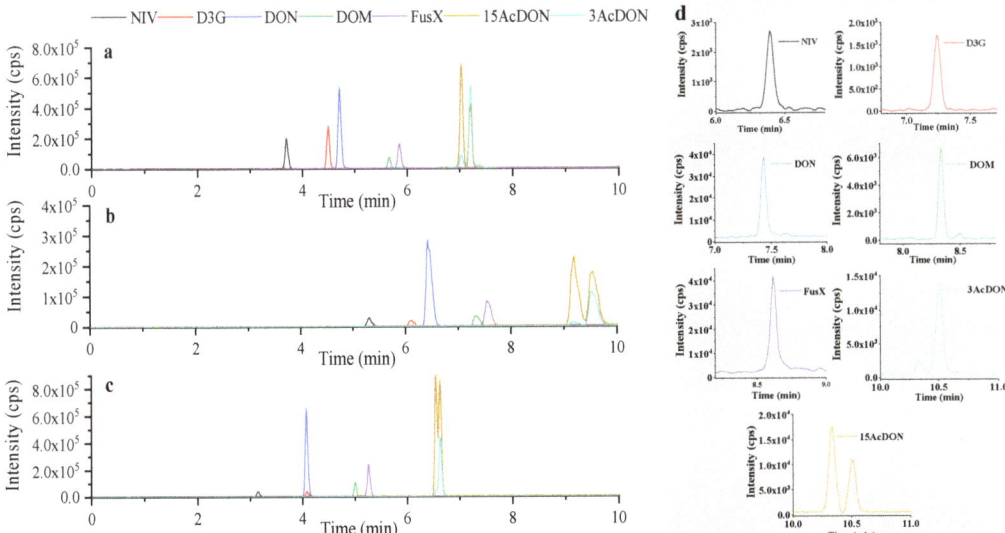

Figure 3. The total ion chromatogram was obtained by the CAPCELL PAK C18 MGII column (**a**), the CAPCELL CORE C18 column (**b**), or the ADME–HR column (**c**). Extracted ion chromatograms of 7 analytes obtained by linking CAPCELLPAK MF C8 SG80 with CAPCELLPAK C18 MGII under optimal conditions (**d**).

In a study, the toxicokinetics of DON, and its acetylated derivatives 3AcDON and 15AcDON, and its main metabolite DOM-1 in chicken and pig plasma were determined by LC-MS/MS after a simple deproteinization step with acetonitrile, followed by evaporation and reconstitution [22]. The method focuses on the analysis of these mycotoxins in animal plasma. However, the difference in sample matrices presents distinct challenges for sample preparation. In contrast, our method utilizes an online SPE using a RAM column for the cleanup of complex cereal-based food matrices. The RAM column allows for the direct injection of samples by trapping small analytes while eluting macromolecules, effectively removing potential interferences from the matrix.

Furthermore, our method achieves satisfactory separation of the analytes, especially the positional isomers 3AcDON and 15AcDON, within a short analysis time using a core-shell analytical column (CAPCELL PAK C18 MGII). Although the two methods are designed for different sample matrices, both demonstrate good performance for the quantitative analysis of DON and its derivatives. Our approach, tailored for cereal-based prepared foods, offers advantages in terms of efficient sample cleanup and enhanced chromatographic separation, making it suitable for the reliable determination of type B trichothecenes in these complex matrices.

3.3. Time of Valve Switching

During 0–1.3 min, the six-port valve is in position A, and the RAM column is performing sample pretreatment. According to the flow rate, column inner diameter, and column length, the system's dead time is calculated to be approximately 1.0 min. Since we want to remove large molecules from the sample through online pretreatment, and these substances are not retained on the RAM column, while also ensuring that the target small molecules can be retained on the RAM column without being eluted, we choose to complete the pretreatment in as short a time as possible and quickly switch the retained target substances to the two-dimensional system to ensure that their recovery is not compromised. Based on the above considerations, we switch the six-port valves to position B at 1.3 min. During 1.3 min–11.1 min, the RAM column is connected in series with the analytical column in the two-dimensional system, and the RAM column adopts a reverse-phase flushing mode (opposite to 0–1.3 min) to backflush the target substances retained on the RAM column after pretreatment to the analytical column (which is in forward-flush mode) for sample separation and detection. After all target components have been effectively analyzed, the six-port valve is switched back to position A at 11.1 min and maintained until 15 min to balance the system and prepare for the analysis of the next sample. The valve switching times are shown in Table S1.

3.4. Method Validation

In this study, the gradient elution program was carefully designed to prevent this possibility, and no carry-over effects were observed for any compounds. The RAM column can be used to extract multiple samples without significant signal loss or the need for replacement. All steps of method optimization, validation, and sample analysis were performed using the same RAM column, with a total of over 1000 injections.

The established SPE–UPLC–MS/MS method is suitable for the quantification of seven type B trichothecenes in whole-grain prepared foods. Therefore, appropriate sensitivity assessment is necessary. As shown in Table 2, with instant brown rice, oatmeal, and whole-wheat flour products (whole-wheat bread) as representative matrices, the LODs and LOQs of the target toxins were 0.05–0.6 µg/kg and 0.15–2 µg/kg, respectively. In the last decade, the target mycotoxins in cereals reported using LC–MS/MS are generally in the range of 0.02–50 µg/kg for LODs and 0.11–200 µg/kg for LOQs [9,22–27], as detailed in Table S2. In comparison, this study established an online automated system that completes purification and enrichment in one step, and the method is sensitive enough to meet the analytical requirements for trace residues of seven trichothecenes, such as DON, in prepared cereal foods.

According to the SANTE guidelines [28], matrix effects (MEs) in the range of −20% to +20% are considered insignificant. As shown in Table 2, matrix effects varied among different compounds, with an overall fluctuation range of −14.4% to 5.4%, but early-eluting compounds appeared to exhibit higher matrix effects than later-eluting compounds. Consistent with previous literature assessments, DON, D3G, and NIV commonly exhibit varying degrees of matrix effects in LC-MS/MS analysis, especially in oat matrices, mainly manifesting as ion suppression. Among them, D3G and NIV are more significantly affected by matrix effects than DON [29]. To reduce the impact of matrix effects, methods such as isotope-labeled internal standards, matrix-matched standard curves, dilution and injection can be adopted. Considering that the pretreatment method provided in this study has greatly reduced the matrix effects, which are not as significant as reported in the above literature (exceeding the range of −20% to +20%), a matrix-matched calibration strategy that balances cost and sensitivity was adopted to minimize matrix effects and ensure accurate quantification. The linear regression data are summarized in Table 2. All relevant mycotoxins had r values greater than 0.999 within the applicable working range, indicating good linearity of the calibration curves.

The intra-day and inter-day precision (expressed as % RSD) in three typical sample matrices met international standards [30,31], as shown in Table S2, with values below

4.29 and 11.7%, respectively, which are acceptable for complex samples [32,33]. At low concentrations (the first point of the calibration curve), the RSD values for the seven compounds were less than 9.5%, indicating good precision of the method, mainly due to the automated control of the online analytical system and the robustness of the RAM column. The accuracy of the method was evaluated through recovery experiments using spiked samples at three concentrations. The recoveries ranged from 89.7% to 103.6% (Table S3). It is noteworthy that the proposed method can achieve good precision and accuracy without the use of isotope-labeled internal standards, which is important in reducing the generation of hazardous waste and greatly reducing funding investment costs.

Quality control (QC) samples were prepared in the initial mobile phase (standard concentration was 10 times the quantification limit of each analyte) and analyzed before and after each batch of samples. After the last QC sample, acetonitrile was injected to clean the system and check for any residual effects before starting the analysis of a new batch of samples. No carry-over effects were observed.

3.5. Application to Real Samples

3.5.1. Occurrence of Mycotoxins in Samples

Application, the established method was used to detect seven type B trichothecene toxins in 160 whole-grain prepared food samples of eight categories collected from the Chinese market. The levels of the seven mycotoxins were obtained, and the results are shown in Figure 4 and Table S3. Whole-grain products retain the germ and bran of the grain and have not undergone deep processing such as peeling and grinding, resulting in a low toxin removal rate. Among the 160 samples, 112 (70.0%) contained at least one toxin. DON had the highest detection rate (70.0%) and the highest maximum detected concentration (1685.2 µg/kg). This residue level is compliant with the Codex Alimentarius Commission standard (2000 µg/kg) and is slightly lower than the European Union (EU) standard (1750 µg/kg). However, it exceeds the standard set by China (1000 µg/kg) [34–36]. NIV, 3AcDON, D3G, and 15AcDON followed, with detection rates of 38.1%, 30.6%, 21.9%, and 8.8%, and maximum detected concentrations of 90.3, 208.1, 28.6, and 47.2 µg/kg, respectively. This result is supported by multiple studies, as DON is usually the trichothecene toxin with the highest detection rate and contamination level in cereal grains such as wheat and oats and their processed products [37,38]. Compared to other trichothecenes such as NIV, *F. graminearum* has a higher capacity to biosynthesize DON, with a faster production rate per unit of fungal biomass. This higher biosynthetic efficiency, coupled with the rapid growth of *F. graminearum* on cereal grains, results in higher levels of DON contamination [39]. Acetylated DON derivatives (3AcDON and 15AcDON) originate from the secondary metabolic processes of specific chemotypes of *F. graminearum* and usually co-contaminate grains with DON, but at relatively lower levels [40]. It is worth noting that the detection rate and content of 3AcDON are usually higher than those of 15AcDON [41], which is confirmed again by the results in this study. In comparison, although the contamination levels of D3G and NIV are lower than those of DON, they should not be ignored. Several studies have demonstrated that grains can be co-contaminated with NIV and D3G, with concentrations ranging from tens to hundreds of µg/kg [42,43]. This suggests that when assessing the risk of trichothecene contamination in cereal products, in addition to focusing on free DON, attention should also be paid to other coexisting analogs [44].

FusX, as an acetylated derivative of NIV, exhibits relatively low toxicity, and current research primarily focuses on the detection of this toxin in grains, which are raw materials for processed foods. A study conducted in Canada from 2008 to 2010 demonstrated that FusX was detected in less than 1% of wheat samples, with the highest concentration being only 30 µg/kg [45]. In contrast, analyses by Bryła and his team of Polish grain samples from 2014 to 2016 found detection rates of FusX in wheat and barley to be 4% and 2%, respectively, with the highest concentration reaching 122 µg/kg [46]. Although these values are higher than those reported in Canada, they remain low compared to the primary trichothecene DON. Similarly, in this study, FusX was detected in 5 out of 160 samples, with the highest concentration found in whole-wheat dumpling wrappers being 17.9 µg/kg. However, a study in Sichuan Province, China, revealed a significantly higher detection rate of FusX in rice samples, at 28.6%, with the highest concentration detected being 455.1 µg/kg [47]. These findings indicate that while the contamination rate of FusX in grains is generally low (less than 5%), the detection rate and level of contamination vary according to region and crop type. Given that contamination in raw materials can migrate to the final processed products, continuous monitoring of FusX contamination levels in grains is crucial.

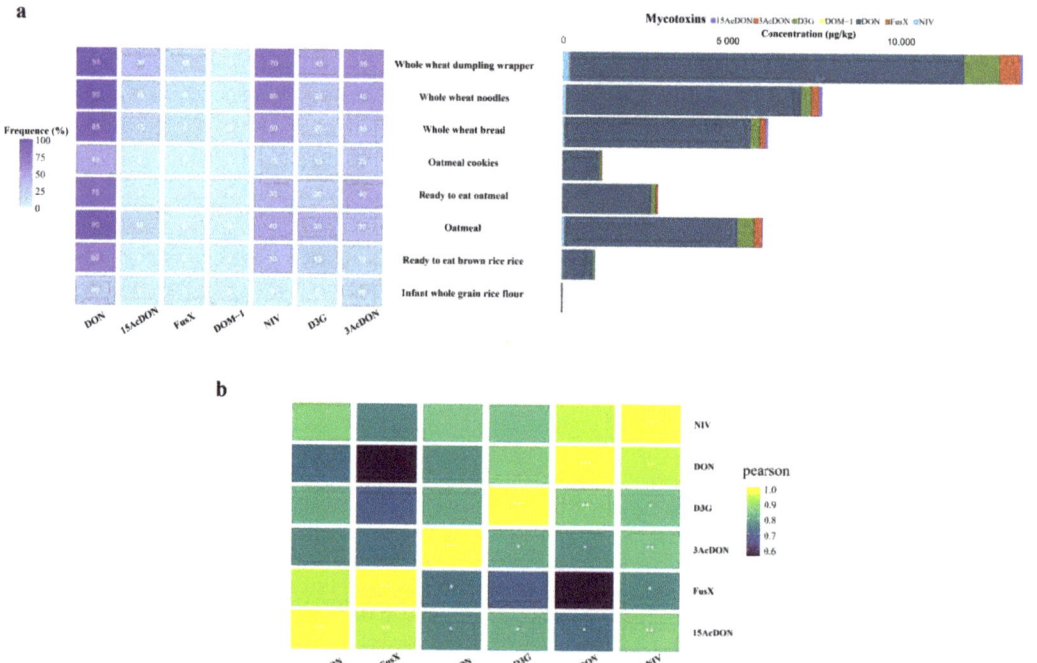

Figure 4. Occurrence of B-type TCNs in 160 whole-grain prepared foods collected across China (**a**). Co–contamination heatmap of the Pearson correlation matrix indicating the prevalence of B-type TCNs combinations (**b**). The color gradient ranges from dark purple to light yellow, corresponding to correlation values from 0.6 to 1.0, respectively. Asterisks indicate statistical significance (* $p < 0.05$, ** $p < 0.01$, and *** $p < 0.001$).

DOM–1 is a de-epoxy derivative of DON. This method monitored its contamination in 160 whole-grain-based foods, and the results showed no detection. DOM–1 mainly originates from the metabolic transformation of DON in animals and is rarely directly detected in grains and their processed products. Broekaert et al. [48] found that the proportion of DOM–1 detected in 190 samples (grains such as wheat, corn, and oats) was only 2.1%, with a maximum detected concentration of 23 µg/kg, which is much lower than DON and other derivatives. Moreover, Payros et al. [49] analyzed various DON derivatives in wheat and its flour products, and DOM–1 residue was not detected in any of the samples. This study further confirms that the risk of direct contamination of this derivative in grains is low.

3.5.2. Contamination Characteristics of Type B Trichothecenes in Different Types of Samples

From Figure 4a, it can be seen that TCNs contamination varies greatly among different food categories. Whole-wheat dumpling wrappers are the most severely contaminated prepared food, followed by whole-wheat noodles, oatmeal, and whole-wheat bread. In contrast, infant whole-grain rice flour is almost uncontaminated, while instant brown rice, instant oats, and oatmeal cookies have lower contamination levels. The reasons for this difference may include the following: First, the quality and contamination status of raw grains differ. Cereals such as wheat and oats are more susceptible to *F. graminearum* infection, while rice has a relatively stronger resistance to infection [50]. Second, product quality standards and regulatory efforts vary. As a special dietary food, infant food has stricter raw material quality control and a higher frequency of self-inspection by enterprises and government supervision, and it is difficult for highly contaminated products to enter the market. Third, there are differences in food processing techniques. High-temperature baking, extrusion puffing, and cooking processes help reduce toxin levels in foods such as oatmeal cookies and instant oats [51]. The moisture content of dumpling wrappers is higher than other cereal products such as bread and biscuits (usually around 35%), and DON has good solubility in moisture, making it easier to accumulate in high-moisture dumpling wrappers. The processing of dumpling wrappers is relatively complex, from dough mixing and resting to rolling and shaping, which takes a long time. The lengthy processing provides more opportunities for residual Fusarium to multiply and produce toxins [52]. Finally, most dumpling wrappers sold in the market are in bulk, and improper storage conditions during the shelf life can easily lead to moisture absorption and mold growth. Residual Fusarium will multiply in large quantities, further increasing the DON content. In addition, the pH value of dumpling wrappers (usually between 5.0–6.0) provides favorable acidic conditions for the stability of DON [53].

Therefore, to reduce DON contamination in whole-wheat dumpling wrappers, it is necessary to control the entire chain from farm to table, improve the quality of whole-wheat flour raw materials, optimize production processes, improve storage and transportation conditions of finished products, and take multiple measures simultaneously to achieve good results.

3.5.3. Co-Contamination Patterns

In the whole-grain prepared food samples in this study, the main contamination patterns of DON + NIV, DON + D3G, and DON + NIV + 3AcDON (Figure 4) are all produced by Fusarium fungi such as *F. graminearum* and *F. culmorum*. It has been confirmed that the biosynthesis of DON and NIV is regulated by the same gene cluster (Trichothecene biosynthesis gene cluster, TRI) [54]. Mutations or deletions of the TRI8 and TRI13 genes in the gene cluster lead to *F. graminearum* synthesizing different types of DON derivatives (3AcDON and D3G) [55], which is further demonstrated by the results of this study. In addition, climate change and global warming have led to more extreme weather conditions with high temperatures and heavy rainfall, providing favorable conditions for the growth and reproduction of Fusarium fungi, which also exacerbates the risk of toxin contamination in these food raw materials.

3.6. Risk Assessment

Considering that DOM–1 was not detected in any of the samples, and infant whole-grain rice flour was almost uncontaminated, we proceeded to conduct a risk assessment for the residues of six trichothecene mycotoxins (TCNs), excluding DOM-1, in seven other categories of whole-grain prepared foods. The hazard quotient (HQ) and hazard index (HI) were calculated using the method recommended by the WHO, acknowledged for its global applicability and comparative risk assessment across various foodstuffs.

As shown in Table 3, whole-wheat dumpling wrappers had the highest average contents of DON and D3G, reaching 590.77 µg/kg and 52.70 µg/kg, respectively. The exposure level (EDI) of DON in whole-wheat dumpling wrappers was 0.9846 µg/kg·day·bw, close to its toxicity reference value (TDI) of 1 µg/kg·day·bw, with a health risk quotient (HQ) as high as 98.462%. Whole-wheat dumpling wrappers also had the highest total health risk index (HI), reaching 136.408%, indicating that the total risk of type B trichothecenes in this food has exceeded the standard. The risk of DON has been previously found in commercially available noodles, steamed buns, and flour in China [56–58], and this study is the first to find it in whole-grain prepared foods, reflecting that DON contamination in whole-grain prepared foods remains a serious food safety issue that urgently needs effective measures to control. The DON contents in oats, instant oats, and oatmeal cookies were relatively low, but still reached 260.36, 133.93, and 55.86 µg/kg, respectively. The HQ value of oats was 43.393%, and the HI value was 60.419%, which also requires attention. In contrast, instant brown rice had the lowest contents and risk levels of various type B trichothecene toxins, and the overall risk was controllable. In addition to DON and D3G, 3AcDON and 15AcDON were co-contaminated in whole-wheat dumpling wrappers and whole–wheat noodles. Although the HQ values were not high, considering that existing studies have found synergistic toxic effects of these acetylated derivatives with DON in in vitro and in vivo experiments such as intestinal epithelial cells, piglets, and zebrafish [59–61], their hazards should not be ignored. However, it is pertinent to acknowledge that this additive approach may not always precisely reflect the interactive complexity of mycotoxin exposure.

Table 3. Dietary exposure risk assessment of trichothecene mycotoxins in grain processed foods in the Chinese population.

Whole Grain Pre-Processed Foods	Type B Trichothecenes	C (µg/kg)	TDI (µg/kg·day·bw)	EDI (µg/kg·day·bw)	HQ (%)	HI (%)
Ready-to-eat brown rice	DON	45.60	1	0.0760	7.600	9.510
	D3G	2.24	0.3	0.0037	1.242	
	NIV	2.06	0.7	0.0034	0.490	
	3AcDON	0.67	1	0.0011	0.112	
	15AcDON	0.25	1	0.0004	0.042	
	FusX	0.10	0.7	0.0002	0.024	
Oatmeal	DON	260.36	1	0.4339	43.393	60.419
	D3G	24.95	0.3	0.0416	13.862	
	NIV	3.93	0.7	0.0066	0.936	
	3AcDON	12.28	1	0.0205	2.046	
	15AcDON	0.96	1	0.0016	0.159	
	FusX	0.10	0.7	0.0002	0.024	
Ready-to-eat oatmeal	DON	133.93	1	0.2232	22.321	27.010
	D3G	6.86	0.3	0.0114	3.808	
	NIV	1.27	0.7	0.0021	0.303	
	3AcDON	3.03	1	0.0050	0.504	
	15AcDON	0.30	1	0.0005	0.050	
	FusX	0.10	0.7	0.0002	0.024	
Oatmeal cookies	DON	55.86	1	0.0931	9.310	11.490
	D3G	2.89	0.3	0.0048	1.606	
	NIV	1.29	0.7	0.0022	0.308	
	3AcDON	1.15	1	0.0019	0.192	
	15AcDON	0.30	1	0.0005	0.050	
	FusX	0.10	0.7	0.0002	0.024	
Whole-wheat bread	DON	279.51	1	0.4659	46.585	57.242
	D3G	13.83	0.3	0.0230	7.681	
	NIV	3.59	0.7	0.0060	0.854	
	3AcDON	8.88	1	0.0148	1.480	
	15AcDON	3.43	1	0.0057	0.572	
	FusX	0.30	0.7	0.0005	0.071	
Whole-wheat noodles	DON	354.05	1	0.5901	59.009	71.100
	D3G	14.47	0.3	0.0241	8.041	
	NIV	5.21	0.7	0.0087	1.241	
	3AcDON	12.13	1	0.0202	2.022	
	15AcDON	4.42	1	0.0074	0.736	
	FusX	0.21	0.7	0.0004	0.051	

Table 3. Cont.

Whole Grain Pre-Processed Foods	Type B Trichothecenes	C (μg/kg)	TDI (μg/kg·day·bw)	EDI (μg/kg·day·bw)	HQ (%)	HI (%)
Whole-wheat dumpling wrapper	DON	590.77	1	0.9846	98.462	136.408
	D3G	52.70	0.3	0.0878	29.277	
	NIV	10.84	0.7	0.0181	2.580	
	3AcDON	31.40	1	0.0523	5.234	
	15AcDON	3.88	1	0.0065	0.647	
	FusX	0.88	0.7	0.0015	0.209	

Note: Whole-grain prepared foods consumption is 100 g/d. C: mean concentration of mycotoxin in samples. Mean body weight is 60 kg. Mycotoxin intake = (Whole-grain prepared foods consumption × C)/(mean body weight × 1000). HQ (Hazard Quotient, %) = mycotoxin intake × 100/TDI. HI (Hazard Index, %) = $\sum$HQ.

4. Conclusions

For the first time, this study established an online SPE–UPLC–MS/MS method for the rapid quantitative determination of seven type B trichothecene toxins in whole-grain prepared foods. By designing a single-valve dual-column system and using a high-pressure six-port valve to connect the RAM purification column and the analytical column in parallel, column switching after sample injection was achieved, simultaneously accomplishing purification and separation. The results showed that this method improves efficiency and speed on the basis of reducing costs (less manual input and no need for internal standards) and has good robustness. After validation, the method was found to be sensitive and accurate, suitable for routine large-scale quantitative analysis of type B trichothecene toxin contamination in whole-grain prepared foods. The practicality of the method was verified by quantifying seven mycotoxins in 160 batches of eight categories of whole-grain prepared foods.

Overall, the total risk of type-B trichothecenes in whole-grain processed foods is a cause for concern. DON is the most prevalent and severe trichothecene toxin in these foods. However, D3G, NIV, and 3AcDON often coexist, and their harmful effects may be added. Currently, relevant standards are not perfect, and the contamination situation is underestimated. It is recommended to strengthen the monitoring of trichothecene toxin contamination in whole-grain raw materials and improve the processing technology of prepared foods. In addition, it is very necessary and urgent to formulate detailed maximum limits for related toxins in these foods.

This study used the recommended daily intake value of whole grains for adults in the Chinese Dietary Guidelines as the food factor (F value) for estimating exposure. This assumption is based on the following considerations: First, whole-grain prepared foods are one of the important sources of whole-grain intake in the diet; second, in the absence of actual survey data, the recommended value in the dietary guidelines can be used as a reference benchmark for assessing potential exposure risks [62]. However, it should be noted that it is crucial to articulate that such risk quantifications incorporate several assumptions. These include standardized consumption data, uniform absorption rates, and constant daily intake over time, which may not capture the nuances of population-specific dietary habits or acute consumption patterns. Moreover, the TDI value for DON is itself based on certain toxicological assumptions that might not encompass all subpopulations' sensitivities. Despite these inherent uncertainties, employing this WHO-recommended approach provides an initial, albeit approximate, framework to gauge potential health risks and guide preventative strategies. The assessment acts as an impetus for more nuanced, targeted studies and supports the necessity for stringent control measures to mitigate DON contamination in whole-grain prepared foods. In the future, it will be necessary to conduct a nationwide consumption survey of whole-grain prepared foods to obtain more accurate food factor data to better assess the exposure level and health risks of the population.

Supplementary Materials: The following supporting information can be downloaded at: https://www.mdpi.com/article/10.3390/toxics12050336/s1, Table S1: A summary of B-type trichothecenes detection in grains via LCMS/MS over the last decade. Table S2: Accuracy and precision data for determination of 7 mycotoxins at three levels in one day ($n = 6$) and three distinct days ($n = 18$). Table S3: The occurrence of 7 TCNs in 160 Whole grain prepared foods samples from 8 food categories collected in Chinese market.

Author Contributions: Conceptualization, X.N., Y.H. and Y.Y.; Data curation, X.N. and Y.H.; Formal analysis, X.N. and Y.Y.; Investigation, S.J., Y.Z. and P.C.; Methodology, X.N., J.C. and P.C.; Software, X.N. and J.L.; Supervision, X.S. and J.C.; Visualization, T.L. and J.J.; Writing—original draft, X.N. and Y.Y.; Writing—review & editing, X.N., J.J., X.S. and J.C. All authors have read and agreed to the published version of the manuscript.

Funding: This research was funded by the National Key Research and Development Program of China (2022YFF1100701), and the Training Fund for academic leaders of NIFDC (2021X5).

Institutional Review Board Statement: Not applicable.

Informed Consent Statement: Not applicable.

Data Availability Statement: All data used in this work is available either within the article or in the Supporting Information File.

Conflicts of Interest: Author Yanchun Hui was employed by the company Sanyo Fine Trading Co. Ltd. The remaining authors declare that the research was conducted in the absence of any commercial or financial relationships that could be construed as a potential conflict of interest.

Abbreviations

Solid phase extraction (SPE), restricted-access media (RAM), trichothecenes (TCNs), deoxynivalenol (DON), 3–acetyldeoxynivalenol (3AcDON), 15–acetyldeoxynivalenol (15AcDON), deoxynivalenol 3–glucuronide (D3G), de-epoxy-deoxynivalenol (DOM–1), fusarenon–X (FusX), nivalenol (NIV), ultra-high-performance liquid chromatography-tandem mass spectrometry (UHPLC–MS/MS), limit of detection (LOD), limit of quantification (LOQ).

References

1. European Food Safety Authority. Risk to human and animal health related to the presence of deoxynivalenol and its acetylated and modified forms in food and feed. *EFSA J.* **2020**. [CrossRef]
2. World Health Organization. *Deoxynivalenol (DON) in Feed and Food*; World Health Organization: Geneva, Switzerland, 2021.
3. You, Y.; Hu, Q.; Liu, N.; Xu, C.; Lu, S.; Xu, T.; Mao, X. Metabolite analysis of *Alternaria* mycotoxins by LC-MS/MS and multiple tools. *Molecules* **2023**, *28*, 3258. [CrossRef]
4. Pavlenko, R.; Berzina, Z.; Reinholds, I.; Bartkiene, E.; Bartkevics, V. An occurrence study of mycotoxins in plant-based beverages using liquid chromatography-mass spectrometry. *Toxins* **2024**, *16*, 53. [CrossRef]
5. Casado, N.; Gañán, J.; Morante-Zarcero, S.; Sierra, I. New Advanced materials and sorbent-based microextraction techniques as strategies in sample preparation to improve the determination of natural toxins in food samples. *Molecules* **2020**, *25*, 702. [CrossRef]
6. Meneely, J.P.; Ricci, F.; van Egmond, H.P.; Elliott, C.T. Current methods of analysis for the determination of trichothecene mycotoxins in food. *TrAC Trends Anal. Chem.* **2011**, *30*, 192–203. [CrossRef]
7. Svahn, O.; Björklund, E. High flow-rate sample loading in large volume whole water organic trace analysis using positive pressure and finely ground sand as a SPE-column in-line filter. *Molecules* **2019**, *24*, 1426. [CrossRef]
8. European Commission. Commission Decision 2002/657/EC of 12 August 2002 Implementing Council Directive 96/23/EC Concerning the Performance of Analytical Methods and the Interpretation of Results. *Off. J. Eur. Communities* **2002**, *50*, 8–36. Available online: https://eur-lex.europa.eu/legal-content/EN/TXT/?uri=CELEX:32002D0657 (accessed on 11 February 2024).
9. Zhao, Z.; Rao, Q.; Song, S.; Liu, N.; Han, Z.; Hou, J.; Wu, A. Simultaneous determination of major type B trichothecenes and deoxynivalenol-3-glucoside in animal feed and raw materials using improved DSPE combined with LC-MS/MS. *J. Chromatogr. B Analyt. Technol. Biomed. Life Sci.* **2014**, *963*, 75–82. [CrossRef]
10. Chinese Nutrition Society. *The Chinese Dietary Guidelines 2022*; People's Medical Publishing House: Beijing, China, 2022.
11. World Health Organization. Towards a harmonised total diet study approach: A guidance document. *EFSA J.* **2011**, *9*, 2450.

12. EFSA Panel on Contaminants in the Food Chain. Risks to Human and Animal Health Related to the Presence of Deoxynivalenol and Its Acetylated and Modified Forms in Food and Feed. *EFSA J.* **2017**, *15*, 4718. Available online: https://www.efsa.europa.eu/en/efsajournal/pub/4718 (accessed on 11 February 2024).
13. EFSA Panel on Contaminants in the Food Chain. Scientific Opinion on Risks for Animal and Public Health Related to the Presence of Nivalenol in Food and Feed. *EFSA J.* **2013**, *11*, 3262. Available online: https://www.efsa.europa.eu/en/efsajournal/pub/3262 (accessed on 12 February 2024). [CrossRef]
14. Aupanun, S.; Poapolathep, S.; Giorgi, M.; Imsilp, K.; Poapolathep, A. An overview of the toxicology and toxicokinetics of fusarenon-X, a type B trichothecene mycotoxin. *J. Vet. Med. Sci.* **2017**, *79*, 6–13. [CrossRef] [PubMed]
15. Wang, Y.J.; Nie, J.Y.; Yan, Z.; Li, Z.X.; Cheng, Y.; Saqib, F. Multi-mycotoxin exposure and risk assessments for Chinese consumption of nuts and dried fruits. *J. Integr. Agri.* **2023**, *164*, 112456. [CrossRef]
16. Ojuri, O.T.; Ezekiel, C.N.; Eskola, M.K.; Šarkanj, B.; Babalola, A.D.; Sulyok, M.; Krska, R. Mycotoxin co-exposures in infants and young children consuming household- and industrially-processed complementary foods in Nigeria and risk management advice. *Food Control* **2019**, *98*, 312–322. [CrossRef]
17. Schaarschmidt, S.; Fauhl-Hassek, C. Mycotoxins during the processes of nixtamalization and tortilla production. *Toxins* **2019**, *11*, 227. [CrossRef]
18. Rahmani, A.; Jinap, S.; Soleimany, F. Qualitative and quantitative analysis of mycotoxins. *Compr. Rev. Food Sci. Food Saf.* **2009**, *8*, 202–251. [CrossRef]
19. Agriopoulou, S.; Stamatelopoulou, E.; Varzakas, T. Advances in analysis and detection of major mycotoxins in foods. *Foods* **2020**, *9*, 518. [CrossRef]
20. Solanki, M.K.; Abdelfattah, A.; Sadhasivam, S.; Zakin, V.; Wisniewski, M.; Droby, S.; Sionov, E. Analysis of stored wheat grain-associated microbiota reveals biocontrol activity among microorganisms against mycotoxigenic Fungi. *J. Fungi* **2020**, *6*, 781. [CrossRef]
21. Chen, J.; Li, P.; Zhang, T.; Xu, Z.; Huang, X.; Wang, R.; Du, L. Review on Strategies and Technologies for Exosome Isolation and Purification. *Front. Bioeng. Biotechnol.* **2020**, *9*, 811971. [CrossRef]
22. Broekaert, N.; Devreese, M.; De Mil, T.; Croubels, S. Development and validation of an LC-MS/MS method for the toxicokinetic study of deoxynivalenol and its acetylated derivatives in chicken and pig plasma. *J. Chromatogr. B* **2014**, *971*, 43–51. [CrossRef]
23. Tahoun, I.F.; Gab-Allah, M.A.; Yamani, R.N.; Shehata, A.B. Development and validation of a reliable LC-MS/MS method for simultaneous determination of deoxynivalenol and T-2 toxin in maize and oats. *Microchem. J.* **2021**, *169*, 106599. [CrossRef]
24. Mohamed, A.; Gab-Allah, K.C.; Byungjoo, K. Accurate determination of type B trichothecenes and conjugated deoxynivalenol in grains by isotope dilution-liquid chromatography tandem mass spectrometry. *Food Control* **2021**, *121*, 107557.
25. Woo, S.Y.; Lee, S.Y.; Park, S.B.; Chun, H.S. Simultaneous determination of 17 regulated and non-regulated Fusarium mycotoxins co-occurring in foodstuffs by UPLC-MS/MS with solid-phase extraction. *Food Chem.* **2024**, *438*, 137624. [CrossRef] [PubMed]
26. Zhang, Y.Y.; Zhao, M.J.; Liu, C.Y.; Ma, K.; Liu, T.Y.; Chen, F.; Wu, L.N.; Hu, D.J.; Lv, G.P. Comparison of two commercial methods with a UHPLC-MS/MS method for the determination of multiple mycotoxins in cereals. *Food Chem.* **2023**, *406*, 135056. [CrossRef] [PubMed]
27. Kresse, M.; Drinda, H.; Romanotto, A.; Speer, K. Simultaneous determination of pesticides, mycotoxins, and metabolites as well as other contaminants in cereals by LC-LC-MS/MS. *J. Chromatogr. B Analyt. Technol. Biomed Life Sci.* **2019**, *1117*, 86–102. [CrossRef] [PubMed]
28. Njumbe Ediage, E.; Van Poucke, C.; De Saeger, S. A multi-analyte LC-MS/MS method for the analysis of 23 mycotoxins in different sorghum varieties: The forgotten sample matrix. *Food Chem.* **2015**, *117*, 397–404. [CrossRef]
29. European Commission. Guidance Document on Analytical Quality Control and Method Validation Procedures for Pesticide Residues Analysis in Food and Feed. Document No. SANTE/11813/2017. 2017. Available online: https://www.eurl-pesticides.eu/userfiles/file/EurlALL/SANTE_11813_2017-fin.pdf (accessed on 8 March 2024).
30. De Colli, L.; Elliott, C.; Finnan, J.; Grant, J.; Arendt, E.K.; McCormick, S.P.; Danaher, M. Determination of 42 mycotoxins in oats using a mechanically assisted QuEChERS sample preparation and UHPLC-MS/MS detection. *J. Chromatogr. B Analyt. Technol. Biomed. Life Sci.* **2020**, *1150*, 122187. [CrossRef] [PubMed]
31. International Union of Pure and Applied Chemistry. Harmonized Guidelines for Single-Laboratory Validation of Methods of Analysis. *Pure Appl. Chem.* **2002**, *74*, 835–855. [CrossRef]
32. Food and Drug Administration. Analytical Procedures and Methods Validation for Drugs and Biologics. 2015. Available online: https://www.fda.gov/regulatory-information/search-fda-guidance-documents/analytical-procedures-and-methods-validation-drugs-and-biologics (accessed on 8 March 2024).
33. López-Serna, R.; Pérez, S.; Ginebreda, A.; Petrović, M.; Barceló, D. Fully automated determination of 74 pharmaceuticals in environmental and waste waters by online solid phase extraction-liquid chromatography-electrospray-tandem mass spectrometry. *Talanta* **2010**, *83*, 410–424. [CrossRef]
34. Gros, M.; Rodríguez-Mozaz, S.; Barceló, D. Rapid analysis of multiclass antibiotic residues and some of their metabolites in hospital, urban wastewater and river water by ultra-high-performance liquid chromatography coupled to quadrupolelinear ion trap tandem mass spectrometry. *J. Chromatogr. A* **2013**, *1292*, 173–188. [CrossRef]
35. Codex Alimentarius Commission. *General Standard for Contaminants and Toxins in Food and Feed (CODEX STAN 193–1995)*; Codex Alimentarius Commission: Rome, Italy, 2015.

36. European Commission. Commission Regulation (EC) No 1881/2006 of 19 December 2006 setting maximum levels for certain contaminants in foodstuffs. *Off. J. Eur. Union* **2006**, *L364*, 5–24.
37. National Health and Family Planning Commission of the People's Republic of China, Standardization Administration of China. *GB 2761-2017 National Food Safety Standard-Maximum Levels of Mycotoxins in Foods*; Standards Press of China: Beijing, China, 2017.
38. Vogelgsang, S.; Beyer, M.; Pasquali, M.; Jenny, E.; Musa, T.; Bucheli, T.D.; Wettstein, F.E.; Forrer, H.R. An eight-year survey of wheat shows distinctive effects of cropping factors on different Fusarium species and associated mycotoxins. *Eur. J. Agron.* **2019**, *105*, 62–77. [CrossRef]
39. Bryła, M.; Waśkiewicz, A.; Podolska, G.; Szymczyk, K.; Jędrzejczak, R.; Damaziak, K.; Sułek, A. Occurrence of 26 mycotoxins in the grain of cereals cultivated in Poland. *Toxins* **2016**, *8*, 160. [CrossRef]
40. Amarasinghe, C.C.; Simsek, S.; Brûlé-Babel, A.; Fernando, W.G. Analysis of deoxynivalenol and deoxynivalenol-3-glucosides content in Canadian spring wheat cultivars inoculated with Fusarium graminearum. *Food Addit. Contam. Part A* **2016**, *33*, 1254–1264. [CrossRef]
41. Ueno, Y.; Hsieh, D.P.H. The toxicology of mycotoxins. *Crit. Rev. Toxicol.* **1985**, *14*, 99–132. [CrossRef]
42. Gruber-Dorninger, C.; Novak, B.; Nagl, V.; Berthiller, F. Emerging mycotoxins: Beyond traditionally determined food contaminants. *J. Agric. Food Chem.* **2017**, *65*, 7052–7070. [CrossRef]
43. Penagos-Tabares, F.; Khiaosa-Ard, R.; Nagl, V.; Faas, J.; Jenkins, T.; Sulyok, M.; Zebeli, Q. Mycotoxins, Phytoestrogens and other secondary metabolites in Austrian pastures: Occurrences, contamination levels and implications of geo-climatic factors. *Toxins* **2021**, *13*, 460. [CrossRef]
44. Zhou, H.; Xu, A.; Liu, M.; Yan, Z.; Qin, L.; Liu, H.; Wu, A.; Liu, N. Mycotoxins in wheat flours marketed in Shanghai, China: Occurrence and dietary risk assessment. *Toxins* **2022**, *14*, 748. [CrossRef]
45. Palacios, S.A.; Erazo, J.G.; Ciasca, B.; Lattanzio, V.M.T.; Reynoso, M.M.; Farnochi, M.C.; Torres, A.M. Occurrence of deoxynivalenol and deoxynivalenol-3-glucoside in durum wheat from Argentina. *Food Chem.* **2017**, *230*, 728–734. [CrossRef]
46. Tittlemier, S.A.; Roscoe, M.; Trelka, R.; Gräfenhan, T. Fusarium damage in small cereal grains from Western Canada. 2. Occurrence of fusarium toxins and their source organisms in durum wheat harvested in 2010. *J. Agr. Food Chem.* **2013**, *61*, 5438–5448. [CrossRef]
47. Chen, X.; Dong, F.; Zhong, L.; Wu, D.; Wang, S.; Xu, J.; Ma, G.; Shi, J. Contamination Pattern of Fusarium Toxinsin Cerealsin Sichuan Province. *J. Sichuan Agri. Univ.* **2021**, *39*, 141–148.
48. Broekaert, N.; Devreese, M.; De Mil, T.; Fraeyman, S.; Antonissen, G.; De Baere, S.; De Backer, P.; Vermeulen, A.; Croubels, S. Oral bioavailability, hydrolysis, and comparative toxicokinetics of 3-acetyldeoxynivalenol and 15-acetyldeoxynivalenol in broiler chickens and pigs. *J. Agric. Food Chem.* **2015**, *63*, 8734–8742. [CrossRef]
49. Payros, D.; Alassane-Kpembi, I.; Pierron, A.; Loiseau, N.; Pinton, P.; Oswald, I.P. Toxicology of deoxynivalenol and its acetylated and modified forms. *Arch Toxicol.* **2016**, *90*, 2931–2957. [CrossRef]
50. Schaarschmidt, S.; Fauhl-Hassek, C. The fate of mycotoxins during the processing of wheat for human consumption. *Compr. Rev. Food Sci. Food Saf.* **2018**, *17*, 556–593. [CrossRef]
51. Karlovsky, P.; Suman, M.; Berthiller, F.; De Meester, J.; Eisenbrand, G.; Perrin, I.; Oswald, I.P.; Speijers, G.; Chiodini, A.; Recker, T.; et al. Impact of food processing and detoxification treatments on mycotoxin contamination. *Mycotoxin Res.* **2016**, *32*, 179–205. [CrossRef]
52. Ovando-Martínez, M.; Ozsisli, B.; Anderson, J.; Whitney, K.; Ohm, J.-B.; Simsek, S. Analysis of deoxynivalenol and deoxynivalenol-3-glucoside in hard red spring wheat inoculated with Fusarium graminearum. *Toxins* **2013**, *5*, 2522–2532. [CrossRef]
53. Wu, Q.; Kuča, K.; Humpf, H.U.; Klímová, B.; Cramer, B. Fate of deoxynivalenol and deoxynivalenol-3-glucoside during cereal-based thermal food processing: A review study. *Mycotoxin Res.* **2017**, *33*, 79–91. [CrossRef]
54. Brown, D.W.; McCormick, S.P.; Alexander, N.J.; Proctor, R.H.; Desjardins, A.E. A genetic and biochemical approach to study trichothecene diversity in Fusarium sporotrichioides and Fusarium graminearum. *Fungal Genet. Biol.* **2001**, *32*, 121–133. [CrossRef]
55. Alexander, N.J.; McCormick, S.P.; Waalwijk, C.; van der Lee, T.; Proctor, R.H. The genetic basis for 3-ADON and 15-ADON trichothecene chemotypes in Fusarium. *Fungal Genet. Biol.* **2011**, *48*, 485–495. [CrossRef]
56. Gao, X.; Mu, P.; Wen, J.; Sun, Y.; Chen, Q.; Deng, Y. Detoxification of trichothecene mycotoxins by a novel bacterium, Eggerthella sp. DII-9. *Food Chem. Toxicol.* **2018**, *112*, 310–319. [CrossRef]
57. Geng, Z.; Yang, D.; Zhou, M.; Zhang, P.; Wang, D. Determination of deoxynivalenol in Chinese steamed bread by HPLC-UV method: A survey of the market in Hebei province, China. *Food Control* **2018**, *92*, 43–49.
58. Peng, W.X.; Marchal, J.L.M.; van der Poel, A.F.B. Strategies to prevent and reduce mycotoxins for compound feed manufacturing. *Ani. Feed Sci. Tech.* **2018**, *237*, 129–153. [CrossRef]
59. Alassane-Kpembi, I.; Kolf-Clauw, M.; Gauthier, T.; Abrami, R.; Abiola, F.A.; Oswald, I.P.; Puel, O. New insights into mycotoxin mixtures: The toxicity of low doses of Type B trichothecenes on intestinal epithelial cells is synergistic. *Toxicol. Appl. Pharmacol.* **2013**, *272*, 191–198. [CrossRef]
60. Alizadeh, A.; Braber, S.; Akbari, P.; Garssen, J.; Fink-Gremmels, J. Deoxynivalenol impairs weight gain and affects markers of gut health after low-dose, short-term exposure of growing pigs. *Toxins* **2015**, *7*, 2071–2095. [CrossRef]

61. Zhou, H.; George, S.; Li, C.; Gurusamy, S.; Sun, X.; Gong, Z.; Qian, H. Combined toxicity of prevalent mycotoxins studied in fish cell line and zebrafish larvae revealed that type of interactions is dose-dependent. *Aquat. Toxicol.* **2017**, *193*, 60–71. [CrossRef]
62. Mann, K.D.; Pearce, M.S.; McKevith, B.; Thielecke, F.; Seal, C.J. Whole grain intake and its association with intakes of other foods, nutrients and markers of health in the National Diet and Nutrition Survey rolling programme 2008–2011. *Br. J. Nutr.* **2015**, *13*, 1595–1602. [CrossRef]

Disclaimer/Publisher's Note: The statements, opinions and data contained in all publications are solely those of the individual author(s) and contributor(s) and not of MDPI and/or the editor(s). MDPI and/or the editor(s) disclaim responsibility for any injury to people or property resulting from any ideas, methods, instructions or products referred to in the content.

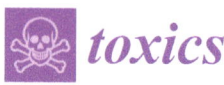

Article

High-Coverage UHPLC-MS/MS Analysis of 67 Mycotoxins in Plasma for Male Infertility Exposure Studies

Xiao Ning [1,2], Lulu Wang [2], Jia-Sheng Wang [3], Jian Ji [1], Shaoming Jin [2], Jiadi Sun [1], Yongli Ye [1], Shenghui Mei [4,5], Yinzhi Zhang [1], Jin Cao [2,*] and Xiulan Sun [1,*]

1. School of Food Science and Technology, International Joint Laboratory on Food Safety, Synergetic Innovation Center of Food Safety and Quality Control, Jiangnan University, Wuxi 214122, China; nx200730079@163.com (X.N.); jijian@jiangnan.edu.cn (J.J.); sunjiadi@jiangnan.edu.cn (J.S.); yyly0222@163.com (Y.Y.); yinzhizhang@jiangnan.edu.cn (Y.Z.)
2. Key Laboratory of Food Quality and Safety for State Market Regulation, National Institute of Food and Drug Control, Beijing 100050, China; wanglulu199805@163.com (L.W.); yjackyming@126.com (S.J.)
3. Department of Environmental Health Science, College of Public Health, University of Georgia, Athens, GA 30602, USA; jswang@uga.edu
4. Department of Pharmacy, Beijing Tiantan Hospital, Capital Medical University, Beijing 100070, China; meishenghui1983@126.com
5. Department of Clinical Pharmacology, School of Pharmaceutical Sciences, Capital Medical University, Beijing 100069, China
* Correspondence: caojin@nifdc.org.cn (J.C.); sxlzzz@jiangnan.edu.cn (X.S.); Tel.: +86-010-6709-5070 (J.C.); +86-0510-8591-2330 (X.S.)

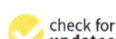

Citation: Ning, X.; Wang, L.; Wang, J.-S.; Ji, J.; Jin, S.; Sun, J.; Ye, Y.; Mei, S.; Zhang, Y.; Cao, J.; et al. High-Coverage UHPLC-MS/MS Analysis of 67 Mycotoxins in Plasma for Male Infertility Exposure Studies. *Toxics* 2024, 12, 395. https://doi.org/10.3390/toxics12060395

Academic Editor: Minjian Chen

Received: 3 April 2024
Revised: 15 May 2024
Accepted: 21 May 2024
Published: 28 May 2024

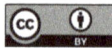

Copyright: © 2024 by the authors. Licensee MDPI, Basel, Switzerland. This article is an open access article distributed under the terms and conditions of the Creative Commons Attribution (CC BY) license (https://creativecommons.org/licenses/by/4.0/).

Abstract: Mycotoxins are a class of exogenous metabolites that are major contributors to foodborne diseases and pose a potential threat to human health. However, little attention has been paid to trace mycotoxin co-exposure situations in vivo. To address this, we devised a novel analytical strategy, both highly sensitive and comprehensive, for quantifying 67 mycotoxins in human plasma samples. This method employs isotope dilution mass spectrometry (IDMS) for approximately 40% of the analytes and utilizes internal standard quantification for the rest. The mycotoxins were classified into three categories according to their physicochemical properties, facilitating the optimization of extraction and detection parameters to improve analytical performance. The lowest limits of detection and quantitation were 0.001–0.5 µg/L and 0.002–1 µg/L, respectively, the intra-day precision ranged from 1.8% to 11.9% RSD, and the intra-day trueness ranged from 82.7–116.6% for all mycotoxins except Ecl, DH-LYS, PCA, and EnA (66.4–129.8%), showing good analytical performance of the method for biomonitoring. A total of 40 mycotoxins (including 24 emerging mycotoxins) were detected in 184 plasma samples (89 from infertile males and 95 from healthy males) using the proposed method, emphasizing the widespread exposure of humans to both traditional and emerging mycotoxins. The most frequently detected mycotoxins were ochratoxin A, ochratoxin B, enniatin B, and citrinin. The incidence of exposure to multiple mycotoxins was significantly higher in infertile males than in healthy subjects, particularly levels of ochratoxin A, ochratoxin B, and citrinin, which were significantly increased. It is necessary to carry out more extensive biological monitoring to provide data support for further study of the relationship between mycotoxins and male infertility.

Keywords: mycotoxin; UHPLC-MS/MS; emerging mycotoxins; male infertility; human biomonitoring

1. Introduction

Mycotoxins are harmful secondary metabolites produced by fungi, commonly found in the environment and food. Strict regulations have been implemented worldwide to establish maximum residue limits for the six types of typical traditional mycotoxins commonly contaminated in food. However, in recent years, some mycotoxins that had received little attention or were newly discovered have been found to have high detection rates in food, such as beauvericin, cyclopiazonic acid, enniatins, and sterigmatocystin [1–5]. These mycotoxins, collectively referred to as emerging mycotoxins, are neither routinely tested nor regulated by legislation [6,7]. Consuming mycotoxin-contaminated foods can lead to acute or chronic diseases. The World Health Organization has identified mycotoxins as major contributors to foodborne illnesses that pose potential threats to human health. Numerous studies have shown that exposure to a mixture of mycotoxins is particularly concerning due to potential synergistic interactions, leading to new and unexpectable effects [8,9]. Therefore, monitoring human exposure to multiple mycotoxins and conducting risk assessments are crucial.

Toxicological studies have indicated that both known and emerging mycotoxins can have negative effects on reproduction [10,11]. Infertility affects about 15% of couples worldwide, with a steady increase [12]. Male factors are responsible for at least 50% of infertility cases [13,14]. The significant decline in sperm quality and human fertility globally has been attributed to various factors [15,16], including the impact of endocrine-disrupting chemicals like mycotoxins [17]. However, the relationship between the development of male infertility and mycotoxin exposure remains unclear due to the lack of reliable data on human internal exposure to mycotoxins. Common biomarkers for mycotoxin exposure involve proteins, DNA adducts, phase I and phase II metabolites, and the parent compounds [18,19]. Only a few methods have effectively detected multiple mycotoxins from different groups in human plasma samples (Table S1). This limited capability has led to underestimations of simultaneous exposure to multiple emerging mycotoxins [20–23]. Therefore, it is important to establish a detection method to trace foodborne mycotoxins in body fluids that can study the concurrent exposure to mycotoxins and investigate their relationship with male infertility.

Typical assessments of mycotoxin exposure usually involve combining data on their occurrence in food with information about food consumption. However, this approach has certain limitations. For example, the distribution of mycotoxins in food products is not homogeneous, and some mycotoxins are chemically activated by the human body and therefore cannot be detected before consumption. Furthermore, the bioavailability and toxicology of mycotoxins can vary depending on the food treatment and inter-individual differences [24]. Therefore, conducting accurate risk assessments based solely on these data is difficult. Human biomonitoring (HBM) offers a more direct method of investigation by combining the levels of substances in internal body fluids with data on external sources of exposure. HBM provides a more reliable assessment as it correlates mycotoxins with specific disorders rather than focusing solely on food contamination. Ultra-high liquid chromatography–tandem mass spectrometry (UHPLC-MS/MS) is a highly selective and sensitive technology that can be used to analyze multiple chemically diverse mycotoxins from complex biological matrices. Optimizing the extraction and clean-up steps is crucial for implementing this multi-mycotoxin analytical method since mycotoxins have different acid/base properties and cover a wide range of polarities [24,25].

The critical aspect of this work is the rational grouping to achieve the simultaneous analysis of as many components of the same class as possible. During biomonitoring studies, the presence of specific mycotoxins is often unpredictable. The availability of a method capable of precisely quantifying a wide range of commonly occurring mycotoxins in the food supply has significantly lowered the cost of individual sample analysis compared to methods that target a single mycotoxin. It allows for monitoring of large number of samples (hundreds or thousands) to identify sub-populations that may exceed recommended exposure guidelines.

The aim of this study was to develop a rapid, sensitive, accurate, and robust strategy for the quantitative identification of 67 mycotoxins in human plasma, employing a combination of isotope dilution and internal standard quantification through UHPLC/MS/MS. Specifically, isotope dilution mass spectrometry (IDMS) was utilized for approximately 40% of the analytes, mainly for those where reference standards were available, while the remaining were quantified using internal standard methods. This approach allowed us to include both traditional and emerging mycotoxins. The applicability of the improved

UHPLC-MS/MS method was then demonstrated by analyzing plasma from 184 males from China, including 89 infertile individuals and 95 fertile individuals. Finally, the study investigated the correlation between male infertility and mycotoxin exposure. To the best of our knowledge, this is the first study in China to evaluate exposure to 67 mycotoxins by analyzing plasma samples from infertile males.

2. Materials and Methods

2.1. Materials and Equipment

The information about the types, molecular formulas, and structures of 67 mycotoxins obtained from Romer Labs (Tulln, Austria) are shown in Tables 1 and S2. LC-MS grade acetonitrile (ACN), 99% formic acid (FA), glacial acetic acid (HAc), ammonium acetate (CH_3COONH_4), and ammonium formate (NH_4HCO_2) were supplied by Fisher Scientific (Waltham, MA, USA). Ultrapure water was generated using a Milli-Q purification system (Millipore, MA, USA). Captiva EMR-Lipid (1 mL) cartridges and Oasis PRiME-HLB (30 mg, 1 mL) cartridges were purchased from Agilent Technologies (Santa Clara, CA, USA) and Waters (Milford, MA, USA), respectively.

Table 1. Group information for 67 mycotoxins and based on the pre-treatment steps.

Groups	Analytes	Abbreviation	Analytes	Abbreviation
A group	aflatoxin B_1	AFB_1	dihydrolysergol	DH-LYS
	aflatoxin B_2	AFB_2	elymoclavine	Ecl
	aflatoxin G_1	AFG_1	Ergine	Ergine
	aflatoxin G_2	AFG_2	ergocornine	Eco
	aflatoxin M_1	AFM_1	ergocorninine	Econ
	aflatoxin M_2	AFM_2	ergocristine	Ecr
	ochratoxin A	OTA	ergocristinine	Ecrn
	ochratoxin B	OTB	dihydroergocristine	DH-Ecr
	fumonisin B_1	FB_1	ergokryptine	Ek
	fumonisin B_2	FB_2	ergokryptinine	Ekn
	fumonisin B_3	FB_3	ergometrine	Em
	T-2 toxin	T2	ergometrinine	Emn
	HT-2 toxin	HT2	ergosinine	Esn
	T-2 triol toxin	T2(OH)3	ergotamine	Et
	beauvericin	BEA	ergotaminine	Etn
	enniatin A	EnA	gliotoxin	GLIO
	enniatin A_1	EnA_1	mycophenolic acid	MPA
	enniatin B	EnB	penicillic acid	PCA
	enniatin B_1	EnB_1	roquefortine C	RC
	neosolaniol	NEO	sterigmatocystin	STG
	15-acetoxyscirpenol	15AS	cyclopiazonic acid	CPA
	4,15-diacetoxyscirpenol	DAS	citrinin	CIT
	agroclavine	Acl		
B group	zearalanone	ZAN	altenuene	ALT
	zearalenone	ZEN	tenuazonic acid	TeA
	alpha-zearalenol	α-ZEL	altertoxin I	AXT I
	beta-zearalenol	β-ZEL	tentoxin	TEN
	alpha-zearalanol	α-ZAL	moniliformin	MON
	beta-zearalanol	β-ZAL	patulin	PAT
	alternariol	AOH	ochratoxin- alpha	OTα
	alternariol monomethyl ether	AME		

Table 1. Cont.

Groups	Analytes	Abbreviation	Analytes	Abbreviation
C group	deoxynivalenol	DON	nivalenol	NIV
	deoxynivalenol 3-glucuronide	D3G	3-acetyldeoxynivalenol	3AcDON
	deepoxy-deoxynivalenol	DOM	15-acetyldeoxynivalenol	15AcDON
	fusarenon-X	FusX		
IS	^{13}C-aflatoxin B$_1$	^{13}C-AFB$_1$	^{13}C-sterigmatocystin	^{13}C-STG
	^{13}C-aflatoxin B$_2$	^{13}C-AFB$_2$	^{13}C-citrinin	^{13}C-CIT
	^{13}C-aflatoxin G$_1$	^{13}C-AFG$_1$	^{13}C-zearalanone	^{13}C-ZEN
	^{13}C-aflatoxin G$_2$	^{13}C-AFG$_2$	^{13}C-patulin	^{13}C-PAT
	^{13}C-aflatoxin M$_1$	^{13}C-AFM$_1$	^{13}C-alternariol	^{13}C-AOH
	^{13}C-ochratoxin A	^{13}C-OTA	^{13}C-alternariol monomethyl ether	^{13}C-AME
	^{13}C-T-2 toxin	^{13}C-T2	^{13}C-tenuazonic acid	^{13}C-TeA
	^{13}C-HT-2 toxin	^{13}C-HT2	tentoxin-d$_3$	TEN-d$_3$
	^{13}C-fumonisin B$_1$	^{13}C-FB$_1$	^{13}C-deoxynivalenol	^{13}C-DON
	^{13}C-fumonisin B$_2$	^{13}C-FB$_2$	^{13}C-deoxynivalenol	^{13}C-D3G
	^{13}C-fumonisin B$_3$	^{13}C-FB$_3$	^{13}C-nivalenol	^{13}C-NIV
	^{13}C-4,15-diacetoxyscirpenol	^{13}C-DAS	^{13}C-3-acetyldeoxynivalenol	^{13}C-3AcDON
	^{13}C-mycophenolic acid	^{13}C-MPA	^{13}C-15-acetyldeoxynivalenol	^{13}C-15AcDON
	^{13}C-roquefortine C	^{13}C-RC		

Analyses were conducted using a SCIEX ExionLCTM AD liquid chromatography-tandem triple QuadTM 7500 mass spectrometry (AB SCIEX, Framingham, MA, USA) system. Data acquisition and processing were performed using the accompanying software (AB SCIEX, Framingham, MA, USA, version 2.2).

2.2. Sampling

This observational study was conducted in the Beijing Obstetrics and Gynecology Hospital, Capital Medical University. Adult males aged 21–49 years who underwent a medical exam or attend an infertility clinic were included in this study. From December 2014 to August 2015, we recruited 184 subjects who met the inclusion and exclusion criteria. The criteria for inclusion in the case ($n = 89$) and the control group ($n = 95$) are detailed in Supplementary Materials. The study was approved by the ethics committee of the Beijing Obstetrics and Gynecology Hospital, Capital Medical University (ethics number 20141201). All participants signed written informed consents. Blood samples were collected after overnight fasting using EDTA vacuum tubes by professional nurses. Plasma samples were separated by centrifugation at $900\times g$ for 15 min. Then, the plasma samples were aliquoted and stored at -80 °C in freezers until analysis.

2.3. Sample Preparation

Group A. The corresponding 10 µL mixed isotope-labeled internal standard (IS) was added to 0.1 mL of homogenized human plasma samples. After being shaken and mixed, the mixture was incubated for 30 min at 25 °C. Next, 0.4 mL of ACN acidified by 0.1% FA was added to the mixture for protein precipitation, ultrasounded for 20 min, and centrifuged at $9600\times g$ for 5 min. Following that, the supernatant was dried under nitrogen at 40 °C and re-dissolved in 0.1 mL of ACN/water (1:9 v/v). The solution was mixed for 30 s using a vortex and centrifuged at $13,800\times g$ for 10 min. The supernatant was then taken for further analysis.

Group B. Initially, 10 µL of mixed isotope-labeled internal standard (IS) was added to 0.1 mL of homogenized human plasma samples. The mixture was vigorously shaken and then incubated at 25 °C for 30 min to ensure thorough integration of the IS. Following incubation, 0.4 mL of ACN/water (84:16, v/v) was added for protein precipitation. This mixture was subjected to ultrasonication for 20 min and subsequently centrifuged at $9600\times g$ for 5 min to separate the supernatant. For purification, the supernatant was processed through Captiva EMR-Lipid cartridges. After the column effluent was collected, 1 mL of ACN/water (4:1, v/v) was passed through the column to elute any remaining analytes. The eluates were combined, dried under nitrogen at 40 °C, and then reconstituted in 0.1 mL of ACN/water (1:9, v/v). The final mixture was vortexed for 30 s and centrifuged at $13,800\times g$ for 10 min. The clear supernatant was then collected for further analysis.

Group C. The sample preparation process for Group C was similar to that of Group B, with the primary difference being the purification step. Instead of Captiva EMR-Lipid cartridges, PRiME-HLB cartridges were used for purifying the supernatants. After collecting the column effluent, 1 mL of ACN was passed through the column to ensure complete elution. The effluents were then combined and processed in the same subsequent steps as in Group B.

2.4. UHPLC-MS/MS Analysis

A Poroshell 120 EC-C18 column (2.1 × 150 mm, 2.7 μm, Agilent, Santa Clara, CA, USA) was selected for chromatographic separation. Detailed information on the applied mobile phase gradients and optimization information about other chromatographic conditions can be found in the Supplementary Materials, including the MS/MS, scheduled multiple reaction monitoring (SMRM), and ion source parameters. Table S3 summarizes the MS parameters of 67 mycotoxins and 27 labeled IS.

2.5. Method Validation

The validation of the method was conducted in compliance with the established guidelines [26–28], and the specific indicators and methodology were as follows.

2.5.1. Selectivity and Limit of Quantitation (LOQ)

The selectivity determination of methodological refer to [29]. The LOQ was determined as the lowest concentration that satisfies a minimum signal-to-noise ratio of 10.

2.5.2. Carry-Over Effect and Linearity

Determination of carry-over effects and acceptable levels refer to the article of Ediage et al. [30]. Matrix-matched calibration curves were prepared daily for the quantification of mycotoxins in plasma, ranging from the LOQ to 100 times the LOQ, with a labeled IS concentration set at 20 times the LOQ. Blank plasma was spiked with a combined standard of mycotoxins to achieve a concentration of 100 times the LOQ for each mycotoxin. The preparation of calibration curve samples, HPLC-MS/MS analysis, and calculations were based on the method proposed by Slobodchikova et al. [31]. The selection of the corresponding IS for each analyte is clearly presented in Table S3.

2.5.3. Trueness and Precision

Accuracy encompasses both trueness and precision, reflecting the influence of both systematic and random errors. The trueness of the method was reflected in the average recovery of 67 analytes at three spiked levels in the blank male plasma. Precision was determined by analyzing the spiked samples for six replicates within a single day (intra-day) and over three consecutive days (inter-day) and expressed in terms of the RSD. The bias and RSD of validation samples should be within ±20% and less than 15%, respectively.

2.5.4. Recovery and Matrix Effect

The quality control (QC) samples were randomly prepared with plasma from 12 control groups and stored at −80 °C before use. Three batches of validation samples at three levels were prepared according to Yang et al. [32]. Briefly, 67 mycotoxins and IS were added in mixed plasma from 12 individuals in control groups (set as A), in water (set as B), and post-protein precipitated in mixed plasma from 12 individuals in control groups (set as C). The three batches were then treated and analyzed based on the optimal methods. The recovery rate was calculated as the percentage of the ratio of A to C, and the matrix effect was calculated as the percentage of the ratio of C to B.

2.5.5. Stability

Stability studies include long-term stability studies and short-term stability studies. In the short-term stability test, the recovery of validation samples at 2-fold and 100-fold LOQ were measured under different time-temperature combination conditions (in plasma: 4 °C or 25 °C for 3 h, 6 h, 1 day, 3 days, and 5 days and three freeze-thaw cycles from −80 °C to 25 °C; post treatment: 4 °C for 120 h). The samples were stored at −80 °C for two months in the long-term stability study, otherwise under the same conditions as in the short-term study.

2.6. Statistical Analysis

Categorical variables were presented as frequencies and percentages. The Shapiro–Wilk test was used to examine the normality of the continuous variables. Each mycotoxin concentration exhibited a skewed distribution; therefore, the median and interquartile range were used to describe the mycotoxin concentrations. Chi-squared or Fisher's exact tests were applied to compare the differences in mycotoxin detection rates between the case and control groups. The concentrations of mycotoxins with positive detection rates of more than 70% were compared, and the concentrations below the detection levels were imputed using 50% of the LOD. The Spearman correlation analysis was used to analyze the correlations between different mycotoxins. All statistical analyses were performed using StataMP version 16.0 and R 4.2.2.

3. Results and Discussion

3.1. Optimization of Mobile Phase

During the quantitative analysis of compounds in complex biological matrices, efficient chromatographic separation is important to avoid ionization interference of the MS source and to enhance the sensitivity and accuracy of the entire analysis. Thus, effects of mobile phase composition on the chromatographic performance were investigated. Figure 1 shows the ratio of the peak area of each analyte under process conditions to the peak area under the final optimization conditions. As shown in Figure 1A, an acidic mobile phase generated abundant hydrogen ions, which assisted the positive ionization and enhanced the sensitivity of detection of most analytes in group A, such as OTs, FBs, and AFs. The FA (green and blue dot) was more effective compared to the weaker acid HAc (orange dot). An increase in FA concentration from 0.1% to 0.2% improved the peak shapes and sensitivity of detection of FBs and some emerging mycotoxins, including ergot alkaloids, MPA, STG, and GLIO. However, this change suppressed the signal intensity of some important mycotoxins, including AFs and OTs. Therefore, the optimal concentration of FA was set as 0.1%. Notably, this mobile phase composition did not lead to sufficient signal intensity for the detection of T2, HT2, and some emerging mycotoxins, such as BEA, enniatins, DAS, NEO, and 15AS.

When NH_4HCO_2 was included in the mobile phase, the signal intensities of the NH_4^+ adducts produced were higher than those of the H^+ adducts. However, higher concentrations of NH_4HCO_2 inhibited the ionization of most regulated mycotoxins, such as AFs, OTs, and FBs, which is consistent with the results of Qiu et al. [33]. Moreover, all mycotoxins exhibited maximum signal intensities when mobile phase (A) consisted of 1 mM NH_4HCO_2 with 0.1% FA in aqueous solution and mobile phase (B) was ACN. Although CPA analysis under neutral conditions led to tailing peaks, sharp peaks and good separations were obtained using the optimized acidic mobile phase. However, the signal intensities of most compounds in group B were suppressed in acid or alkaline media. Previous studies reported that the addition of CH_3COONH_4 in the mobile phase could improve the sensitivity of detection of ZEN and its derivatives and peak shapes of several Alternaria toxins [34,35]. Results showed that the combination of 0.1 mM CH_3COONH_4

(A) and ACN (B) markedly enhanced the signal intensities of most target components and eliminated the tailing peaks of TeA and PAT (Figure 1C). Thus, 0.1 mM CH$_3$COONH$_4$ and ACN were selected as the mobile phase with the best-balanced performance.

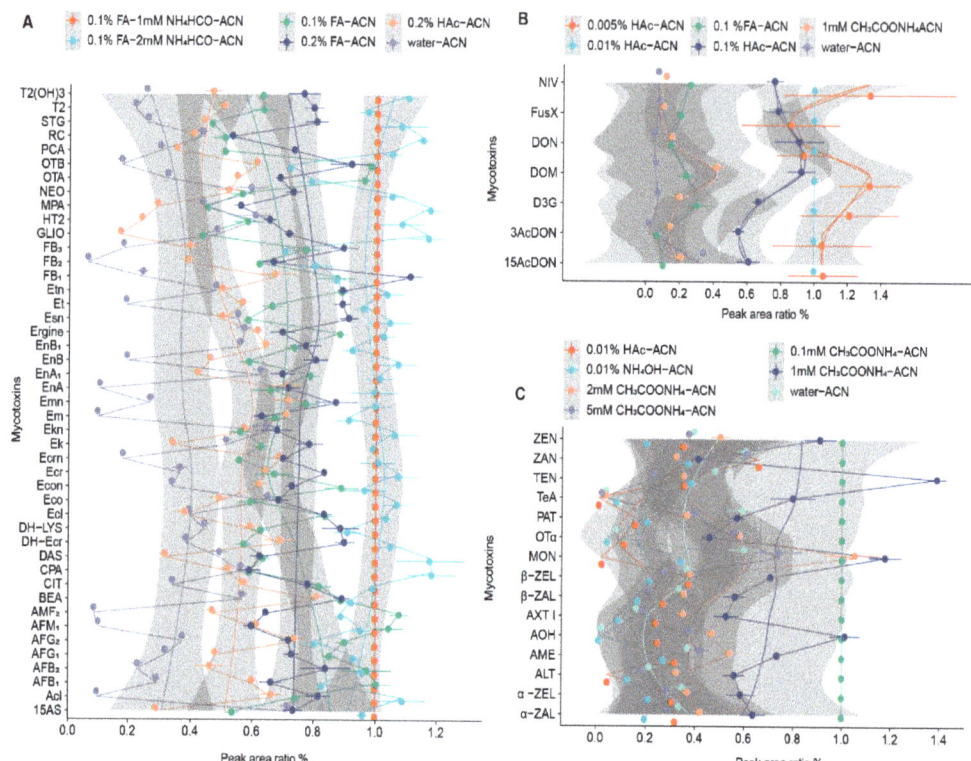

Figure 1. Effects of different mobile phase conditions on peak areas. (**A**) 45 mycotoxins of group A. (**B**) 15 mycotoxins of group B. (**C**) 7 mycotoxins of group C ($n = 3$). The concentrations of mycotoxins in the samples were as follows: Acl, Ecl, Em, Esn, CPA, STG, EnA1, EnB, EnB1, Ergine, Econ, Etn, OTA, OTB, AFM1, and AFM2: 0.5 ng/mL. Ek, Ekn, Emn, MPA, NEO, RC, T2, DH-Ecr, EnA, and BEA: 1 ng/mL. 15AS, AFB1, AFB2, AFG1, AFG2, Ecr, Ecrn, Eco, T2(OH)$_3$, AME, ZEN, AXT I, OTα, DAS, DH-LYS, Et, and FB3: 5 ng/mL. ALT, TeA, FB1, FB2, HT2, PCA, CIT, AOH, TEN, α-ZAL, β-ZAL, α-ZEL, β-ZAL, ZAN, and D3G: 10 ng/mL. 3AcDON, FusX, NIV, GLIO, DON, DOM, and MON: 50 ng/mL. PAT, and 15AcDON: 100 ng/mL.

Regarding group C compounds, when HAc was used instead of FA at the same concentration of 0.1%, the intensity of the analytes increased from 1.7-fold (for D3G) to 6.0-fold (for 3AcDON) (Figure 1B). The [M+CH$_3$COO]$^-$ provided by HAc greatly enhanced the ionization of the analytes. Upon reducing the concentration of HAc from 0.1% to 0.01%, the signal intensity of 3AcDON increased by 1.8-fold. A further decrease from 0.01% to 0.005% improved all signal intensities, except for DON and FusX. However, the use of 0.005% HAc resulted in poor precision for all analytes, with the RSD of the peak area for the tested mycotoxins ($n = 3$) ranging between 11% and 32%. On the other hand, the RSD was between 1% and 4% when 0.01% HAc was used, and the signal intensities of all analytes improved, while the peaks of NIV and D3G became sharper. Therefore, a 0.01% HAc aqueous solution was chosen as mobile phase (A), and ACN was used as mobile phase (B) for the group C compounds.

3.2. Optimization of Ion Source Parameters

To further enhance performance, we manually optimized the key parameters that impact the ionization procedure, such as ionization mode and the curtain gas, in a stepwise manner. We conducted tests on the ion spray voltage (ISV) ranging from 1400 to 2600 V, the source temperature ranging from 350 to 650 °C, and the pressures of the nebulizer gas (gas1) and auxiliary gas (gas2) ranging from 30 to 80 ps. These ion source parameters had varying effects on the peak areas of the 67 mycotoxins.

As shown in Figure 2A, the peak areas of FBs, T2, HT2, T2(OH)$_3$, cyclohexaester peptides (BEA and enniatins), and diacetoxyscirpenols (DAS, NEO, and 15AS) substantially increased with each increment of ISV. Conversely, the peak areas of AFs, STG, CPA, MPA, CIT, PCA, and RC slightly decreased. Regarding OTs, ergot alkaloids, and their respective inin-epimers, their optimal ISV value was achieved at 2000 V, with the peak areas diminishing at both higher and lower ISV values. Hence, 2000 V was chosen as the ISV for analyzing group A mycotoxins. While most analytes exhibited an increase in signal intensity with rising temperature, T2, HT2, T2(OH)$_3$, cyclohexaester peptides, diacetoxyscirpenols, and GLIO displayed a significant decrease when the temperature surpassed 450 °C. Therefore, 450 °C was selected as the optimum temperature.

The peak areas of T2, HT2, T2(OH)$_3$, diacetoxyscirpenols, and GLIO were directly proportional to the pressure of gas1, whereas other analytes showed optimal sensitivity when the pressure of gas1 reached 40 psi. As the pressure of gas2 increased, the peak areas of most analytes also increased, except for cyclohexaester peptides and diacetoxyscirpenols, which showed a decrease in sensitivity. To cater to the requirements of most mycotoxins, the pressure of gas1 was maintained at 40 psi, while gas2 was kept at 80 psi. These conditions provided adequate sensitivity of detection for all analytes. Concerning group B mycotoxins, increasing the ISV value resulted in a uniform increase and subsequent decrease in the peak area of all analytes (Figure 2B). The optimum performance was achieved at an ISV of −1800 V at 500 °C, with gas1 and gas2 pressures set at 40 and 80 psi, respectively. For compounds in group C, the relationships between the ion source parameters and the response values of the analytes were similar to those in group B. Most compounds in group C exhibited a slight increase in peak areas with increasing gas2 pressure, except for 15AcDON, which saw a decrease in the peak area (Figure 2B). Therefore, a moderate value of 50 psi was used for the pressure of gas2.

3.3. Optimization of the Pre-Treatment Methods

Enhanced Matrix Removal-Lipid (EMR-Lipid) cartridges and PRiME Hydrophile-Lipophile Balance (PRiME-HLB) cartridges are two novel polymer-based sorbent technologies that promise highly selective removal of phospholipids and proteins from complex matrices [36]. The extraction solvent was optimized by considering the physical interactions of mycotoxins with lipids and/or proteins in serum, as well as the wide range of log p values (ranging from −1.9 to 4.74) of the 67 mycotoxins. Additionally, a SPE (PRiME-HLB or EMR-Lipid) clean-up step was included to assess the efficiency of the combined extraction steps in inhibiting the matrix interference and achieving satisfactory recovery for all mycotoxins.

Concerning group A compounds, complex acidic analytes such as FBs and OTs necessitated a higher water content or a lower pH for efficient extraction. However, a higher water content impeded the extraction of other analytes, leading to the conclusion that pH adjustment is a preferable approach for optimizing extraction [37]. The use of FA-acidified ACN as an extraction solvent significantly improved the recoveries of strongly polar analytes such as FBs and OTA, which qualitatively matched the findings reported by Arce-López et al. [36]. Nonetheless, FA concentrations exceeding 0.1% decreased the extraction efficiency. Notably, mycotoxins such as RC, STG, DAS, Ecl, Ergine, and PCA exhibited recoveries below 80% or above 120%. The M_E evaluation of these mycotoxins indicated that these variations in recovery were a result of ionization suppression or enhancement, rather than poor extraction. Satisfactory recoveries for these analytes were obtained after performing IS corrections, underscoring the necessity for quantitation using IS. Figure 3 presents a comparison of the R_A and M_E values obtained from different sample preparation protocols for 45 group A mycotoxins.

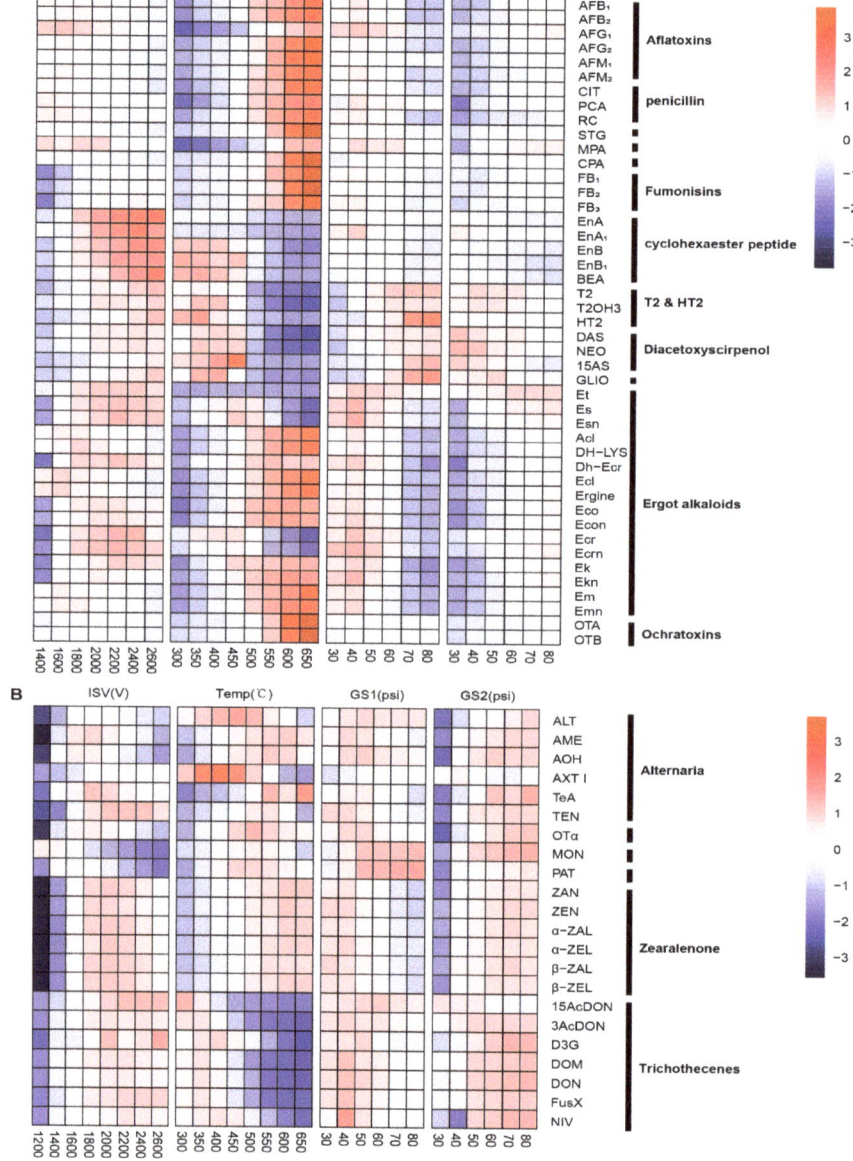

Figure 2. Evaluation of the effects of ion source parameters on detection sensitivity. The values were presented as the ratio of the peak area under the noted conditions to the peak area under initial conditions. (**A**) Group A analytes. (**B**) group B analytes. (n = 3). The concentration of each mycotoxin is described in the legend of Figure 1.

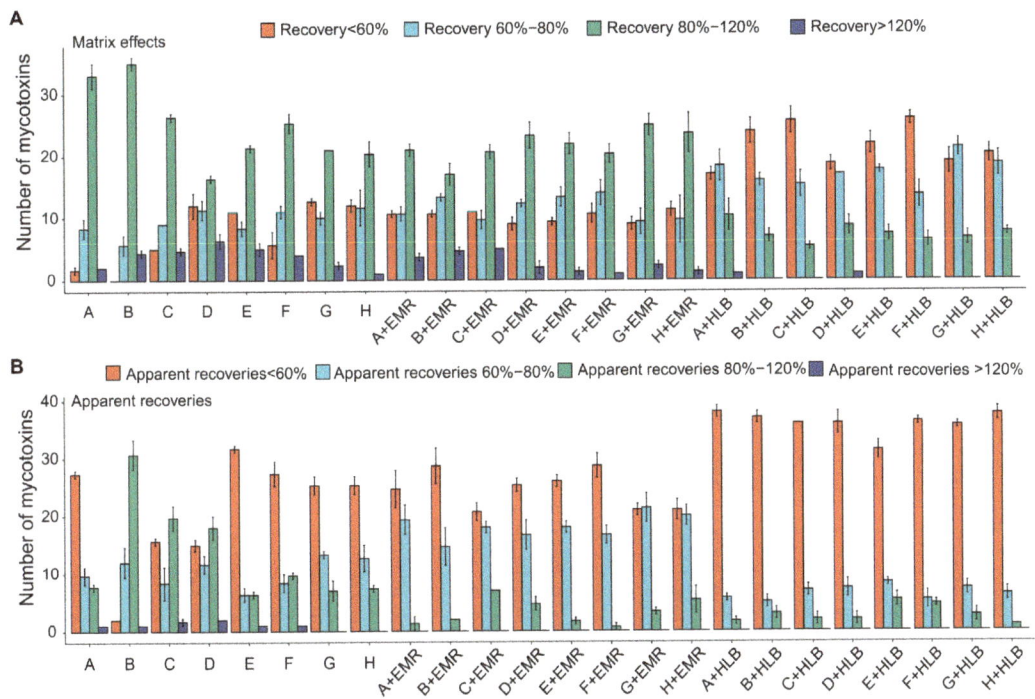

Figure 3. Assessment of the effects of solid-phase extraction purification on the matrix effects (**A**) and apparent recovery values (**B**) of 45 mycotoxins in group A. The abbreviations in the illustration are as follows: A: ACN; B: 0.1% FA ACN; C: 0.5% FA ACN; D: 1% FA ACN; E: water-ACN (16:84, v/v); F: 0.1% FA ACN (16:84, v/v); G: 0.5% FA ACN (16:84, v/v); H: 1% FA ACN (16:84, v/v). The concentration of each mycotoxin is described in the legend of Figure 1.

Regarding the analytes monitored in the negative ion mode for groups B and C, it was found that an acidic extraction solvent was not suitable, and the lack of FA resulted in substantial ME. To address this issue, an SPE cartridge was used to filter out impurities in plasma, which improved the ionization of target mycotoxins by reducing the matrix effect. However, a single column was not appropriate for both groups. The unsatisfactory recovery rates (<70%) of ZAN (28–63%), AOH (10–33%), TeA (6–57%), MON (13–45%), and PAT (8–61%) using PRiME-HLB (HLB) could be attributed to factors such as non-specific adsorption and the limited retention capacity of reversed-phase hydrophobic sorbents for highly polar analytes. In Figure S1, it can be observed that when ACN/water (84/16, v/v) was used as the extraction solvent in combination with an EMR-Lipid SPE clean-up step, the recoveries of all compounds in group B were above 70% before IS correction, except for AOH (52.4%) and PAT (48.3%). Similarly, when ACN was used as an extraction solvent followed by purification with an HLB cartridge, the recoveries of DON and its derivatives were higher than 70% except for NIV (42.4%). These results indicate that most mycotoxins exhibit poor recoveries due to their suppression of ionization, except for AOH, PAT, and NIV, which had low extraction efficiency. Additionally, no interfering peaks were detected at retention times and m/z channels that were similar to the mycotoxins (Figure S2), demonstrating the selectivity of the method and absence of interference from endogenous substances.

3.4. Methodology Validation

3.4.1. LOQ and Selectivity

Supplementary Figure S2 shows the typical UHPLC-MS/MS chromatograms of the validation samples prepared by spiking blank plasma at LOQ levels. The presence of a labeled IS did not impart any measurable influence on the quantification of all analytes. Despite the observation of some interfering peaks at the elution time of analytes, their responses were significantly lower, and they accounted for far less than 20% of the response shown at the LOQ level for each analyte. The labeled IS did not have any significant effect on the quantification of all analytes. The signal-to-noise ratios of LOQ samples were more than 11.3. The LODs ranged between 0.001 µg/L (Acl, Ecl, Em, Esn, EnA1, EnB, EnB1, CPA, and STG) and 0.5 µg/L (PAT), with corresponding LOQs ranging between 0.002 and 1 µg/L. Compared to previously reported methods of mycotoxin analysis, our method allows for the detection of the largest number of analytes while also offering the highest reported sensitivity. Notably, the LODs of FusX, OTB, NIV, T2, HT2, NEO, ZAN, and STG attained with the proposed method were lower compared to those attained with a single method that employed a clean-up step using EMR-Lipid [34]. This finding demonstrates the need to design sample preparation methods that consider the physicochemical properties of mycotoxins.

3.4.2. Carry-Over Effect and Linearity

There was no carry-over effect for all analytes. Satisfactory linearities were obtained for all mycotoxins (R^2 range of 0.9902–0.9999).

3.4.3. Trueness and Precision

As shown as Table S4, at three validation levels, the mean intra-day trueness ranged from 82.7% to 116.6%, and intra-day precision ranged from 1.8% to 11.9% RSD, except for Ecl (66.4% to 78.7%), DH-LYS (75.2% to 78.2%), PCA (72.5% to 77.4%), and EnA (117.1% to 129.8%). The analysis of 63 out of 67 mycotoxins met the trueness requirement and precision. The inter-day trueness ranged between 80.2–117.7%, while the precision ranged from 3.1–13.8% RSD. The results indicate that this method effectively analyzes trace concentrations of mycotoxins.

3.4.4. Recovery and Matrix Effect

In Figure S1, when ACN/water (84/16, v/v) was used as the extraction solvent in combination with an EMR-Lipid SPE clean-up step, the recoveries of all compounds in group B were greater than 70% before IS correction, except for AOH (52.4%) and PAT (48.3%). Similarly, when ACN was used as an extraction solvent followed by purification with an HLB cartridge, the recoveries of DON and its derivatives in group C were higher than 70%, except for NIV (42.4%). These results suggest that most mycotoxins show poor recoveries due to their suppression of ionization, except for the low extraction efficiency of AOH, PAT, and NIV. Due to the complexity of the matrix, the matrix effect values ranged between 62.5% and 155.6%, while recovery values ranged between 59.6% and 146.4%, indicating the need for IS compensation for accurate mycotoxins analysis. For the analytes without commercially available standards, IS that showed comparable recovery values were chosen as reference IS.

3.4.5. Stability

Data obtained from the short-term stability studies revealed an almost insignificant degradation (<10%) of the different analytes at the different time-temperature combinations, except for CIT, AFM_1, AFB_1, AFG_1, and AFG_2 for which the two-fold LOQ spiked analyte concentrations were unstable after 6 h at 25 °C, and 10% to 20% of the initially spiked analyte concentrations was lost (Figure S3). This result is in agreement with the study by Ediage et al. [30]. The 120 h stability shows that very long analytical batches, suitable for exposure monitoring studies, can be accommodated using the current method.

Further short-term stability investigations carried out at temperatures of 4 °C and 25 °C for durations of 1, 3, and 5 days revealed notable losses (Table S5). Specifically, samples stored at 25 °C for 5 days exhibited a reduction of at least 20% in their initial analyte concentrations. The analytes that underwent the most degradation were CIT, T2 toxins, HT2, AFM1, AFB1, AFG1, AFG2, DON, and DOM (Figure S3). Remarkably, less than 30% of the initial T2 toxin and AFG1 concentrations were retained after 5 days, regardless of the storage temperature. In contrast, the non-polar analytes within the group (including ZAN, ZEN, OTA, and their derivatives) demonstrated minimal degradation compared to the polar analytes such as DON and its derivatives, across all time-temperature combinations.

In response to concerns regarding the potential effects of long-term storage on our samples, it is crucial to note that our methodology required plasma samples to be thawed on ice and promptly processed to mitigate degradation. For the long-term stability test, minimal degradation (<5%) was observed in the various analytes after 2 months of storage at -80 °C. This minimal change was corroborated by applying identical collection and storage protocols to both control and case groups in the latter part of our study. This approach was designed to ensure that any potential degradation effects were systematically controlled and consistent across all samples, thus providing a reliable basis for our comparative analysis. This synchronization in handling and storage mitigates the variability that might otherwise arise from differential treatment of samples, allowing us to draw more accurate inferences about the correlation between mycotoxin exposure and male infertility.

3.5. Detection of Mycotoxin Levels in Plasma Samples

Mycotoxins are lipophilic and can attach to proteins in plasma, allowing them to persist in organisms for long periods of time after chronic exposure [38]. The presence of mycotoxins in urine is usually a sign of recent ingestion, whereas the presence of mycotoxins in plasma is more closely associated with long-term exposure [39]. Therefore, compared to urine, plasma samples are more suitable for biological monitoring, permitting the generation of more comprehensive and reliable data for the creation of risk assessments. The UPLC-MS/MS chromatograms of blank plasma samples and plasma matrices spiked with standards representing the 67 mycotoxins are presented in Figure S2. The mycotoxin contents in plasma from 184 human male subjects are shown in Table S6. Among the 67 analyzed mycotoxins, 16 of the 28 traditional mycotoxins and 24 of the 39 emerging mycotoxins were detected in the plasma samples. The most prevalent mycotoxins included both traditional mycotoxins (OTB at 100% and OTA at 98.4%) and emerging mycotoxins (CIT at 79.3%, EnB at 77.2%, BEA at 68.5%, and CPA at 44.6%), suggesting the widespread exposure of both traditional and emerging mycotoxins in male plasma.

The prevalence of these analytes in various foods has become increasingly well established. Globally, OTA contamination has been frequently documented in raw agricultural products, including grain, coffee, peas, and meat [40,41]. In 2017, a report on OTA contamination detection in rice samples from various regions in Africa showed that out of 4000 samples, the OTA content in raw and processed grains exceeded 38% and 29%, respectively, with the highest level of OTA content being 1164 µg/kg [42]. A study performed in Tehran, Iran, reported similar results, with 69 out of 100 rice samples containing OTA. In previous studies, CIT has been detected in various plant-based food commodities, particularly in cereals, fruit, and vegetables [43]. Qiu et al. revealed that more than 80% of the 13 types of food samples in the 6th China Total Dietary Study were contaminated with mycotoxins [33]. In our results, the most frequently detected mycotoxins were BEA and EnB.

In Figure 4, it is observed that OTs, FBs, and DONs were identified as the most abundant traditional mycotoxins, with an average combined contribution ratio from 12.0% to 69.2% of the total of traditional mycotoxins. Additionally, penicillins (CIT, PAT, and PCA), cyclohexaester peptides (EnB, BEA, EnB$_1$, and EnA$_1$), MPA, and GLIO were the predominant emerging mycotoxins, with a combined average contribution ratio of 12.5–43.3%. Apart from these mycotoxins, which consistently occurred at relatively high concentrations, the remaining detectable mycotoxins were present in low concentrations, collectively contributing to less than 6% of the total mycotoxin burden. Despite their low concentrations, some mycotoxins, including two emerging mycotoxins (ergot alkaloids at 50.5% and CPA at 44.6%), were detected more frequently, suggesting their widespread occurrence in common foods. The high detection rate of ergot alkaloids was mainly derived from Esn (23.9%), Acl (14.1%), and DH-LYS (13.6%), whereas CPA was detected individually.

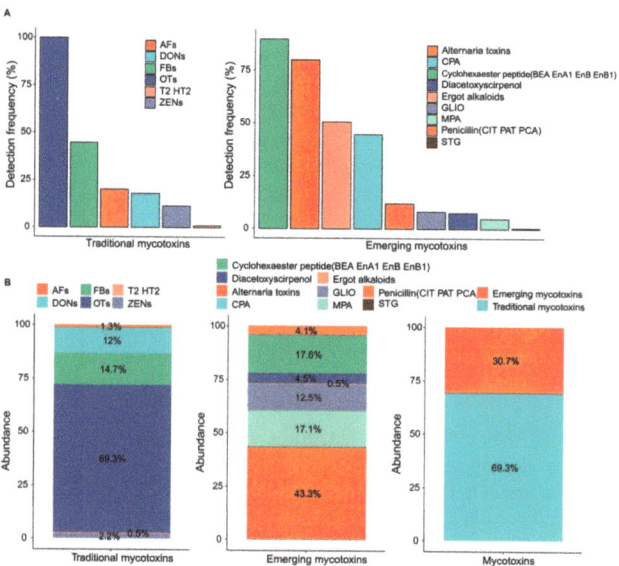

Figure 4. Prevalence and composition profiles of mycotoxins in plasma samples collected from 184 Chinese males. (**A**) Detection frequency of both traditional and emerging mycotoxins. (**B**) Abundance levels of traditional and emerging mycotoxins.

3.6. Analysis of Major Co-Exposure Mycotoxins

Figure S4 shows representative MRM chromatograms of the positive samples. The results indicate that all participants were exposed to a minimum of two different mycotoxins. Interestingly, the plasma from one infertile participant was found to contain at least 14 mycotoxins. The established mycotoxins OTA, AFB_1, FB_1, and DON are known to induce negative reproductive effects, including reductions in the weight of reproductive organs, daily sperm production, epididymal sperm count, and the numbers of viable and motile sperm [44–47]. The emerging mycotoxins CIT and CPA have exhibited similar effects. CPA has been shown to decrease the sperm quality and rates of in vitro fertilization success in mice, and it has been found to induce p53-dependent apoptosis in the testis of mice [48–50]. Among all the detected mycotoxins, OTA, OTB, EnB, and CIT exhibited detection frequencies higher than 70%.

As shown in Figure 5A, positive concentration correlations were observed between OTA and OTB ($r = 0.72$, $p < 0.01$), OTA and EnB ($r = 0.36$, $p < 0.01$), OTA and CIT ($r = 0.21$, $p < 0.01$), OTB and CIT ($r = 0.22$, $p < 0.01$), OTB and EnB ($r = 0.33$, $p < 0.01$), and EnB and CIT ($r = 0.17$, $p < 0.05$), indicating that these mycotoxins co-migrate in some common food sources. These results were consistent with Gupta et al., who determined that *Penicillium* and *Aspergillus* spp. can produce both OTs and CIT. This co-production means that co-exposure to these mycotoxins is common in foods. Out of 250 grain samples, five contained OTA (147 ± 7.9 µg/kg), CIT (49 ± 1.9 µg/kg), and OTB (1.2 ± 0.7 µg/kg) [48]. Previous studies have also reported that fungi of the genus *Penicillium* can degrade CIT, leading to the production of OTA. Consequently, the European Union and other interntional organizations have warned that the chronic toxicity of such emerging toxins and the synergistic toxicity of co-exposure with traditional toxins may pose a threat to human health.

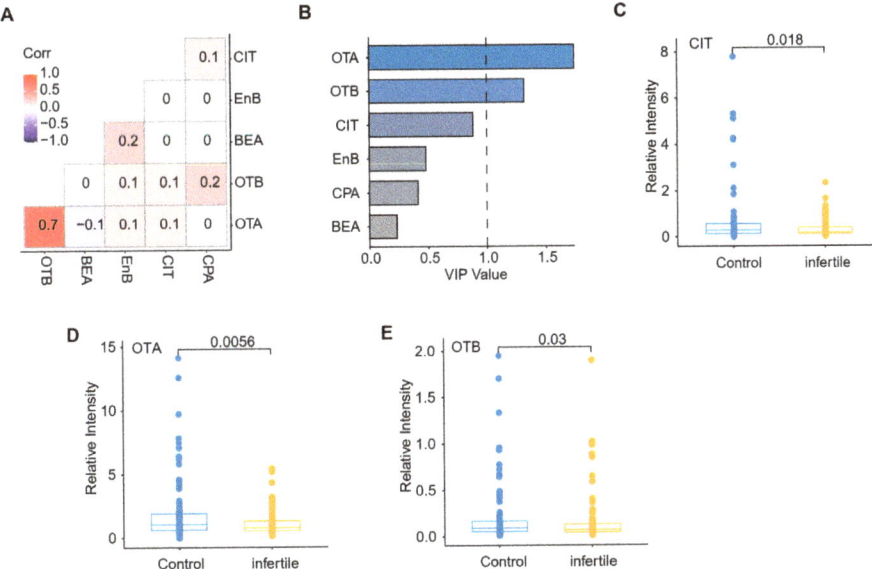

Figure 5. Multivariate statistical analysis of mycotoxin levels in plasma samples. (**A**) Heatmaps for Spearman's correlation coefficients between concentrations of metabolites in plasma samples. (**B**) VIP bar plot of mycotoxins based on the OPLS-DA model. (**C**–**E**) Boxplot of the plasma levels of mycotoxins (CIT, OTA, and OTB) with a high (>70%) incidence between normal and infertile male plasma.

The mean OTA concentration (0.904 µg/L) and range (0.117–14.103 µg/L) observed in infertile males in this study were similar to those reported in a survey on rural residents aged 18 to 66 years in China and to those observed in ill children in Spain [36,51]. OTα, a metabolite of OTA, was not detected in plasma; the same results were reported in studies of Chinese, German, and Belgian populations [24,51,52]. This is not surprising because OTα is mainly excreted in urine as glucuronide or sulfate conjugates [49,50]. Furthermore, little attention has been paid to OTB exposure, mainly because previous studies have reported a relatively low incidence of 11.4% [37]. In contrast, our results suggest that the incidence of exposure to OTB is 100%, with our method exhibiting an LOD for OTB detection that is approximately 200-fold lower compared to that of the method used by López et al. [37]. It is possible that the relative insensitivity of their method resulted in a high number of false negative results in Spanish children. It should be noted that the mean concentrations obtained in the two studies were similar, 0.22 and 0.57 µg/L, respectively.

The incidences of DON and its derivatives were low in plasma samples, except for FusX, even though their LODs were improved by choosing $[M+CH_3COO]^-$ as the precursor ion. This result is consistent with previous studies on German subjects, in which DON and especially its phase II metabolites were often detectable in urine [53,54], suggesting a rapid excretion of these compounds. To our knowledge, our study is the first to report on plasma exposure to FusX. FusX was detectable because the LOD of our method (0.05 µg/L) is substantially lower than that of the method described by Arce-López et al. (1.95 µg/L) [37]. In addition, it may be that FusX is either produced internally from DON or obtained directly from food or the environment, as it readily accumulates in the plasma and is excreted from the body relatively slowly.

Several HBM studies have revealed a high incidence of CIT in plasma. For example, a study on plasma samples from 104 young adult patients in Bangladesh revealed an incidence of 90%, with a mean plasma concentration of 0.22 µg/L [55]. Similarly, a study in the Czech Republic showed that 100% of subjects with renal tumors were CIT-positive, with a mean concentration of 0.061 µg/L. In a study on subjects from Tunisia, the prevalence was slightly lower at 36%, whereas in our study, the mean concentration was higher at 0.49 µg/L. Our study aligns more closely with a high prevalence of CIT exposure [56]. The high incidence of EnB observed in our study was also consistent with a study on healthy German volunteers [52]. Thus, the present study confirms the emergence of CIT and EnB as critical toxins in plasma and provides novel information on other emerging mycotoxins such as BEA and CPA.

3.7. Analysis of Potential Correlation between Mycotoxin Exposure and Infertility

Co-exposure to multiple mycotoxins was frequent among both control and infertile subjects. The most common result was co-exposure to 7–14 mycotoxins. Notably, this finding occurred more frequently among individuals in the infertility group (60%) compared to those in the control group (44%), indicating a strong correlation between multi-exposure and infertility. According to the variable importance of the projection values (VIP) bar plot of mycotoxins selected based on the orthogonal partial least square discriminant analysis (OPLS-DA) model, OTA, OTB and CIT exposure contributed the most to infertility outcome (Figure 5B). The prevalence levels of FusX, ergot alkaloids, Esn, and MPA in the infertility group (19%, 59%, 34%, and 9%, respectively) were notably elevated compared to those observed in the control group (8%, 43%, 15%, and 1%, respectively; $p < 0.05$). However, as these mycotoxins were monitored in a human biological matrix for the first time, the relationship between their occurrence or levels and specific diseases has not been well-studied. It is worth noting that the rate of detection of CPA in infertile male samples (47.2%) was higher than in fertile male samples (42.1%). Additionally, as mentioned above, several studies have demonstrated the harmful effects of CPA on spermatogenesis. Therefore, further studies on the dose-effect relationship of CPA exposure and the pathogenesis of male infertility are warranted.

The Mann–Whitney U test was used to conduct inter-group comparisons of the plasma levels of mycotoxins that were found in more than 70% of the samples (Figure 5B–D). The median values of OTB, OTA, and CIT levels in the infertility group (0.095, 1.070, and 0.329 µg/L, respectively) were higher than those in the control group (0.066, 0.760, and 0.198 µg/L, respectively). All these three mycotoxins showed the highest levels in samples from the infertility group. When the concentrations were analyzed as continuous variables, significant differences were observed between the two groups (all $p < 0.05$). Interestingly, OTB, OTA, and CIT, which were elevated in infertile male subjects, are known to induce reproductive and significant renal toxicities. They have been reported as the cause of kidney diseases in humans and animal models [57–60]. The apparent toxicity of these mycotoxins, coupled with their high prevalence and concentrations in infertile male subjects, necessitates further research on the toxicity of OTs and CIT alone and in combination in infertile men. As for EnB, another mycotoxin with a high incidence, measured concentrations ranged between 0.002 and 0.037 µg/L in the infertility group and 0.002 and 0.147 µg/L in the control group. No statistical difference was observed between the two groups, suggesting that EnB does not significantly contribute to male infertility.

4. Conclusions

This study has successfully developed a comprehensive UHPLC-MS/MS method for the quantitative analysis of 67 mycotoxins in plasma, showcasing its sensitivity, accuracy, and robustness. Our findings underscore the significance of investigating the link between mycotoxin exposure and male infertility, particularly focusing on specific reproductive toxins that could impair reproductive health. Despite the potential association suggested by our results, establishing a definitive connection requires more conclusive evidence.

The role of environmental factors in male fertility is critical, as adverse conditions can significantly impact reproductive capabilities [61]. It is essential to acknowledge that male infertility likely results from the complex interplay of multiple environmental factors, rather than mycotoxins alone. Consequently, further research is needed to validate our findings, understand the underlying mechanisms, and assess the broader impact of environmental toxins on fertility. Expanding the scope of our study to include diverse sample types and larger populations from various geographic regions will help provide a more comprehensive understanding of these interactions and support more definitive conclusions.

Supplementary Materials: The following supporting information can be downloaded at: https://www.mdpi.com/article/10.3390/toxics12060395/s1, Figure S1: RA and ME assessment of mycotoxins pre-purification and post-purification by SPE (HLB or EMR). Part (B1) and (B2) are the 15 analytes from group B, and Part (C) is the 7 analytes from group C; Figure S2: LC-MS/MS extracted ion chromatograms of bank plasma samples and plasma matrices at their respective LOQ; Figure S3: Short term stability study at 4 °C and 25 °C for 3 h, 6 h, 1 day, 3 days and 5 days storage period (%); Figure S4: Representative S-MRM chromatograms of positive plasma samples; Table S1: A summary of mycotoxins HBM in human plasma, serum, and blood using LC-MS/MS; Table S2: Chemical properties of 67 mycotoxins analyzed in this study; Table S3: MS parameters of 67 mycotoxins; Table S4: Evaluation of the developed method for sensitivity, ME, RM, linearity, and precision of 67 mycotoxins; Table S5: Short term stability study at 4 °C and 25 °C for 3 h, 6 h, 1 day, 3 days, and 5 days storage period (%); Table S6: Comparison between previously reported LODs and LODs determined in this study for mycotoxins; Table S7: Mycotoxins levels in individual plasma samples using the UHPLC-MS/MS method. The references [62–67] are cited in the Supplementary materials.

Author Contributions: Conceptualization, X.N., L.W. and Y.Y.; Data curation, X.N. and L.W.; Formal analysis, X.N. and Y.Y.; Investigation, S.J., Y.Z. and J.S.; Methodology, X.N., J.C. and S.M.; Software, X.N. and J.J.; Supervision, J.-S.W., X.S. and J.C.; Visualization, X.N. and S.M.; Writing—original draft, X.N. and Y.Y.; Writing—review & editing, X.N., J.-S.W., X.S. and J.C. All authors have read and agreed to the published version of the manuscript.

Funding: This work was supported by the National Key Research and Development Program of China (2021YFC2401100), Fundamental Research Funds for the Central Universities (JUSRP222001), and Collaborative Innovation Center of Food Safety and Quality Control in Jiangsu Province, Jiangnan University.

Institutional Review Board Statement: Not applicable.

Informed Consent Statement: Not applicable.

Data Availability Statement: All data used in this work is available either within the article or in the supporting information file.

Conflicts of Interest: The authors declare that they have no known competing financial interests or personal relationships that could have appeared to influence the work reported in this paper.

References

1. Ekwomadu, T.I.; Dada, T.A.; Nleya, N.; Gopane, R.; Sulyok, M.; Mwanza, M. Variation of Fusarium free, masked, and emerging mycotoxin metabolites in maize from agriculture regions of South Africa. *Toxins* **2020**, *12*, 149. [CrossRef] [PubMed]
2. Jajić, I.; Dudaš, T.; Krstović, S.; Krska, R.; Sulyok, M.; Bagi, F.; Savić, Z.; Guljaš, D.; Stankov, A. Emerging fusarium mycotoxins fusaproliferin, beauvericin, enniatins, and moniliformin in Serbian maize. *Toxins* **2019**, *11*, 357. [CrossRef] [PubMed]
3. EFSA. Scientific opinion on the risks for animal and public health related to the presence of Alternaria toxins in feed and food. *EFSA J.* **2011**, *9*, 2407. [CrossRef]
4. EFSA. Scientific opinion on the risks for public and animal health related to the presence of citrinin in food and feed. *EFSA J.* **2012**, *10*, 2605.
5. EFSA. Scientific opinion on risks for animal and public health related to the presence of nivalenol in food and feed. *EFSA J.* **2013**, *11*, 3262. [CrossRef]
6. EFSA. Scientific opinion on the risks to human and animal health related to the presence of beauvericin and enniatins in food and feed. *EFSA J.* **2014**, *12*, 3802.

7. EFSA Panel on Contaminants in the Food Chain (CONTAM); Knutsen, H.K.; Alexander, J.; Barregård, L.; Bignami, M.; Brüschweiler, B.; Ceccatelli, S.; Cottrill, B.; Dinovi, M.; Grasl-Kraupp, B.; et al. Risks to human and animal health related to the presence of moniliformin in food and feed. *EFSA J.* **2018**, *16*, e05082. [PubMed]
8. Braun, D.; Eva, S.; Doris, M.; Benedikt, W. Longitudinal assessment of mycotoxin co-exposures in exclusively breastfed infants. *Environ. Inter.* **2020**, *142*, 105845. [CrossRef] [PubMed]
9. Kokeb, T.; Alemayehu, A.; Giles, T.H.-C.; Seifu, H.G.; Patrick, K.; Tefera, B.; Van de Mario, V.; De Sarah, S.; De Marthe, B.; Carl, L. Multiple mycotoxin exposure during pregnancy and risks of adverse birth outcomes: A prospective cohort study in rural Ethiopia. *Environ. Inter.* **2022**, *160*, 107052.
10. Khoury, D.E.; Fayjaloun, S.; Nassar, M.; Sahakian, J.; Aad, P.Y. Updates on the effect of mycotoxins on male reproductive efficiency in mammals. *Toxins* **2019**, *11*, 515. [CrossRef]
11. Chiminelli, I.; Spicer, L.J.; Maylem, E.R.S.; Caloni, F. Emerging mycotoxins and reproductive effects in animals: A short review. *J. Appl. Toxicol.* **2022**, *42*, 1901–1909. [CrossRef] [PubMed]
12. Esteves, S.C.; Hamada, A.; Kondray, V.; Pitchika, A.; Agarwal, A. What every gynecologist should know about male infertility: An update. *Arch. Gynecol. Obstet.* **2012**, *286*, 217–229. [CrossRef] [PubMed]
13. Sharlip, I.D.; Jarow, J.P.; Belker, A.M.; Lipshultz, L.I.; Sigman, M.; Thomas, A.J.; Schlegel, P.N.; Howards, S.S.; Nehra, A.; Damewood, M.D.; et al. Best practice policies for male infertility. *Fertil. Steril.* **2002**, *77*, 873–882. [CrossRef] [PubMed]
14. Li, W.N.; Jia, M.M.; Peng, Y.Q.; Ding, R.; Fan, L.Q.; Liu, G. Semen quality pattern and age threshold: A retrospective cross-sectional study of 71,623 infertile men in China, between 2011 and 2017. *Reprod. Biol. Endocrinol.* **2019**, *17*, 107. [CrossRef] [PubMed]
15. Rolland, M.; Le Moal, J.; Wagner, V.; Royère, D.; De Mouzon, J. Decline in semen concentration and morphology in a sample of 26,609 men close to general population between 1989 and 2005 in France. *Hum. Reprod.* **2012**, *28*, 462–470. [CrossRef] [PubMed]
16. Rosa-Villagrán, L.; Barrera, N.; Montes, J.; Riso, C.; Sapiro, R. Decline of semen quality over the last 30 years in Uruguay. *Basic Clin. Androl.* **2021**, *31*, 8. [CrossRef] [PubMed]
17. Eze, U.A.; Okonofua, F.E. High prevalence of male infertility in Africa: Are mycotoxins to blame? *Afr. J. Reprod. Health* **2015**, *19*, 9–17. [PubMed]
18. Wipfler, R.; McCormick, S.P.; Proctor, R.H.; Teresi, J.M.; Hao, G.; Ward, T.J.; Alexander, N.; Vaughan, M.M. Synergistic phytotoxic effects of culmorin and trichothecene mycotoxins. *Toxins* **2019**, *11*, 555. [CrossRef] [PubMed]
19. Vejdovszky, K.; Hahn, K.; Braun, D.; Warth, B.; Marko, D. Synergistic estrogenic effects of Fusarium and Alternaria mycotoxins in vitro. *Arch. Toxicol.* **2016**, *91*, 1447–1460. [CrossRef]
20. Malachová, A.; Stránská, M.; Václavíková, M.; Elliott, C.T.; Black, C.; Meneely, J.; Hajšlová, J.; Ezekiel, C.N.; Schuhmacher, R.; Krska, R. Advanced LC-MS-based methods to study the co-occurrence and metabolization of multiple mycotoxins in cereals and cereal-based food. *Anal. Bioanal. Chem.* **2018**, *410*, 801–825. [CrossRef]
21. Rausch, A.K.; Brockmeyer, R.; Schwerdtle, T. Development and validation of a liquid chromatography tandem mass spectrometry multi-method for the determination of 41 free and modified mycotoxins in beer. *Food Chem.* **2021**, *338*, 127801. [CrossRef] [PubMed]
22. Coppa, C.F.S.C.; Cirelli, A.C.; Gonçalves, B.L.; Barnabé, E.M.B.; Khaneghah, A.M.; Corassin, C.H.; Oliveira, C.A.F. Dietary exposure assessment and risk characterization of mycotoxins in lactating women: Case study of São Paulo state, Brazil. *Food Res. Int.* **2020**, *134*, 109272. [CrossRef] [PubMed]
23. Chen, T.; Tan, T.; Zhu, W.; Gong, L.; Yan, Y.; Li, Q.; Xiao, D.; Li, Y.; Yang, X.; Hao, L.; et al. Exposure assessment of urinary deoxynivalenol in pregnant women in Wuhan, China. *Food Chem. Toxicol.* **2022**, *167*, 113289. [CrossRef] [PubMed]
24. Heyndrickx, E.; Sioen, I.; Huybrechts, B.; Callebaut, A.; De Henauw, S.; De Saeger, S. Human biomonitoring of multiple mycotoxins in the Belgian population: Results of the BIOMYCO study. *Environ. Int.* **2015**, *84*, 82–89. [CrossRef] [PubMed]
25. Warth, B.; Fruhmann, P.; Wiesenberger, G.; Kluger, B.; Sarkanj, B.; Lemmens, M.; Hametner, C.; Fröhlich, J.; Adam, G.; Krska, R.; et al. Deoxynivalenol-sulfates: Identification and quantification of novel conjugated (masked) mycotoxins in wheat. *Anal. Bioanal. Chem.* **2014**, *407*, 1033–1039. [CrossRef] [PubMed]
26. FDA. Guidance for Industry: Bioanalytical Method Validation. 2013. Available online: http://www.fda.gov/ucm/groups/fdagov-public/@fdagov-drugs-gen/documents/document/ucm368107.pdf (accessed on 1 June 2023).
27. EMEA. Committee for Medicinal Products for Human Use, Guideline on Bioanalytical Method Validation. EMEA/CHMP/EWP/192217/2009 Rev. 1 Corr. 2**. 21 July 2011. Available online: http://www.ema.europa.eu/docs/en_GB/document_library/Scientific_guideline/2011/08/WC500109686.pdf (accessed on 3 June 2023).
28. CLSI. Mass Spectrometry in the Clinical Laboratory: General Principles and Guidance; Approved Guideline. 2007. Available online: http://shop.clsi.org/c.1253739/site/Sample_pdf/C50A_sample.pdf (accessed on 24 July 2023).
29. Mei, S.; Shi, X.; Du, Y.; Cui, Y.; Zeng, C.; Ren, X.; Yu, K.; Zhao, Z.; Lin, S. Simultaneous determination of plasma methotrexate and 7-hydroxy methotrexate by UHPLC–MS/MS in patients receiving high-dose methotrexate therapy. *J. Pharm. Biomed. Anal.* **2018**, *158*, 300–306. [CrossRef] [PubMed]
30. Ediagea, E.N.; Mavungua, J.D.D.; Songa, S.; Wub, A.; Peteghema, C.V.; Saeger, S.D. A direct assessment of mycotoxin biomarkers in human urine samples by liquid chromatography tandem mass spectrometry. *Anal. Chim. Acta* **2012**, *741*, 58–69. [CrossRef] [PubMed]
31. Slobodchikova, I.; Vuckovic, D. Liquid chromatography—High resolution mass spectrometry method for monitoring of 17 mycotoxins in human plasma for exposure studies. *J. Chromatogr. A* **2018**, *1548*, 51–63. [CrossRef] [PubMed]

32. Yang, H.; Zhang, D.; Mei, S.; Zhao, Z. Simultaneous determination of plasma lamotrigine, lamotrigine N2-glucuronide and lamotrigine N2-oxide by UHPLC-MS/MS in epileptic patients. *J. Pharm. Biomed. Anal.* **2022**, *220*, 115017. [CrossRef]
33. Qiu, N.; Sun, D.; Zhou, S.; Li, J.; Zhao, Y.; Wu, Y. Rapid and sensitive UHPLC-MS/MS methods for dietary sample analysis of 43 mycotoxins in China total diet study. *J. Adv. Res.* **2021**, *39*, 15–47. [CrossRef]
34. Yogendrarajah, P.; Van Poucke, C.; De Meulenaer, B.; De Saeger, S. Development and validation of a QuEChERS based liquid chromatography tandem mass spectrometry method for the determination of multiple mycotoxins in spices. *J. Chromatogr. A* **2013**, *1297*, 1–11. [CrossRef] [PubMed]
35. Tölgyesi, Á.; Stroka, J.; Tamosiunas, V.; Zwickel, T. Simultaneous analysis of Alternaria toxins and citrinin in tomato: An optimised method using liquid chromatography-tandem mass spectrometry. *Food Addit. Contam. Part A* **2015**, *32*, 1512–1522. [CrossRef] [PubMed]
36. Arce-López, B.; Lizarraga, E.; Flores-Flores, M.; Irigoyen, Á.; González-Peñas, E. Development and validation of a methodology based on Captiva EMR-lipid clean-up and LC-MS/MS analysis for the simultaneous determination of mycotoxins in human plasma. *Talanta* **2020**, *206*, 120193. [CrossRef] [PubMed]
37. Arce-López, B.; Lizarraga, E.; Lopez de Mesa, R.; González-Peñas, E. Assessment of exposure to mycotoxins in Spanish children through the analysis of their levels in plasma samples. *Toxins* **2021**, *13*, 150. [CrossRef]
38. Sirot, V.; Fremy, J.-M.; Leblanc, J.-C. Dietary exposure to mycotoxins and health risk assessment in the second French total diet study. *Food Chem. Toxicol.* **2012**, *52*, 1–11. [CrossRef] [PubMed]
39. Marín, S.; Cano-Sancho, G.; Sanchis, V.; Ramos, A.J. The role of mycotoxins in the human exposome: Application of mycotoxin biomarkers in exposome-health studies. *Food Chem. Toxicol.* **2018**, *121*, 504–518. [CrossRef]
40. Pleadin, J.; Zadravec, M.; Lešić, T.; Vahčić, N.; Frece, J.; Mitak, M.; Markov, K. Co-occurrence of ochratoxin A and citrinin in unprocessed cereals established during a three-year investigation period. *Food Addit. Contam. Part B Surveill.* **2018**, *11*, 20–25. [CrossRef]
41. Taniwaki, M.H.; Pitt, J.I.; Copetti, M.V.; Teixeira, A.A.; Iamanaka, B.T. nderstanding mycotoxin contamination across the food chain in Brazil: Challenges and opportunities. *Toxins* **2019**, *11*, 411. [CrossRef] [PubMed]
42. Lee, H.J.; Ryu, D. Worldwide occurrence of mycotoxins in cereals and cereal-derived food products: Public health perspectives of their co-occurrence. *J. Agric. Food Chem.* **2017**, *65*, 7034–7051. [CrossRef]
43. Elfadil, D.; Silveri, F.; Palmieri, S.; Della Pelle, F.; Sergi, M.; Del Carlo, M.; Amine, A.; Compagnone, D. Liquid-phase exfoliated 2D graphene nanoflakes electrochemical sensor coupled to molecularly imprinted polymers for the determination of citrinin in food. *Talanta* **2023**, *253*, 124010. [CrossRef]
44. Csenki, Z.; Garai, E.; Faisal, Z.; Csepregi, R.; Garai, K.; Sipos, D.K.; Szabó, I.; Kőszegi, T.; Czéh, Á.; Czömpöly, T.; et al. The individual and combined effects of ochratoxin A with citrinin and their metabolites (ochratoxin B, ochratoxin C, and dihydrocitrinone) on 2D/3D cell cultures, and zebrafish embryo models. *Food Chem. Toxicol.* **2021**, *158*, 112674. [CrossRef] [PubMed]
45. Peraica, M.; Domijan, A.-M.; Šarić, M. Mycotoxic and aristolochic acid theories of the development of endemic nephropathy. *Arch. Ind. Hyg. Toxicol.* **2008**, *59*, 59–65. [CrossRef]
46. Ostry, V.; Malir, F.; Ruprich, J. Producers and important dietary sources of ochratoxin A and citrinin. *Toxins* **2013**, *5*, 1574–1586. [CrossRef]
47. Supriya, C.; Girish, B.P.; Reddy, P.S. Aflatoxin b1-induced reproductive toxicity in male rats: Possible mechanism of action. *Int. J. Toxicol.* **2014**, *33*, 155–161. [CrossRef] [PubMed]
48. Bonyadi, F.; Hasanzadeh, S.; Malekinejad, H. Cyclopiazonic acid induced p53-dependent apoptosis in the testis of mice: Another male related risk factor of infertility. *Environ. Toxicol.* **2021**, *36*, 903–913. [CrossRef] [PubMed]
49. Bonyadi, F.; Hasanzadeh, S.; Malekinejad, H.; Najafi, G. Cyclopiazonic acid decreases sperm quality and in vitro fertilisation rate in mice. *World Mycotoxin J.* **2018**, *11*, 599–610. [CrossRef]
50. Da Silva, E.O.; Bracarense, A.P.F.L.; Oswald, I.P. Mycotoxins and oxidative stress: Where are we? *World Mycotoxin J.* **2018**, *11*, 113–134. [CrossRef]
51. Fan, K.; Xu, J.; Jiang, K.; Liu, X.; Meng, J.; Di Mavungu, J.D.; Guo, W.; Zhang, Z.; Jing, J.; Li, H.; et al. Determination of multiple mycotoxins in paired plasma and urine samples to assess human exposure in Nanjing, China. *Environ. Pollut.* **2019**, *248*, 865–873. [CrossRef]
52. Osteresch, B.; Viegas, S.; Cramer, B.; Humpf, H.-U. Multi-mycotoxin analysis using dried blood spots and dried serum spots. *Anal. Bioanal. Chem.* **2017**, *409*, 3369–3382. [CrossRef]
53. Gerding, J.; Cramer, B.; Humpf, H. Determination of mycotoxin exposure in Germany using an LC-MS/MS multibiomarker approach. *Mol. Nutr. Food Res.* **2014**, *58*, 2358–2368. [CrossRef]
54. Warth, B.; Sulyok, M.; Krska, R. LC-MS/MS-based multibiomarker approaches for the assessment of human exposure to mycotoxins. *Anal. Bioanal. Chem.* **2013**, *405*, 5687–5695. [CrossRef]
55. Ali, N.; Hossain, K.; Degen, G.H. Blood plasma biomarkers of citrinin and ochratoxin A exposure in young adults in Bangladesh. *Mycotoxin Res.* **2017**, *34*, 59–67. [CrossRef] [PubMed]
56. Ouhibi, S.; Vidal, A.; Martins, C.; Gali, R.; Hedhili, A.; De Saeger, S.; De Boevre, M. LC-MS/MS methodology for simultaneous determination of patulin and citrinin in urine and plasma applied to a pilot study in colorectal cancer patients. *Food Chem. Toxicol.* **2020**, *136*, 110994. [CrossRef] [PubMed]

57. Jagdale, P.R.; Dev, I.; Ayanur, A.; Singh, D.; Arshad; Ansari, K.M. Safety evaluation of ochratoxin A and citrinin after 28 days repeated dose oral exposure to Wistar rats. *Regul. Toxicol. Pharmacol.* **2020**, *115*, 104700. [CrossRef]
58. Rašić, D.; Mladinić, M.; Želježić, D.; Pizent, A.; Stefanović, S.; Milićević, D.; Konjevoda, P.; Peraica, M. Effects of combined treatment with ochratoxin A and citrinin on oxidative damage in kidneys and liver of rats. *Toxicon* **2018**, *146*, 99–105. [CrossRef]
59. Ghallab, A.; Hassan, R.; Myllys, M.; Albrecht, W.; Friebel, A.; Hoehme, S.; Hofmann, U.; Seddek, A.-L.; Braeuning, A.; Kuepfer, L.; et al. Subcellular spatio-temporal intravital kinetics of aflatoxin B_1 and ochratoxin A in liver and kidney. *Arch. Toxicol.* **2021**, *95*, 2163–2177. [CrossRef]
60. Echodu, R.; Malinga, G.M.M.; Kaducu, J.M.; Ovuga, E.; Haesaert, G. Prevalence of aflatoxin, ochratoxin and deoxynivalenol in cereal grains in Northern Uganda: Implication for food safety and health. *Toxicol. Rep.* **2019**, *6*, 1012–1017. [CrossRef]
61. Kumar, N.; Singh, A.K. Impact of environmental factors on human semen quality and male fertility: A narrative review. *Environ. Sci. Eur.* **2022**, *34*, 6. [CrossRef]
62. De Santis, B.; Brera, C.; Mezzelani, A.; Soricelli, S.; Ciceri, F.; Moretti, G.; Debegnach, F.; Bonaglia, M.C.; Villa, L.; Molteni, M.; et al. Role of mycotoxins in the pathobiology of autism: A first evidence. *Nutr. Neurosci.* **2019**, *22*, 132–144. [CrossRef]
63. Malir, F.; Louda, M.; Ostry, V.; Toman, J.; Ali, N.; Grosse, Y.; Malirova, E.; Pacovsky, J.; Pickova, D.; Brodak, M.; et al. Analyses of biomarkers of exposure to nephrotoxic mycotoxins in a cohort of patients with renal tumours. *Mycotoxin Res.* **2019**, *35*, 391–403. [CrossRef]
64. Mauro, T.; Hao, L.; Pop, L.C.; Buckley, B.; Schneider, S.H.; Bandera, E.V.; Shapses, S.A. Circulating zearalenone and its metabolites differ in women due to body mass index and food intake. *Food Chem. Toxicol.* **2018**, *116*, 227–232. [CrossRef] [PubMed]
65. Cao, X.; Li, X.; Li, J.; Niu, Y.; Shi, L.; Fang, Z.; Zhang, T.; Ding, H. Quantitative determination of carcinogenic mycotoxins in human and animal biological matrices and animal-derived foods using multi-mycotoxin and analyte-specific high performance liquid chromatography-tandem mass spectrometric methods. *J. Chromatogr. B* **2018**, *1073*, 191–200. [CrossRef] [PubMed]
66. De Santis, B.; Raggi, M.E.; Moretti, G.; Facchiano, F.; Mezzelani, A.; Villa, L.; Bonfanti, A.; Campioni, A.; Rossi, S.; Camposeo, S.; et al. Study on the Association among Mycotoxins and other Variables in Children with Autism. *Toxins* **2017**, *9*, 203. [CrossRef]
67. Osteresch, B.; Cramer, B.; Humpf, H.U. Analysis of ochratoxin A in dried blood spots—Correlation between venous and finger-prick blood, the influence of hematocrit and spotted volume. *J. Chromatogr. B* **2016**, *1020*, 158–164. [CrossRef]

Disclaimer/Publisher's Note: The statements, opinions and data contained in all publications are solely those of the individual author(s) and contributor(s) and not of MDPI and/or the editor(s). MDPI and/or the editor(s) disclaim responsibility for any injury to people or property resulting from any ideas, methods, instructions or products referred to in the content.

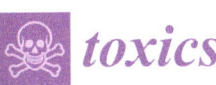

Article

Multi-Omics Analysis Reveals the Toxicity of Polyvinyl Chloride Microplastics toward BEAS-2B Cells

Chengzhi Liu [1], Shuang Chen [1], Jiangliang Chu [1], Yifan Yang [1], Beilei Yuan [1,*] and Huazhong Zhang [2,3,*]

1. College of Safety Science and Engineering, Nanjing Tech University, Nanjing 210009, China; 18005194475@163.com (C.L.); chenshuangs28@163.com (S.C.); 18734001211@163.com (J.C.); yangyifan917@163.com (Y.Y.)
2. Department of Emergency Medicine, The First Affiliated Hospital of Nanjing Medical University, Nanjing 210029, China
3. Institute of Poisoning, Nanjing Medical University, Nanjing 211100, China
* Correspondence: yuanbeilei@163.com (B.Y.); zhanghuazhong313@163.com (H.Z.)

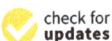

Citation: Liu, C.; Chen, S.; Chu, J.; Yang, Y.; Yuan, B.; Zhang, H. Multi-Omics Analysis Reveals the Toxicity of Polyvinyl Chloride Microplastics toward BEAS-2B Cells. *Toxics* **2024**, *12*, 399. https://doi.org/10.3390/toxics12060399

Academic Editor: David R. Wallace

Received: 27 April 2024
Revised: 18 May 2024
Accepted: 28 May 2024
Published: 30 May 2024

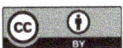

Copyright: © 2024 by the authors. Licensee MDPI, Basel, Switzerland. This article is an open access article distributed under the terms and conditions of the Creative Commons Attribution (CC BY) license (https://creativecommons.org/licenses/by/4.0/).

Abstract: Polyvinyl chloride microplastics (PVC-MPs) are microplastic pollutants widely present in the environment, but their potential risks to human lung health and underlying toxicity mechanisms remain unknown. In this study, we systematically analyzed the effects of PVC-MPs on the transcriptome and metabolome of BEAS-2B cells using high-throughput RNA sequencing and untargeted metabolomics technologies. The results showed that exposure to PVC-MPs significantly reduced the viability of BEAS-2B cells, leading to the differential expression of 530 genes and 3768 metabolites. Further bioinformatics analyses showed that PVC-MP exposure influenced the expression of genes associated with fluid shear stress, the MAPK and TGF-β signaling pathways, and the levels of metabolites associated with amino acid metabolism. In particular, integrated pathway analysis showed that lipid metabolic pathways (including glycerophospholipid metabolism, glycerolipid metabolism, and sphingolipid metabolism) were significantly perturbed in BEAS-2B cells following PVC-MPs exposure. This study provides new insights and targets for a deeper understanding of the toxicity mechanism of PVC-MPs and for the prevention and treatment of PVC-MP-associated lung diseases.

Keywords: microplastics; polyvinyl chloride; BEAS-2B; multi-omics; lipid metabolism

1. Introduction

Plastic products are widely used in a variety of fields, including healthcare, construction, and textiles, due to their low weight, durability, ease of processing, and low cost [1–4]. The global production of plastics is increasing dramatically each year, reaching 400 million tons in 2020, a figure that is expected to double over the next 20 years [5,6]. Because plastics typically take hundreds to thousands of years to degrade, they tend to accumulate in the environment, stemming from various sources [7,8]. Microplastics (MPs) are plastic particles with a diameter of less than 5 mm [9] that may come from the natural decomposition of plastic waste [10] or the use of daily necessities [11]. Reports from the World Health Organization (WHO) indicate the ubiquitous presence of microplastics in the ocean, air, soil, food, and beverages [12]. This could have long-term impacts on the environment and human health, creating a global cause for concern [13].

Currently, most studies have focused on microplastics in the marine environment, while relatively few studies have been conducted on atmospheric MPs [14]. Recently, attention has been focused on atmospheric microplastics, especially in light of concerns about human lung health and exposure outcomes. It has been reported that the per capita inhalation of 26–130 MPs particles per day from the air can pose a significant health risk to humans, especially for vulnerable groups like newborns and children [15]. Some exposure models have shown that moderately active males inhale up to 272 MPs particles per day [16]. After entering the human body, MPs may cause a number of chronic respiratory diseases [17]; affect gastrointestinal peristalsis [18]; and deposit on the surface of tissues or within cells, stimulating an inflammatory response, which can threaten human health [19]. Polyvinyl chloride (PVC), a prominent type of MP, is extensively used in toys, food packaging and cling film, squeeze bottles, shampoo bottles, detergent and cleaner bottles, medical supplies, construction products, etc. [20], with rising atmospheric levels due to atmospheric transport [21]. Recent studies have shown that exposure to PVC affects liver function, intestinal flora, lipid metabolism, and oxidative stress [22,23]. However, the molecular mechanisms underlying PVC-MP-induced cytotoxicity remain largely unknown.

Finite-element computer simulation approaches [24] and nanotechnology techniques [25] have been used to monitor the distribution and behavior of microplastics in the environment. However, these techniques have certain limitations, such as the need for large datasets associated with computationally costly resources or the complexity of the calibration step prior to data collection, respectively. In the face of these challenges, high-throughput techniques offer new solutions. Compared to traditional methods, high-throughput techniques are able to process large numbers of samples much more quickly, thus enabling the systematic analysis of toxicants in toxicology. Transcriptomics can identify alterations in total transcripts and screen key genes and pathways under stress [26]. Metabolomics allows the study of small-molecule metabolites and chemical reactions in cells or organisms, reflecting cellular physiology and revealing the biochemical dimension of biological information [27]. Metabolomics is the most accurate phenotypic-histologic approach and contains all the information on genetic regulation and expression regulation [28]. The integration of transcriptomics and metabolomics offers a comprehensive characterization of cellular responses and helps to reveal the mechanisms of action of toxicants [29]. Utilizing these two approaches, it was found that polystyrene MPs caused endothelial cell (EC) injury and led to abnormal changes in alanine, aspartate, glutamate, and sphingolipid metabolism [30]. Similarly, multi-omics techniques revealed that human hepatic cells are affected by the toxicity of anthracene and its chlorides [31]. These studies demonstrate that multi-omics analyses are effective in identifying and linking molecules affected by chemical substances, revealing the underlying toxicological mechanisms.

In this study, we utilized a multi-omics approach to investigate the toxicity of PVC-MPs toward BEAS-2B cells, a respiratory cell line that is a major exposure target and toxicity model for MPs [19,32,33]. We revealed the key factors of PVC-MPs affecting cytotoxicity by integrating transcriptomics and metabolomics data.

2. Materials and Methods

2.1. PVC-MPs Characterization

PVC-MPs were purchased from Xingxiang New Materials Co., Ltd. (Dongguan, China). The morphology of PVC-MPs was examined via scanning electron microscopy (SEM) (SU5000, Hitachi, Japan). The average hydrodynamic size and zeta potential of PVC-MPs were measured using a Malvern Zetasizer Nano ZSP (Malvern Panalytical Ltd., Malvern, PA, USA).

2.2. Cell Culture and Cytotoxicity Testing

The BEAS-2B cell line was purchased from the American Type Culture Collection (ATCC). Cells were cultured at 37 °C and in 5% CO_2 in a complete medium containing 10% fetal bovine serum (FBS), 4.5 g/L of D-glucose and L-glutamine, and 110 mg/L of sodium pyruvate. The effects of different concentrations of PVC-MPs on BEAS-2B cell viability after 24 h of exposure were assessed using a CCK-8 Cell Counting Kit (Vazyme, A311-02, Nanjing, China). The CCK-8 assay is more convenient and sensitive than the NRU assay and MTT assay. In this assay, the optical density (OD) value of methylated waste is measured at 450 nm using an enzyme marker, allowing for rapid assessment of cellular activity [34,35]. However, the CCK-8 assay can only be performed at a single time point, and colored drugs may interfere with the readings [36].

2.3. Transcriptomics Analysis

Total RNA was extracted from BEAS-2B cells in treated (800 μg/mL) and control groups with three biological replicates ($n = 3$) using TRIzol Reagent (LifeTechnologies, Carlsbad, CA, USA) according to the manufacturer's instructions. The concentration and integrity of RNA were determined using a NanoDrop 2000 (Thermo Fisher Scientific, Wilmington, DE, USA) and an Agilent Bioanalyzer 2100 system (Agilent Technologies, Santa Clara, CA, USA) to detect the concentration, purity, and integrity of RNA. A total of 1 μg per sample was used to start library construction. Then, sequencing libraries were generated using the Hieff NGS Ultima Dual-mode mRNA Library Prep Kit for Illumina (Yeasen Biotechnology (Shanghai) Co., Ltd., Shanghai, China) with a dual-mode approach: firstly, mRNA enrichment with magnetic beads was used to enrich mRNA; then, USER enzyme was used to cut the hairpin loop structure; and, finally, PCR amplification and magnetic beads were used for purification. Paired-end sequencing was performed by using the Illumina NovaSeq platform to generate a 150-bp sequence. Differential expression analysis was performed on both groups using DESeq2, differentially expressed genes were identified using a negative binomial distribution model, and p-values were corrected using the Benjamini and Hochberg method. Differentially expressed genes (DEGs) were screened for fold change ≥ 1.5 and p-value < 0.05. Functional and pathway analyses of DEGs were conducted using the GO and KEGG databases.

2.4. Untargeted Metabolomics Analysis

Metabolites were extracted from BEAS-2B cells and divided into treated (800 μg/mL) and control groups with 6 biological replicates each ($n = 6$). To the samples, 1000 uL of extraction solution (methanol, acetonitrile, and water = 2:2:1 (v/v)) containing an isotope-labeled internal standard mixture was added. The samples were frozen in liquid nitrogen for 1 min and then thawed and vortexed at 4 °C for 30 s. The procedure was repeated 2–3 times, followed by sonication in an ice-water bath for 10 min, resting at -40 °C for 1 h, and centrifugation at 12,000 rpm for 15 min at 4 °C, and the supernatant was extracted for the assay. A Waters ACQUITY UPLC BEH Amide column was used as the chromatographic column on a Vanquish ultra-performance liquid chromatograph. The primary and secondary mass spectral data were obtained using an Orbitrap Exploris 120 mass spectrometer. Data were converted to the appropriate format using ProteoWizard software (Palo Alto, CA, USA), and peak localization, peak extraction, peak alignment, and integration were performed using the R program package. The data were normalized using internal standards (ISs). Data were logarithmically (LOG) transformed and centered (CTR) using SIMCA software (V16.0.2, Sartorius Stedim Data Analytics AB, Umea, Sweden). VIP > 1 and p-value < 0.05 were used as criteria to screen for differentially expressed metabolites (DEMs) between groups. Pathway enrichment analysis was performed using the MetaboAnalyst 5.0 platform (http://www.metaboanalyst.ca/) (accessed on 20 March 2024).

2.5. Multi-Omics Analysis

Transcriptomics and metabolomics data were jointly analyzed using the Joint Pathway Analysis Module of MetaboAnalyst 5.0, and p-value < 0.05 was used as a screening criterion for significant enrichment of pathways. Metabolome–gene networks were displayed using Metascape software 3.5.

2.6. Statistical Analysis

The data were statistically analyzed using Zetasizer software (version 7.01) and GraphPad Prism software (version 10.2.3), and the results were presented as means ± SDs. Differences were assessed using the Student's t-test or one-way analysis of variance (ANOVA) with Tukey's post hoc test. p-value < 0.05 was considered significant.

3. Results

3.1. Characterization of PVC-MPs

In this study, we examined the morphology, size, and zeta potential of PVC-MPs to characterize them. The SEM images showed that PVC-MPs were spherical and aggregated into different sizes (Figure 1A). The average hydrodynamic size of the PVC-MPs in the medium was 1232 ± 70 nm (Figure 1B). The specific characterization results regarding the zeta potential of PVC-MPs are shown in Table 1. PVC-MPs of different concentrations showed negative charges in DMEM medium, indicating that they tend to repel each other and do not auto-aggregate.

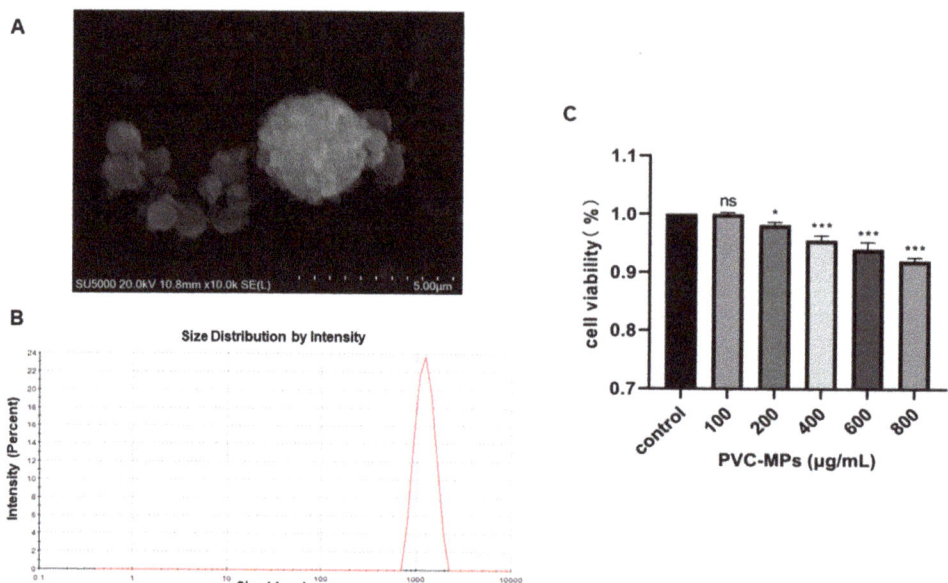

Figure 1. Characterization of PVC-MPs in suspension. (**A**) SEM images of PVC-MPs. (**B**) The physicochemical characterization of particle size. (**C**) Change in cell viability after exposure to different concentrations of PVC-MPs for 24 h. Results are shown as means ± SDs (n = 3 samples per treated group). ns (non-significant); * p-value < 0.05; *** p-value < 0.001.

Table 1. Zeta potentials of different concentrations of PVC-MP dispersions in DMEM medium.

Concentration (µg/mL)	Zeta Potential (mV)
100	−27.53
200	−25.17
400	−25.10
600	−25.52
800	−31.83

3.2. Cytotoxicity Effects of PVC-MPs on BEAS-2B Cells

We evaluated the toxicity of PVC-MPs toward BEAS-2B cells with different doses (100, 200, 400, 600, and 800 µg/mL) for 24 h. As shown in Figure 1C, cell viability experiments showed that PVC-MPs significantly induced cytotoxicity at 200 µg/mL in a dose-dependent manner (p-value < 0.05). Overall, the above results indicated that the PVC-MPs adversely affected the BEAS-2B cells.

3.3. Transcriptomics Analysis of BEAS-2B Samples Exposed to PVC-MPs

3.3.1. Screening and Analysis of Differentially Expressed Genes

In this study, transcriptomic techniques were employed to analyze the gene expression changes in BEAS-2B cells following their exposure to PVC-MPs. After screening, we obtained a total of 530 DEGs, of which 282 were up-regulated and 248 were down-regulated (Figure 2A). The results showed that PVC-MPs had a significant effect on gene expression in BEAS-2B cells. Euclidean clustering analysis of the DEGs showed that there was a significant difference in gene expression patterns between the PVC-MP-exposed and control groups (Figure 2B).

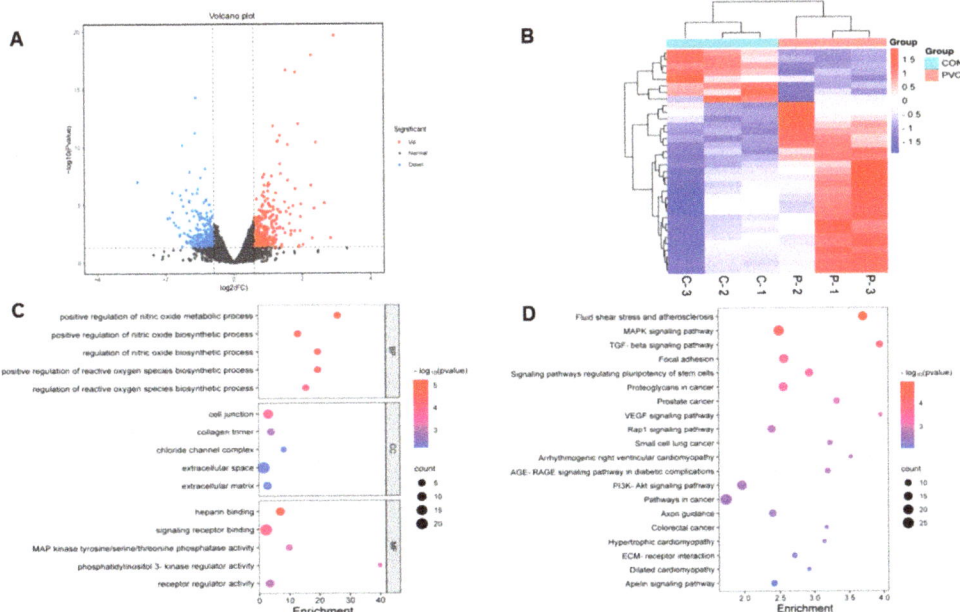

Figure 2. Transcriptomic analysis of BEAS-2B cells after their exposure to 800 μg/mL of PVC-MPs for 24 h. (**A**) Volcano plot of DEGs (blue, downregulated genes; red, upregulated genes). (**B**) Hierarchical clustering based on DEGs (blue, downregulated; red, upregulated). (**C**) GO enrichment analysis of DEGs. (**D**) KEGG pathway enrichment analysis of DEGs.

3.3.2. GO and KEGG Analysis

Gene Ontology (GO) analysis, a gene ontology-based method, categorizes genes into biological processes (BPs), cellular components (CCs), and molecular functions (MFs), aiding in the understanding of gene functions and interactions [37]. Figure 2C shows the enrichment of DEGs in the three GO categories. In the BP category, DEGs were mainly enriched in positive regulation of the nitric oxide metabolic process and positive regulation of the reactive oxygen species biosynthetic process. In the CC category, DEGs were mainly enriched in cell junction and collagen trimer, and in the MF category, DEGs were mainly enriched in heparin binding and signaling receptor binding. Furthermore, to explore the relationship between DEGs and cellular functions, we performed an enrichment analysis of the Kyoto Encyclopedia of Genes and Genomes (KEGG) pathway. KEGG is a database that collects and provides chemical, genomic, and functional information about biological systems, enabling the annotation of gene functions and metabolic pathways [38]. In this analysis, the q-value was used to indicate enrichment significance, with a lower q-value denoting higher significance. The results showed that DEGs were mainly involved in 20 pathways, among which the fluid shear stress and atherosclerosis pathway was the most highly enriched (Figure 2D). In addition, the MAPK signaling pathway and TGF-beta signaling pathway were also significantly enriched.

3.4. Metabolomics Analysis of BEAS-2B Samples Exposed to PVC-MPs

3.4.1. Multivariate Analysis

In this study, we analyzed the control and treated groups using untargeted metabolomics. First, we downscaled the data using principal component analysis (PCA) to show the overall characteristics of the data and sources of variation. As shown in Figure 3A, the PCA scatterplot clearly showed the differences between the two sample groups. Then, we used OPLS-DA to screen for metabolites associated with categorical variables. Similarly, the OPLS-DA plot showed significant differences between the PVC-MP metabolomics dataset and the control group (Figure 3B). Finally, we verified the quality of the model using a permutation test (n = 200). The results showed that the OPLS-DA model exhibited values of Q^2 = 0.849 and R^2Y = 0.988 (Figure 3C), indicating that the model had high stability and reliability.

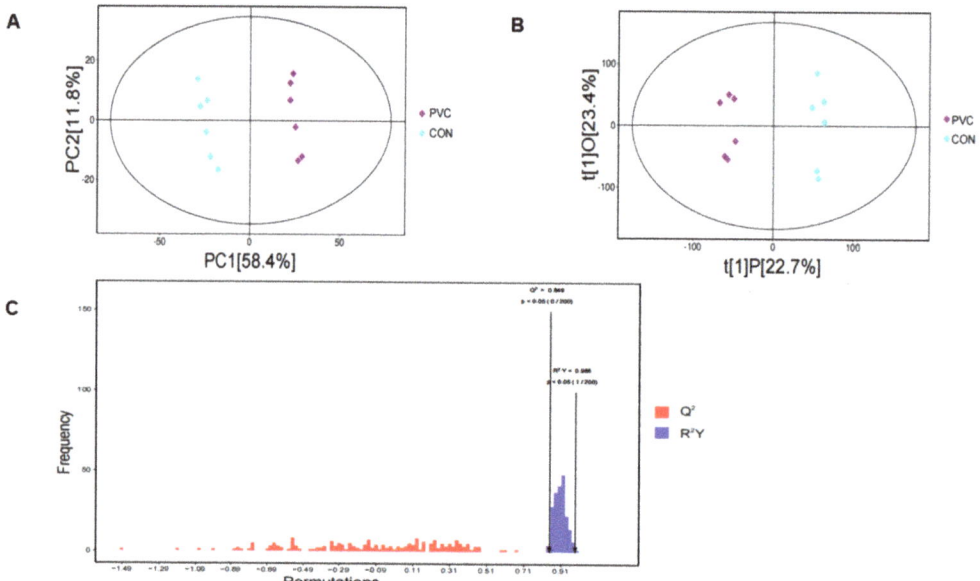

Figure 3. Multivariate analysis of metabolomics data on BEAS-2B cells after 24 h of exposure to PVC-MPs. (**A**) Scatter plot of PCA for metabolomics data. (**B**) Plot of OPLS-DA scores for metabolomics data. (**C**) Plot of the results of the permutation test for OPLS-DA modeling.

3.4.2. Screening and Analysis of Differentially Expressed Metabolites

We used a p-value < 0.05 and VIP > 1 as screening criteria for DEMs and used volcano plots to demonstrate metabolite changes and significance. As shown in Figure 4A, 3768 DEMs were significantly changed, among which 1918 were up-regulated and 1850 were down-regulated. We also analyzed the expression patterns of DEMs using the Euclidean distance matrix and fully interlocked clustering and found that there were significant differences between groups (Figure 4B).

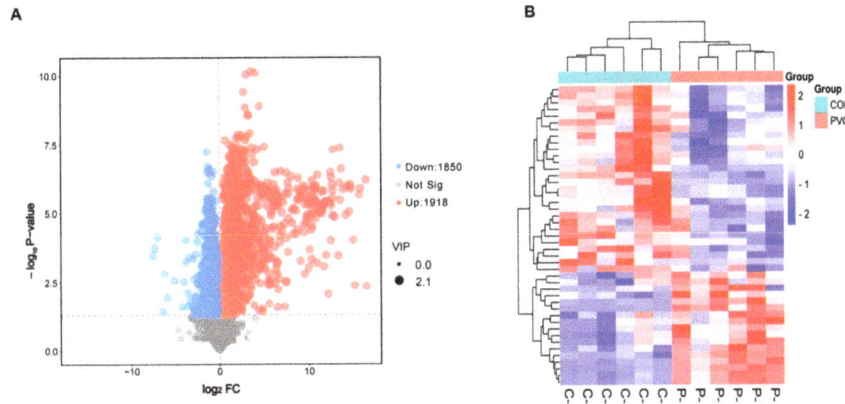

Figure 4. DEMs of BEAS-2B cells affected by exposure to PVC-MPs. (**A**) Volcano plot of DEMs (blue, downregulated metabolites; red, upregulated metabolites). (**B**) Hierarchical clustering of DEMs (blue, downregulated; red, upregulated).

3.4.3. Metabolic Pathway Analysis

Using the KEGG Pathway database, we performed enrichment analysis of DEMs and used bubble plots to show the enrichment results regarding the metabolic pathways (Figure 5A). The results showed that these DEMs were enriched in 43 pathways (Table S1). Of these, valine, leucine, and isoleucine biosynthesis; glycolysis or gluconeogenesis; and pyruvate metabolism were the top three significantly enriched pathways, all of which are related to amino acid metabolism. To further explore the interactions between metabolic pathways, we also conducted a network enrichment analysis based on DEMs, including metabolic pathways, modules, enzymes, reactions, and metabolites (Figure 5B), reflecting the interactions and effects occurring between metabolic pathways as well as the propagation and targeting of perturbations at the pathway level.

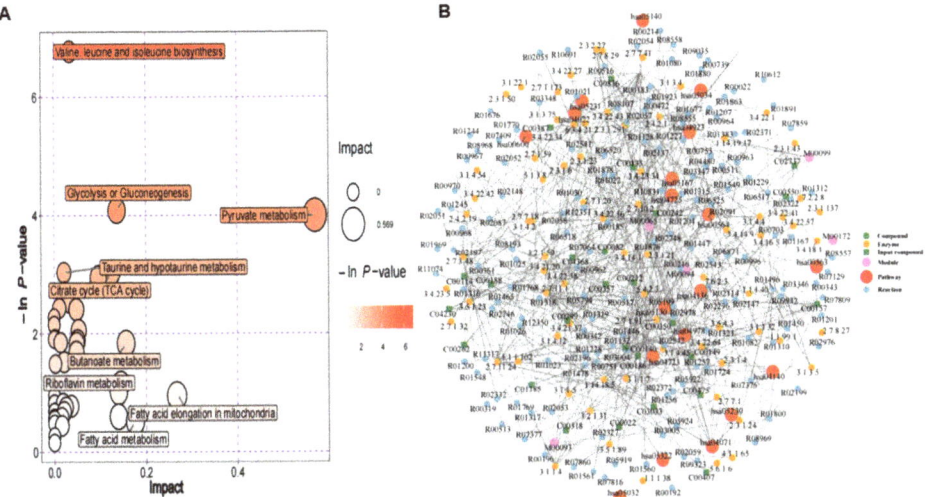

Figure 5. Pathway analysis of BEAS-2B cells exposed to PVC-MPs. (**A**) KEGG pathway enrichment analysis of DEMs. Bubble color indicates the p-value of enrichment analysis, and bubble size indicates the size of influencing factors in topology analysis. (**B**) Diagram of regulatory network analysis.

3.5. Integrated Analysis of Transcriptomics and Metabolomics

To explore the biological significance of DEGs and DEMs, we utilized the Joint Pathway Analysis module of MetaboAnalyst 5.0 for a comprehensive analysis. This analysis revealed key metabolic pathways in PVC-MP-exposed BEAS-2B cells. We calculated the p-value for each pathway using the hypergeometric test and illustrated the top 20 metabolic pathways that DEGs and DEMs jointly mapped to, as shown in Figure 6A. This analysis identified significant involvement of DEGs and DEMs in seven metabolic pathways (Table 2, $p < 0.05$): glycerophospholipid metabolism; glycerolipid metabolism; valine, leucine, and isoleucine biosynthesis; sphingolipid metabolism; terpenoid backbone biosynthesis; synthesis and degradation of ketone bodies; and pyruvate metabolism. Among these, glycerophospholipid metabolism was particularly perturbed, prompting us to construct and visualize the metabolome–gene network for this pathway using Metscape software (version 4.08) (Figure 6B). Additionally, we analyzed changes in matching metabolites within glycerophospholipid metabolism by generating a heat map through Euclidean clustering analysis (Figure 7).

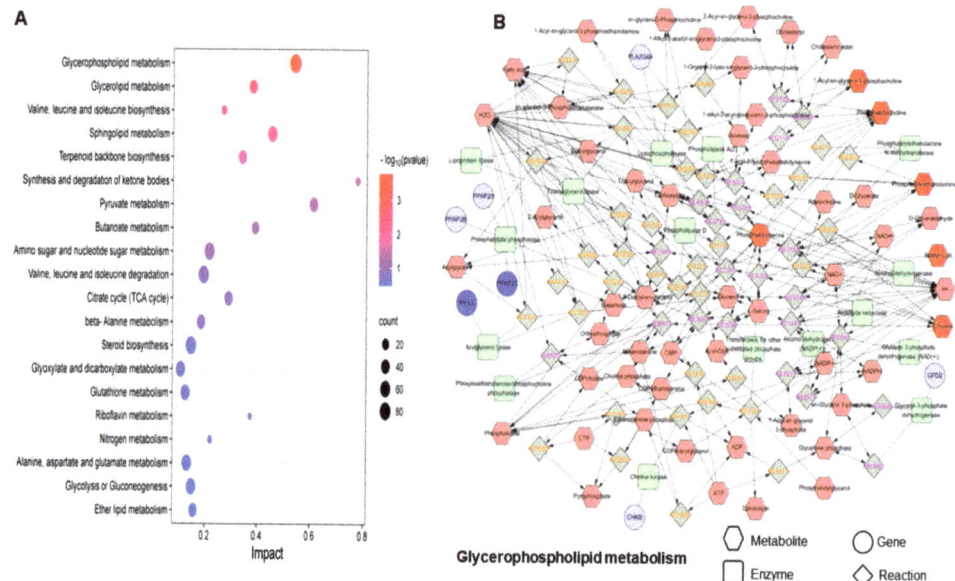

Figure 6. Association analysis of multi-omics data. (**A**) Joint pathway analysis of DEMs and DEGs using MetaboAnalyst 5.0. (**B**) Metabolite–gene network for glycerophospholipid metabolism (from Metscape).

Table 2. Significant enrichment pathways for DEGs and DEMs.

KEGG ID	Pathway	p-Value
ko00564	Glycerophospholipid metabolism	0.0001756
hsa00561	Glycerolipid metabolism	0.0033649
ko00290	Valine, leucine, and isoleucine biosynthesis	0.0046556
map00600	Sphingolipid metabolism	0.0068775
map00900	Terpenoid backbone biosynthesis	0.021066
ko00072	Synthesis and degradation of ketone bodies	0.034016
ko00620	Pyruvate metabolism	0.043594

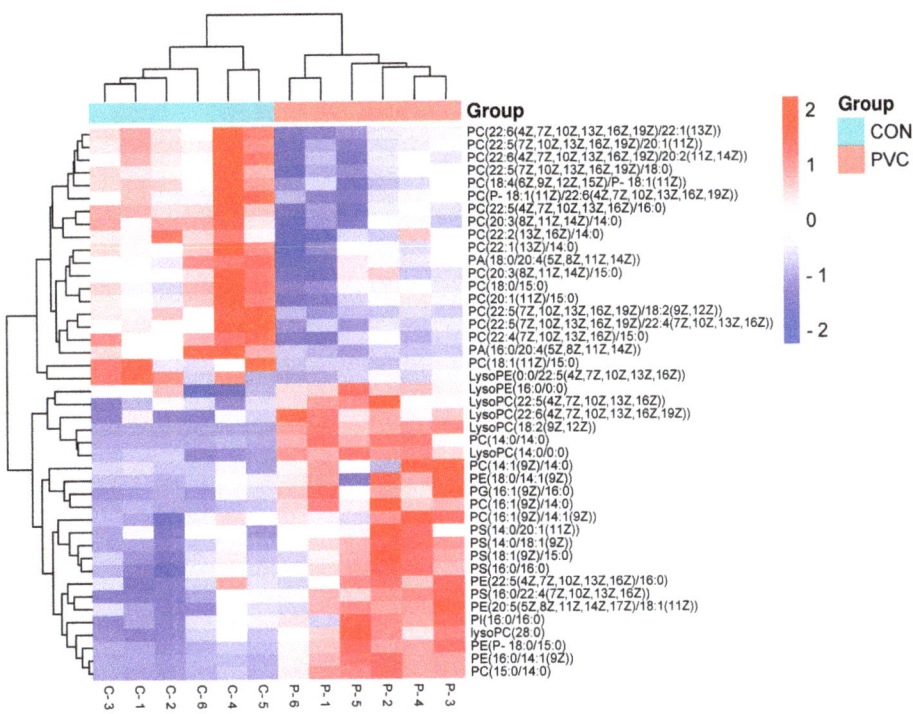

Figure 7. Heatmap of 43 target glycerophospholipids generated via Euclidean clustering analysis.

4. Discussion

Microplastics, emerging environmental pollutants, are widespread worldwide. Studies have shown that airborne microplastic particles are capable of entering human lung tissue [39]. The total amount of microplastics ingested and inhaled by humans from the environment can be as high as 700–1050 µg per week [40]. In addition, numerous reports indicate that microplastics may contribute to the development of lung diseases, especially in individuals exposed to high levels over long periods of time [41]. Therefore, considering the total number of MPs accumulated and ingested in the human body over a long period of time, we chose 800 µg/mL of PVC-MPs as the exposure concentration for our experiment. At this concentration, BEAS-2B cells were exposed to PVC-MPs, and a detailed exploration of the specific effects of PVC-MPs at the cellular molecular level was conducted through high-throughput RNA sequencing and untargeted metabolomics analysis. We found that PVC-MPs could induce a decrease in cell viability in a dose-dependent manner. Previous studies have shown that PVC particles induce apoptosis in various cell types, such as normal human lung fibroblast cells (IMR 90) [42], enterocytes and hepatocytes [43], BHK-21 cells [44], and human lymphocytes [45]. Apoptosis has been reported to be a complex process regulated by multiple cell-signaling pathways, involving the expression and function of numerous genes and proteins [46]. Our study highlighted that the MAPK signaling pathway and the TGF-beta signaling pathway are the primary pathways through which PVC-MPs induce cellular responses. These two signaling pathways play pivotal roles in proliferation, differentiation, and apoptosis across various cell lines [47–51]. TGF-beta regulates the transcription of target genes by binding to their specific receptors and activating downstream SMAD proteins [52]. Meanwhile, there is clear crosstalk between the TGF-β and MAPK pathways and SMAD [53]. A study has demonstrated that both MAPK- and TGF-β-related signaling pathways are activated in pristine graphene-treated cells, leading to macrophage apoptosis [46]. In addition, in PVC-MP-treated cells, we observed an increase in the number of apoptotic genes in the MAPK signaling pathway and TGF-beta signaling pathway, which confirms that PVC-MPs may affect apoptosis in BEAS-2B cells at the transcriptome level.

Metabolomics analysis revealed the effects of environmental pollutants on organisms, in which endogenous metabolites, as end products of gene expression, directly reflect abnormal phenotypes of organisms [54]. In this study, we identified 3768 DEMs in PVC-MP-induced BEAS-2B cells, which were mainly involved in regulating amino acid metabolism. Amino acid metabolism can affect cellular metabolism and cellular processes at multiple levels, involving multiple metabolic pathways and regulatory mechanisms [55]. In particular, the branched-chain amino acid (BCAA) biosynthetic pathway plays an important role in protein synthesis and cell growth regulation [56,57]. Research has demonstrated that BCAA can promote the survival of eukaryotic cells and prolong the lifespan of Saccharomyces cerevisiae [58]. Furthermore, glycolysis and gluconeogenesis serve as the primary pathways for the cellular utilization and production of glucose, a crucial energy source. During glycolysis, glucose is metabolized into pyruvate, which can either enter the mitochondria to engage in the tricarboxylic acid (TCA) cycle, producing acetyl coenzyme A in the presence of oxygen, or be converted into lactate anaerobically through lactate dehydrogenase [59]. However, many diseased cells rely on aerobic glycolysis, known as the "Warburg effect" [60]. A study found that excessive glycolysis led to mitochondrial dysfunction and promoted the production of reactive oxygen species (ROS) [61], which led to cellular oxidative stress and consequently affected cellular autophagy and apoptosis [62]. Another report showed that elevated levels of leucine, isoleucine, valine, and phenylalanine in a Mycobacterium tuberculosis (MTB)-infected C57Bl/6 mouse model suggested that disorders of amino acid metabolism may be associated with alterations in multiple metabolic pathways [63]. These results suggest that disrupted amino acid metabolism may lead to imbalanced energy metabolism and apoptosis.

Multi-omics analysis is essential for understanding the biological mechanisms of diseases and identifying biomarkers by revealing the interactions between genes, proteins, metabolites, and microbiota [64]. This analytical approach dominates the study of cellular function and has enabled the systematic and comprehensive elucidation of complex biological processes by integrating different levels of biomolecular data [65]. In this study, the integrated transcriptomics and metabolomics analysis conducted revealed that lipid metabolism, encompassing glycerophospholipid metabolism, glyceride metabolism, and sphingolipid metabolism, was the most critical pathway for metabolic changes in BEAS-2B cells following exposure to PVC-MPs. Previous studies have demonstrated that lipid metabolism is closely linked to processes such as cell growth, apoptosis, and inflammation [66], influencing the characteristics of cell membranes, leading to the onset and progression of several diseases, including cancer [67]. Glycerophospholipid (GPL) is the major structural lipid of cell membranes [68], and its synthesis and metabolism in eukaryotes involve a variety of intermediates, such as phosphatidylcholine (PC), phosphatidylethanolamine (PE), and lysophosphatidic acid (LPA), which play important roles in cell signaling [69]. Moreover, alterations in GPL levels are important biological indicators of lipid metabolism disorders [70]. In this study, we found that exposure to PVC-MPs resulted in disturbed GPL metabolism in BEAS-2B cells, as evidenced by fluctuations in the content of multiple glycerophospholipids in PC and PE intermediates, as shown in Figure 7.

Environmental factors have had an important impact on lipid metabolism, with air pollution, as an important environmental factor, being capable of disturbing lipid metabolism, leading to lipid peroxidation, oxidative stress, and inflammatory responses, which can increase the risk of developing chronic diseases [71]. Disturbances in GPL metabolism have been observed following gastrointestinal exposure to airborne PM2.5 [72], as well as perturbations in arachidonic acid and glycerolipid metabolism due to the exposure of human bronchial epithelial cells to PM [73]. Furthermore, ceramide, a key molecule in sphingolipid metabolism, has been shown in various IR models to be strongly associated with apoptosis induced by mitochondrial damage [74]. Recent studies have also demonstrated that abnormal sphingolipid metabolism induces apoptosis in a variety of cells, including CNE-2 cells and breast cancer cells [75–77]. In this study, we found that the levels of sphingomyelin (SM) were upregulated in sphingolipid metabolic pathways, including SM (d16:1/24:1(15Z)), SM (d18:1/12:0), SM (d18:0/14:0), and SM (d18:1/14:0). SM is a key sphingolipid essential for processes such as apoptosis, proliferation, and migration and plays a central role in maintaining plasma membrane stability and signaling [78,79]. Additionally, PC, PE, SM, and cholesterol constitute the main components of biological membranes [80]. In this study, exposure to PVC-MPs resulted in changes in PC, PE, and SM levels in BEAS-2B cells, indicating possible damage to the cell membrane that could affect cell survival and metabolic processes.

There are several limitations of our present study. Primarily, MPs are encountered as intricate mixtures in the environment [81]. Our methodology involved the utilization of a singular concentration and type of MPs, which might not encapsulate the comprehensive spectrum of biological responses elicited by varying concentrations and types of MPs on BEAS-2B cells. Additionally, the cytotoxicity evaluation executed via the CCK-8 assay potentially neglected the detection of MPs at diminished concentrations. Thirdly, while pivotal biological pathways were delineated through multi-omics analysis, an in-depth exploration of the specific mechanisms governing these pathways was not conducted. Collectively, these limitations indicate the direction of our future research.

5. Conclusions

We analyzed changes in the transcriptome and metabolome of BEAS-2B cells after their exposure to PVC-MPs. Through a comprehensive analysis of transcriptomics and metabolomics data, we identified disruptions of lipid metabolism in PVC-MP-exposed BEAS-2B cells. The results reveal that PVC-MPs interfere with the metabolic mechanism of BEAS-2B cells and provide new potential targets for the prevention and treatment of PVC-MP-induced lung diseases.

Supplementary Materials: The following supporting information can be downloaded at https://www.mdpi.com/article/10.3390/toxics12060399/s1. Table S1: DEMs enrichment pathways.

Author Contributions: Conceptualization, C.L. and B.Y.; methodology, S.C.; software, J.C.; formal analysis, C.L.; investigation, Y.Y. and S.C.; data curation, J.C. and Y.Y.; writing—original draft preparation, C.L.; writing—review and editing, B.Y. and H.Z.; visualization, C.L.; supervision, H.Z.; project administration, B.Y.; funding acquisition, B.Y. and H.Z. All authors have read and agreed to the published version of the manuscript.

Funding: This work was supported by the National Natural Science Foundation of China [grant numbers No. 81803274]. Jiangsu Province Practice Innovation Program (No. SJCX23-0465). Jiangsu Province Practice Innovation Program (No. SJCX24-0526). The Young Scholars Fostering Fund of the First Affiliated Hospital of Nanjing Medical University.

Institutional Review Board Statement: Not applicable.

Informed Consent Statement: Not applicable.

Data Availability Statement: The data presented in this study are available on request from the corresponding author.

Acknowledgments: The authors would like to thank all the collaborators and colleagues involved in this project for the useful discussions.

Conflicts of Interest: The authors declare no conflicts of interest.

References

1. Joseph, B.; James, J.; Kalarikkal, N.; Thomas, S. Recycling of medical plastics. *Adv. Ind. Eng. Polym. Res.* **2021**, *4*, 199–208. [CrossRef]
2. Romeo, J. Do No Harm: Plastics are playing a major role in giving healthcare professionals the tools and capabilities they need to battle the COVID pandemic. *Plast. Eng.* **2020**, *76*, 41. [CrossRef]
3. Ahmed, N. Utilizing plastic waste in the building and construction industry: A pathway towards the circular economy. *Constr. Build. Mater.* **2023**, *383*, 131311. [CrossRef]
4. Xu, C.; Zhou, G.; Lu, J.; Shen, C.; Dong, Z.; Yin, S.; Li, F. Spatio-vertical distribution of riverine microplastics: Impact of the textile industry. *Environ. Res.* **2022**, *211*, 112789. [CrossRef] [PubMed]
5. Fellner, J.; Brunner, P.H. Plastic waste management: Is circular economy really the best solution? *J. Mater. Cycles Waste Manag.* **2022**, *24*, 1–3. [CrossRef]
6. Walker, T.R.; Fequet, L. Current trends of unsustainable plastic production and micro (nano) plastic pollution. *TrAC Trends Anal. Chem.* **2023**, *160*, 116984. [CrossRef]
7. Chamas, A.; Moon, H.; Zheng, J.; Qiu, Y.; Tabassum, T.; Jang, J.H.; Abu-Omar, M.; Scott, S.L.; Suh, S. Degradation rates of plastics in the environment. *ACS Sustain. Chem. Eng.* **2020**, *8*, 3494–3511. [CrossRef]
8. Klein, S.; Dimzon, I.K.; Eubeler, J.; Knepper, T.P. Analysis, occurrence, and degradation of microplastics in the aqueous environment. In *Freshwater Microplastics: Emerging Environmental Contaminants*; Springer: Berlin/Heidelberg, Germany, 2018; pp. 51–67.
9. Thompson, R.C.; Olsen, Y.; Mitchell, R.P.; Davis, A.; Rowland, S.J.; John, A.W.; McGonigle, D.; Russell, A.E. Lost at sea: Where is all the plastic? *Science* **2004**, *304*, 838. [CrossRef] [PubMed]
10. Arthur, C.; Baker, J.E.; Bamford, H.A. *Proceedings of the International Research Workshop on the Occurrence, Effects, and Fate of Microplastic Marine Debris, Tacoma, WA, USA, 9–11 September 2008*; University of Washington Tacoma: Tacoma, WA, USA, 2009.
11. Hernandez, L.M.; Yousefi, N.; Tufenkji, N. Are there nanoplastics in your personal care products? *Environ. Sci. Technol. Lett.* **2017**, *4*, 280–285. [CrossRef]
12. World Health Organization. *Dietary and Inhalation Exposure to Nano-and Microplastic Particles and Potential Implications for Human Health*; World Health Organization: Geneva, Switzerland, 2022.
13. MacLeod, M.; Arp, H.P.H.; Tekman, M.B.; Jahnke, A. The global threat from plastic pollution. *Science* **2021**, *373*, 61–65. [CrossRef]
14. Allen, S.; Allen, D.; Moss, K.; Le Roux, G.; Phoenix, V.R.; Sonke, J.E. Examination of the ocean as a source for atmospheric microplastics. *PLoS ONE* **2020**, *15*, e0232746. [CrossRef] [PubMed]
15. Prata, J.C. Airborne microplastics: Consequences to human health? *Environ. Pollut.* **2018**, *234*, 115–126. [CrossRef] [PubMed]
16. Vianello, A.; Jensen, R.L.; Liu, L.; Vollertsen, J. Simulating human exposure to indoor airborne microplastics using a Breathing Thermal Manikin. *Sci. Rep.* **2019**, *9*, 8670. [CrossRef] [PubMed]
17. Chen, R.; Hu, B.; Liu, Y.; Xu, J.; Yang, G.; Xu, D.; Chen, C. Beyond PM2.5: The role of ultrafine particles on adverse health effects of air pollution. *Biochim. Biophys. Acta* **2016**, *1860*, 2844–2855. [CrossRef] [PubMed]
18. Liu, K.; Wang, X.; Fang, T.; Xu, P.; Zhu, L.; Li, D. Source and potential risk assessment of suspended atmospheric microplastics in Shanghai. *Sci. Total Environ.* **2019**, *675*, 462–471. [CrossRef] [PubMed]
19. Dong, C.D.; Chen, C.W.; Chen, Y.C.; Chen, H.H.; Lee, J.S.; Lin, C.H. Polystyrene microplastic particles: In vitro pulmonary toxicity assessment. *J. Hazard. Mater.* **2020**, *385*, 121575. [CrossRef]
20. Bajt, O. From plastics to microplastics and organisms. *FEBS Open Bio* **2021**, *11*, 954–966. [CrossRef] [PubMed]
21. Zhang, Y.; Kang, S.; Allen, S.; Allen, D.; Gao, T.; Sillanpää, M. Atmospheric microplastics: A review on current status and perspectives. *Earth-Sci. Rev.* **2020**, *203*, 103118. [CrossRef]
22. Chen, X.; Zhuang, J.; Chen, Q.; Xu, L.; Yue, X.; Qiao, D. Chronic exposure to polyvinyl chloride microplastics induces liver injury and gut microbiota dysbiosis based on the integration of liver transcriptome profiles and full-length 16S rRNA sequencing data. *Sci. Total Environ.* **2022**, *839*, 155984. [CrossRef]
23. Zhuang, J.; Chen, Q.; Xu, L.; Chen, X. Combined exposure to polyvinyl chloride and polystyrene microplastics induces liver injury and perturbs gut microbial and serum metabolic homeostasis in mice. *Ecotoxicol. Environ. Saf.* **2023**, *267*, 115637. [CrossRef] [PubMed]
24. Pilechi, A.; Mohammadian, A.; Murphy, E. A numerical framework for modeling fate and transport of microplastics in inland and coastal waters. *Mar. Pollut. Bull.* **2022**, *184*, 114119. [CrossRef] [PubMed]
25. Marcuello, C. Present and future opportunities in the use of atomic force microscopy to address the physico-chemical properties of aquatic ecosystems at the nanoscale level. *Int. Aquat. Res.* **2022**.
26. Lowe, R.; Shirley, N.; Bleackley, M.; Dolan, S.; Shafee, T. Transcriptomics technologies. *PLoS Comput. Biol.* **2017**, *13*, e1005457. [CrossRef] [PubMed]
27. Galal, A.; Talal, M.; Moustafa, A. Applications of machine learning in metabolomics: Disease modeling and classification. *Front. Genet.* **2022**, *13*, 1017340. [CrossRef] [PubMed]
28. Shah, N.J.; Sureshkumar, S.; Shewade, D.G. Metabolomics: A Tool Ahead for Understanding Molecular Mechanisms of Drugs and Diseases. *Indian J. Clin. Biochem.* **2015**, *30*, 247–254. [CrossRef] [PubMed]
29. Ritchie, M.D.; Holzinger, E.R.; Li, R.; Pendergrass, S.A.; Kim, D. Methods of integrating data to uncover genotype–phenotype interactions. *Nat. Rev. Genet.* **2015**, *16*, 85–97. [CrossRef] [PubMed]

30. Zhang, M.; Shi, J.; Huang, Q.; Xie, Y.; Wu, R.; Zhong, J.; Deng, H. Multi-omics analysis reveals size-dependent toxicity and vascular endothelial cell injury induced by microplastic exposure in vivo and in vitro. *Environ. Sci. Nano* **2022**, *9*, 663–683. [CrossRef]
31. Luo, Y.; Geng, N.; Sun, S.; Cheng, L.; Chen, S.; Zhang, H.; Chen, J. Integration approach of transcriptomics and metabolomics reveals the toxicity of Anthracene and its chlorinated derivatives on human hepatic cells. *Sci. Total Environ.* **2023**, *905*, 166886. [CrossRef] [PubMed]
32. Kyung, S.; Zheng, T.; Park, Y.; Lee, J.; Kim, H. Potential toxicity of polystyrene microplastics with different particle size and surface charge in human lung epithelial BEAS-2B cells. *Toxicol. Lett.* **2022**, *368*, S135–S136. [CrossRef]
33. Wu, Y.; Wang, J.; Zhao, T.; Sun, M.; Xu, M.; Che, S.; Pan, Z.; Wu, C.; Shen, L. Polystyrene nanoplastics lead to ferroptosis in the lungs. *J. Adv. Res.* **2024**, *56*, 31–41. [CrossRef] [PubMed]
34. Lou, J.; Chu, G.; Zhou, G.; Jiang, J.; Huang, F.; Xu, J.; Zheng, S.; Jiang, W.; Lu, Y.; Li, X.; et al. Comparison between two kinds of cigarette smoke condensates (CSCs) of the cytogenotoxicity and protein expression in a human B-cell lymphoblastoid cell line using CCK-8 assay, comet assay and protein microarray. *Mutat. Res. Toxicol. Environ. Mutagen.* **2010**, *697*, 55–59. [CrossRef]
35. Zhang, Y.; Li, W.-Y.; Lan, R.; Wang, J.-Y. Quality monitoring of porous zein scaffolds: A novel biomaterial. *Engineering* **2017**, *3*, 130–135. [CrossRef]
36. Cai, L.; Qin, X.; Xu, Z.; Song, Y.; Jiang, H.; Wu, Y.; Ruan, H.; Chen, J. Comparison of cytotoxicity evaluation of anticancer drugs between real-time cell analysis and CCK-8 method. *ACS Omega* **2019**, *4*, 12036–12042. [CrossRef] [PubMed]
37. Gene Ontology Consortium. Gene ontology consortium: Going forward. *Nucleic Acids Res.* **2015**, *43*, D1049–D1056. [CrossRef] [PubMed]
38. Aoki, K.F.; Kanehisa, M. Using the KEGG database resource. *Curr. Protoc. Bioinform.* **2005**, *11*, 1–12. [CrossRef] [PubMed]
39. Amato-Lourenço, L.F.; Carvalho-Oliveira, R.; Júnior, G.R.; dos Santos Galvão, L.; Ando, R.A.; Mauad, T. Presence of airborne microplastics in human lung tissue. *J. Hazard. Mater.* **2021**, *416*, 126124. [CrossRef] [PubMed]
40. Choi, D.; Hwang, J.; Bang, J.; Han, S.; Kim, T.; Oh, Y.; Hwang, Y.; Choi, J.; Hong, J. In vitro toxicity from a physical perspective of polyethylene microplastics based on statistical curvature change analysis. *Sci. Total Environ.* **2021**, *752*, 142242. [CrossRef] [PubMed]
41. Winiarska, E.; Jutel, M.; Zemelka-Wiacek, M. The potential impact of nano-and microplastics on human health: Understanding human health risks. *Environ. Res.* **2024**, *251*, 118535. [CrossRef] [PubMed]
42. Mahadevan, G.; Valiyaveettil, S. Comparison of genotoxicity and cytotoxicity of polyvinyl chloride and poly (methyl methacrylate) nanoparticles on normal human lung cell lines. *Chem. Res. Toxicol.* **2021**, *34*, 1468–1480. [CrossRef] [PubMed]
43. Stock, V.; Laurisch, C.; Franke, J.; Dönmez, M.H.; Voss, L.; Böhmert, L.; Braeuning, A.; Sieg, H. Uptake and cellular effects of PE, PP, PET and PVC microplastic particles. *Toxicol. Vitr.* **2021**, *70*, 105021. [CrossRef] [PubMed]
44. Mahadevan, G.; Valiyaveettil, S. Understanding the interactions of poly (methyl methacrylate) and poly (vinyl chloride) nanoparticles with BHK-21 cell line. *Sci. Rep.* **2021**, *11*, 2089. [CrossRef] [PubMed]
45. Salimi, A.; Alavehzadeh, A.; Ramezani, M.; Pourahmad, J. Differences in sensitivity of human lymphocytes and fish lymphocytes to polyvinyl chloride microplastic toxicity. *Toxicol. Ind. Health* **2022**, *38*, 100–111. [CrossRef] [PubMed]
46. Li, Y.; Liu, Y.; Fu, Y.; Wei, T.; Le Guyader, L.; Gao, G.; Liu, R.-S.; Chang, Y.-Z.; Chen, C. The triggering of apoptosis in macrophages by pristine graphene through the MAPK and TGF-beta signaling pathways. *Biomaterials* **2012**, *33*, 402–411. [CrossRef]
47. Zhang, W.; Liu, H.T. MAPK signal pathways in the regulation of cell proliferation in mammalian cells. *Cell Res.* **2002**, *12*, 9–18. [CrossRef] [PubMed]
48. Junttila, M.R.; Li, S.P.; Westermarck, J. Phosphatase-mediated crosstalk between MAPK signaling pathways in the regulation of cell survival. *FASEB J.* **2008**, *22*, 954–965. [CrossRef]
49. Sun, Q.Y.; Breitbart, H.; Schatten, H. Role of the MAPK cascade in mammalian germ cells. *Reprod. Fertil. Dev.* **1999**, *11*, 443–450. [CrossRef] [PubMed]
50. Moustakas, A.; Pardali, K.; Gaal, A.; Heldin, C.-H. Mechanisms of TGF-β signaling in regulation of cell growth and differentiation. *Immunol. Lett.* **2002**, *82*, 85–91. [CrossRef] [PubMed]
51. Lee, J.-H.; Mellado-Gil, J.M.; Bahn, Y.J.; Pathy, S.M.; Zhang, Y.E.; Rane, S.G. Protection from β-cell apoptosis by inhibition of TGF-β/Smad3 signaling. *Cell Death Dis.* **2020**, *11*, 184. [CrossRef] [PubMed]
52. Heldin, C.-H.; Miyazono, K.; Ten Dijke, P. TGF-β signalling from cell membrane to nucleus through SMAD proteins. *Nature* **1997**, *390*, 465–471. [CrossRef] [PubMed]
53. ten Dijke, P.; Miyazono, K.; Heldin, C.-H. Signaling inputs converge on nuclear effectors in TGF-β signaling. *Trends Biochem. Sci.* **2000**, *25*, 64–70. [CrossRef] [PubMed]
54. Wang, X.; Jiang, S.; Liu, Y.; Du, X.; Zhang, W.; Zhang, J.; Shen, H. Comprehensive pulmonary metabolome responses to intratracheal instillation of airborne fine particulate matter in rats. *Sci. Total Environ.* **2017**, *592*, 41–50. [CrossRef]
55. Ling, Z.N.; Jiang, Y.F.; Ru, J.N.; Lu, J.H.; Ding, B.; Wu, J. Amino acid metabolism in health and disease. *Signal Transduct. Target. Ther.* **2023**, *8*, 345. [CrossRef] [PubMed]
56. Holeček, M. Branched-chain amino acids in health and disease: Metabolism, alterations in blood plasma, and as supplements. *Nutr. Metab.* **2018**, *15*, 33. [CrossRef] [PubMed]

57. Ruiz-Canela, M.; Toledo, E.; Clish, C.B.; Hruby, A.; Liang, L.; Salas-Salvado, J.; Razquin, C.; Corella, D.; Estruch, R.; Ros, E. Plasma branched-chain amino acids and incident cardiovascular disease in the PREDIMED trial. *Clin. Chem.* **2016**, *62*, 582–592. [CrossRef] [PubMed]
58. Alvers, A.L.; Fishwick, L.K.; Wood, M.S.; Hu, D.; Chung, H.S.; Dunn, W.A., Jr.; Aris, J.P. Autophagy and amino acid homeostasis are required for chronological longevity in Saccharomyces cerevisiae. *Aging Cell* **2009**, *8*, 353–369. [CrossRef] [PubMed]
59. Liao, X.; Liu, S.; Chen, S.; Shan, X.; He, J.; Li, C. Transcriptomic analysis reveals the role of Glycolysis pathway in Litopenaeus vannamei during DIV1 infection. *Fish Shellfish Immunol.* **2023**, *141*, 109036. [CrossRef] [PubMed]
60. DeBerardinis, R.J.; Thompson, C.B. Cellular metabolism and disease: What do metabolic outliers teach us? *Cell* **2012**, *148*, 1132–1144. [CrossRef] [PubMed]
61. Shi, D.Y.; Xie, F.Z.; Zhai, C.; Stern, J.S.; Liu, Y.; Liu, S.L. The role of cellular oxidative stress in regulating glycolysis energy metabolism in hepatoma cells. *Mol. Cancer* **2009**, *8*, 32. [CrossRef] [PubMed]
62. Gao, L.; Loveless, J.; Shay, C.; Teng, Y. Targeting ROS-mediated crosstalk between autophagy and apoptosis in cancer. In *Reviews on New Drug Targets in Age-Related Disorders*; Springer: Berlin/Heidelberg, Germany, 2020; pp. 1–12.
63. Weiner, J., 3rd; Parida, S.K.; Maertzdorf, J.; Black, G.F.; Repsilber, D.; Telaar, A.; Mohney, R.P.; Arndt-Sullivan, C.; Ganoza, C.A.; Fae, K.C.; et al. Biomarkers of inflammation, immunosuppression and stress with active disease are revealed by metabolomic profiling of tuberculosis patients. *PLoS ONE* **2012**, *7*, e40221. [CrossRef] [PubMed]
64. Ding, Z.; Chen, W.; Wu, H.; Li, W.; Mao, X.; Su, W.; Zhang, Y.; Lin, N. Integrative network fusion-based multi-omics study for biomarker identification and patient classification of rheumatoid arthritis. *Chin. Med.* **2023**, *18*, 48. [CrossRef] [PubMed]
65. Yan, J.; Risacher, S.L.; Shen, L.; Saykin, A.J. Network approaches to systems biology analysis of complex disease: Integrative methods for multi-omics data. *Briefings Bioinform.* **2018**, *19*, 1370–1381. [CrossRef]
66. Huang, C.; Freter, C. Lipid metabolism, apoptosis and cancer therapy. *Int. J. Mol. Sci.* **2015**, *16*, 924–949. [CrossRef] [PubMed]
67. Santos, C.R.; Schulze, A. Lipid metabolism in cancer. *FEBS J.* **2012**, *279*, 2610–2623. [CrossRef]
68. Dolce, V.; Rita Cappello, A.; Lappano, R.; Maggiolini, M. Glycerophospholipid synthesis as a novel drug target against cancer. *Curr. Mol. Pharmacol.* **2011**, *4*, 167–175. [CrossRef] [PubMed]
69. Vance, D.E. Glycerolipid biosynthesis in eukaryotes. In *New Comprehensive Biochemistry*; Elsevier: Amsterdam, The Netherlands, 1996; Volume 31, pp. 153–181.
70. Wang, X.; Xu, Y.; Song, X.; Jia, Q.; Zhang, X.; Qian, Y.; Qiu, J. Analysis of glycerophospholipid metabolism after exposure to PCB153 in PC12 cells through targeted lipidomics by UHPLC-MS/MS. *Ecotoxicol. Environ. Saf.* **2019**, *169*, 120–127. [CrossRef] [PubMed]
71. Feng, J.; Cavallero, S.; Hsiai, T.; Li, R. Impact of air pollution on intestinal redox lipidome and microbiome. *Free Radic. Biol. Med.* **2020**, *151*, 99–110. [CrossRef] [PubMed]
72. Zhang, Y.; Li, M.; Pu, Z.; Chi, X.; Yang, J. Multi-omics data reveals the disturbance of glycerophospholipid metabolism and linoleic acid metabolism caused by disordered gut microbiota in PM2.5 gastrointestinal exposed rats. *Ecotoxicol. Environ. Saf.* **2023**, *262*, 115182. [CrossRef] [PubMed]
73. Wang, J.; Zeng, Y.; Song, J.; Zhu, M.; Zhu, G.; Cai, H.; Chen, C.; Jin, M.; Song, Y. Perturbation of arachidonic acid and glycerolipid metabolism promoted particulate matter-induced inflammatory responses in human bronchial epithelial cells. *Ecotoxicol. Environ. Saf.* **2023**, *256*, 114839. [CrossRef] [PubMed]
74. Novgorodov, S.A.; Gudz, T.I. Ceramide and mitochondria in ischemic brain injury. *Int. J. Biochem. Mol. Biol.* **2011**, *2*, 347–361. [PubMed]
75. Nagahara, Y.; Shinomiya, T.; Kuroda, S.; Kaneko, N.; Nishio, R.; Ikekita, M. Phytosphingosine induced mitochondria-involved apoptosis. *Cancer Sci.* **2005**, *96*, 83–92. [CrossRef] [PubMed]
76. Li, J.; Wen, J.; Sun, C.; Zhou, Y.; Xu, J.; MacIsaac, H.J.; Chang, X.; Cui, Q. Phytosphingosine-induced cell apoptosis via a mitochondrially mediated pathway. *Toxicology* **2022**, *482*, 153370. [CrossRef] [PubMed]
77. Zhao, J.; Tian, X.C.; Zhang, J.Q.; Li, T.T.; Qiao, S.; Jiang, S.L. Tribulus terrestris L. induces cell apoptosis of breast cancer by regulating sphingolipid metabolism signaling pathways. *Phytomedicine* **2023**, *120*, 155014. [CrossRef] [PubMed]
78. D'Angelo, G.; Moorthi, S.; Luberto, C. Role and Function of Sphingomyelin Biosynthesis in the Development of Cancer. *Adv. Cancer Res.* **2018**, *140*, 61–96. [CrossRef] [PubMed]
79. Guo, Y.; Chang, L.; Zhang, G.; Gao, Z.; Lin, H.; Zhang, Y.; Hu, L.; Chen, S.; Fan, B.; Zhang, S.; et al. The role of Sphingomyelin synthase 2 (SMS2) in platelet activation and its clinical significance. *Thromb. J.* **2021**, *19*, 27. [CrossRef] [PubMed]
80. Bian, X.; Liu, R.; Meng, Y.; Xing, D.; Xu, D.; Lu, Z. Lipid metabolism and cancer. *J. Exp. Med.* **2021**, *218*. [CrossRef] [PubMed]
81. Choi, D.; Kim, C.; Kim, T.; Park, K.; Im, J.; Hong, J. Potential threat of microplastics to humans: Toxicity prediction modeling by small data analysis. *Environ. Sci. Nano* **2023**, *10*, 1096–1108. [CrossRef]

Disclaimer/Publisher's Note: The statements, opinions and data contained in all publications are solely those of the individual author(s) and contributor(s) and not of MDPI and/or the editor(s). MDPI and/or the editor(s) disclaim responsibility for any injury to people or property resulting from any ideas, methods, instructions or products referred to in the content.

The Cytotoxicity of Tungsten Ions Derived from Nanoparticles Correlates with Pulmonary Toxicity

Jun Yao [1], Pengfei Zhou [1], Xin Zhang [1], Beilei Yuan [1,2,*], Yong Pan [1,2,*] and Juncheng Jiang [2,3,*]

1 College of Safety Science and Engineering, Nanjing Tech University, Nanjing 211816, China
2 Jiangsu Key Laboratory of Hazardous Chemicals Safety and Control, Nanjing Tech University, Nanjing 211816, China
3 School of Environment and Safety Engineering, Changzhou University, Changzhou 213164, China
* Correspondence: yuanbeilei@163.com (B.Y.); yongpan@njtech.edu.cn (Y.P.); jcjiang_njtech@163.com (J.J.)

Abstract: Tungsten carbide nanoparticles (nano-WC) are prevalent in composite materials, and are attributed to their physical and chemical properties. Due to their small size, nano-WC particles can readily infiltrate biological organisms via the respiratory tract, thereby posing potential health hazards. Despite this, the studies addressing the cytotoxicity of nano-WC remain notably limited. To this purpose, the BEAS-2B and U937 cells were cultured in the presence of nano-WC. The significant cytotoxicity of nano-WC suspension was evaluated using a cellular LDH assay. To investigate the cytotoxic impact of tungsten ions (W^{6+}) on cells, the ion chelator (EDTA-2Na) was used to adsorb W^{6+} from nano-WC suspension. Subsequent to this treatment, the modified nano-WC suspension was subjected to flow cytometry analysis to evaluate the rates of cellular apoptosis. According to the results, a decrease in W^{6+} could mitigate the cellular damage and enhance cell viability, which indicated that W^{6+} indeed exerted a significant cytotoxic influence on the cells. Overall, the present study provides valuable insight into the toxicological mechanisms underlying the exposure of lung cells to nano-WC, thereby reducing the environmental toxicant risk to human health.

Keywords: tungsten carbide nanoparticles; epithelial cells; macrophages; cytotoxicity

1. Introduction

Recently, in the field of nanomaterials, there has been a notable trend of development and a substantial increase in research, leading to the continuous introduction of engineered nanomaterials into the market. The impact of nanoparticle exposure on occupational health has garnered significant attention within the field of occupational health and safety [1]. Among various nanomaterials, tungsten carbide nanoparticles (nano-WC) are recognized for their unique properties that contribute to the enhancement of metal hardness and stability [2,3]. Nano-WC is typically sprayed onto heavy machinery, drill bits, and saw blades, substantially enhancing their strength, durability, and wear resistance [4]. These properties, which are used for maintaining the sharpness of saw blades and drill bits in the mining and drilling industries, render nano-WC especially valued in these sectors. However, as the industrial-scale production and application of nano-WC increases, the dust generated from cutting, grinding, and polishing of WC-based materials poses significant occupational health risks to workers [5,6].

Epidemiological and toxicological studies have shown that nano-WC adversely affects respiratory and cardiovascular systems. Exposure to hard metal dust containing nano-WC is associated with an increased risk of occupational asthma and hard metal lung disease (HMLD) [7], which is characterized by difficulty breathing, reduced lung capacity, progressive lung inflammation, and pulmonary fibrosis [8–11]. Additionally, studies have found that tungsten element present in nano-WC has adverse impact on cell viability [12]. It also interferes with the voltage-gated sodium channels in neurons [13], thereby inducing cell apoptosis [6] and inflammation [14]. However, current in vitro studies on WC are limited to fish cell lines [15], and the cytotoxicity of nano-WC has not been reported.

Macrophages are utilized to clear infectious, toxic, or allergenic particles from the airways, while epithelial cells serve to protect underlying tissues from damage. However, nanoparticles (NPs), when exposed to macrophages and epithelial cells, can induce cytotoxicity due to their internalization, subsequently leading to serious lung diseases [16,17]. Reports suggested that in animal model studies, small nanoparticles (NPs) deposited in the respiratory tract easily infiltrate into epithelial and interstitial sites [18,19]. Large NPs can attenuate or inhibit the phagocytic action of macrophages in the alveoli [20]; thus, the phagocytosis of NPs by epithelial cells or macrophages may depend on their size. In vitro experiments have shown that NPs loaded with 2 µg WC can cause significant toxicity to alveolar macrophages with 24 h of exposure at concentrations ranging from 50 to 1667 µg/mL. Furthermore, mouse peritoneal macrophages exposed to between 50 and 300 µg/mL NPs with 2 to 4 µg WC showed signs of toxicity within 6 h of exposure [21]. In a recent study [22], a co-culture model of lung epithelial cells and macrophages was established to simulate the microenvironment of the lung, and examine the toxic and inflammatory effects of tungsten carbide cobalt (WCCo) nanoparticles (NPs). Furthermore, mechanisms underlying lung toxicity due to NPs need to be investigated.

Studies show that the slow release of ions in vivo or in cells is the main cause of cytotoxicity. Song et al. [23] found that dissolved Zn^{2+} plays a major role in mediating the toxic effect of ZnO particles by generating large amounts of reactive oxygen species (ROS) in the cells. Yosuke et al. [24] evaluated the effects of indium tin oxide nanoparticles (ITO NPs), indium chloride ($InCl_3$) and tin chloride ($SnCl_3$) on A549 cells, revealing that the accumulation of indium ions in cells induces oxidative stress, proinflammatory response and DNA damage. In addition, in vitro experiments have also confirmed that indium ions released from ITO particles are the primary source of cytotoxicity and genotoxicity [25–28]. In vitro studies on mammalian cells have shown that the effects on different organs and developmental physiology are dose-dependent [29]. However, the underlying mechanism of nano-WC-induced cytotoxicity is still unrevealed.

In this study, we evaluated the solubility and cytotoxic effects of nano-WC on macrophage and lung epithelial cells. We investigated the apoptosis of U937 macrophage and BEAS-2B epithelial caused by a nano-WC suspension. Furthermore, the metal ion chelator of EDTA-2Na was used to reduce W^{6+} from nano-WC. Subsequently, the rates of cellular apoptosis was measured before or after chelation treatment, thereby validating the effect of W^{6+} on cytotoxicity. Our findings provide a reference for subsequent in vivo studies on the mechanisms of nano-WC toxicity.

2. Materials and Methods

2.1. Materials

Nano-WC (purity $\geq$ 99.99%) were obtained from Boxin Wear-Resisting Alloy Material Co., Ltd. (Xingtai, China). The hydroclynamic size of nano-WC is around 60 nm as shown in Figure S1. In addition, the zeta potential test indicates that the nano-WC is electrically negative at test conditions (Figure S2). They were tested with a Zetasizer Nano ZS ZEN3600 (Malvern, Worcestershire, UK) electrokinetic analyzer. After weighing and autoclaving at 121 °C and 0.12 MPa for 30 min, a nano-WC suspension (200 µg/mL) was prepared in high glucose DMEM (Cytiva, Shanghai, China, for culturing BEAS-2B cells) and RPMI-1640 (ThermoFisher, Shanghai, China, for culturing U937 cells) media, and stored at 4 °C. Before each experiment, the suspension was dispersed in a sonicator for 15 min and then diluted to the required concentration.

2.2. Cell Lines

The human lung epithelial cell line BEAS-2B and the human macrophage cell line U937 were purchased from American Type Culture Collection (ATCC), Shanghai Cell Bank. The cells were cultured in DMEM (Cytiva, Shanghai, China) and RPMI-1640 (ThermoFisher,

Shanghai, China) medium supplemented with 10% (v/v) fetal bovine serum (Gibco, Shanghai, China) and 1% (v/v) penicillin–streptomycin solution (ThermoFisher, Shanghai, China) at 37 °C in an incubator with 5% CO_2, respectively.

2.3. Cell Culture and Measurement of Tungsten Ion Release

BEAS-2B and U937 cells were cultured for 12 h in 24-well plates (1×10^5 cells per well), and washed thrice with PBS to remove non-adherent cells. The cells were then treated with nano-WC of 200 µg/mL for 1, 2, 6, 12, and 24 h. The supernatants were then centrifuged thrice, and the concentration of W^{6+} was measured by inductively coupled plasma mass spectrometry (ICP-MS). A Thermo Electron X Series X7 quadrupole ICP-MS (ELEMENT 2, Shanghai, China) was used. Samples were introduced into the ICP torch using a quartz C-type nebulizer (OpalMist, Beijing, China) and the impact bead spray chamber was cooled to 2 °C. In order to obtain the maximum sensitivity of tungsten, ICP-MS is generally tuned to 1600–1700 V. The retention time of each sample is 10 s, and the concentration of the target element of the measured sample is less than 1 ppm. After the measurement, the system was cleaned with 2–4% dilute nitric acid for 5–10 s, and the concentration and relative standard deviation (RSD) were checked and recorded.

2.4. Transmission Electron Microscopy

BEAS-2B and U937 cells were put in 24-well plates at a density of 1×10^5 cells/well. 50 µg/mL nano-WC suspension was treated as test group. Each group of cells were fixed with 2.5% glutaraldehyde in 0.1 mol/L phosphate buffer (pH = 7.2) for 1 h at ice temperature and post-fixed with 1% OsO_4 in the same buffer for 2 h at room temperature. After fixation, cells were dehydrated with acetone (30%, 50%, 70%, 80% and 90%) and embedded in Spurr resin. Thin sections of 50 nm were cut at the ultramicrotome (RMC POWERTOME XL, RMC, USA) and deposited on 200 mesh copper grids. Fixed samples were stained with uranyl acetate and lead citrate at room temperature for 10 and 12 min, respectively. The cell membrane, chromatin, nucleus, and intracellular particle size distribution were characterized using a 200 kV field emission transmission electron microscope (JEM-2100F) by Japan JEOL.

2.5. Cytotoxicity Analysis

LDH release was analyzed by using the LDH Cytotoxicity Assay Kit (C0016, Beyotime, Shanghai, China) in accordance with the manufacturer's instructions. Briefly, the cells were put in 96-well culture plates at a density of 1×10^5 cells/well and incubated for 12 h. Background blank wells, sample control wells, sample maximum enzyme activity control wells and sample wells were set up. We added 200 µL supernatant to each sample well for another 1 h incubation. Until 1 h before detection, 13 µL of LDH release reagent was added to the "sample maximum enzyme activity control well". Then, 60 µL of LDH detection reagent was added and incubated for 30 min. The supernatant medium was placed in 96-well culture plates, and the absorbance at 490 nm was measured by a microplate reader (EPOCH2, BioTek, Vermont, USA). Mortality is calculated by the following formula:

$$M = \frac{A_{treated} - A_{control}}{A_{activecontrol} - A_{control}} \times 100\% \qquad (1)$$

where M is cellular mortality; $A_{treated}$ is the absorbance of samples exposed to nano-WC; $A_{control}$ is absorbance of untreated control wells; and $A_{active\ control}$ is absorbance of maximum enzyme activity of cells.

To validate the cytotoxicity derived from W^{6+} rather than nano-WC, we conducted cell viability experiments using EDTA-2Na (50 µg/mL) adsorbed W^{6+} as a comparison. BEAS-2B and U937 cells were seeded into 96-well plates at a density of 10^5 cells/well and cultured for 12 h. They were then divided into control, WC, and WC + EDTA-2Na groups, and exposed to nano-WC at a concentration of 200 µg/mL. The Annexin V- Phycoerythrin (PE) 7- amino-actinomycin D (7-AAD) apoptosis detection kit (cat. no. KGA1017; KeyGEN

Bio TECH, Nanjing, China) was used to detect cell death according to the manufacturer's protocol. Cells were resuspended in 100 μL of staining solution at a concentration of 1×10^5 cells/100 μL and incubated in the dark at ambient temperature for 10 min. They were then added to 400 μL of binding buffer. A flow cytometer (Beckman FC-500, Brea, CA, USA) was employed to determine the excitation wavelength at 488 nm. The excitation wavelength at 578 or 647 nm was used to detect PE or 7-AAD fluorescence for cell apoptosis, respectively. The cells can be divided into three subgroups. The viable cells only showed very low intensity of background fluorescence, the early apoptotic cells only showed strong orange-red fluorescence, and the late apoptotic cells showed the double staining of the orange-red and red fluorescence. Samples (n = 10) were randomly selected from each group, and the apoptotic rate was calculated as the percentage of early apoptotic cells or late apoptotic cells.

2.6. Statistical Analysis

Origin 8.0 was used for all statistical analyses. The data were presented as mean ± standard deviation (SD) and the comparison between the two groups was performed using the Student's t-test (for parametric data). p values < 0.05 were considered statistically different.

3. Results

3.1. Decrease in the Viability of Lung Epithelial Cells and Macrophages by Nano-WC

Compared to the untreated BEAS-2B cells (Figure 1A–C), those treated with nano-WC particles show indistinct organelles, indistinct mitochondrial profiles and lysosomes, numerous vesicles, and a condensed nucleoplasm around the nuclear membrane (Figure 1E,F), although the overall cell structure is intact (Figure 1D). Similarly, the control U937 cells have an intact cell membrane and nuclear membrane, along with multiple mitochondria (Figure 2A–C). While the overall structure of these cells is unaffected by nano-WC (Figure 2D), they exhibit an irregular nuclear membrane and a solid nucleolus, large vacuoles, multiple mitochondria (Figure 2E), and segment extracellular lysosomes (black arrows; Figure 2F).

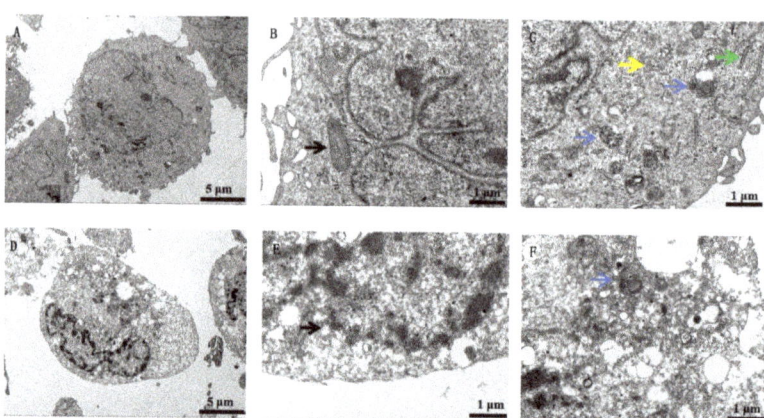

Figure 1. TEM images of BEAS-2B cells in the control group. (**A**) The cell membrane and the nuclear membrane are intact. (**B**) Mitochondria are clear and intact (black arrows) with clear ridges. (**C**) The lysosomes (blue arrows), Golgi apparatus (yellow arrows), and endoplasmic reticulum (green arrows) are clear and intact. Sonicated WC solution was added to BEAS-2B cells and incubated for 24 h. TEM images of BEAS-2B cells exposed to nano-WC. (**D**) The cytosol and nucleus with a nuclear membrane are largely intact. The nucleoplasm is condensed around the nuclear membrane, and there are numerous intracellular vacuoles. (**E**) Mitochondria (black arrows) are poorly defined. (**F**) There are numerous intracellular vacuoles and the lysosomes (blue arrows) are poorly defined.

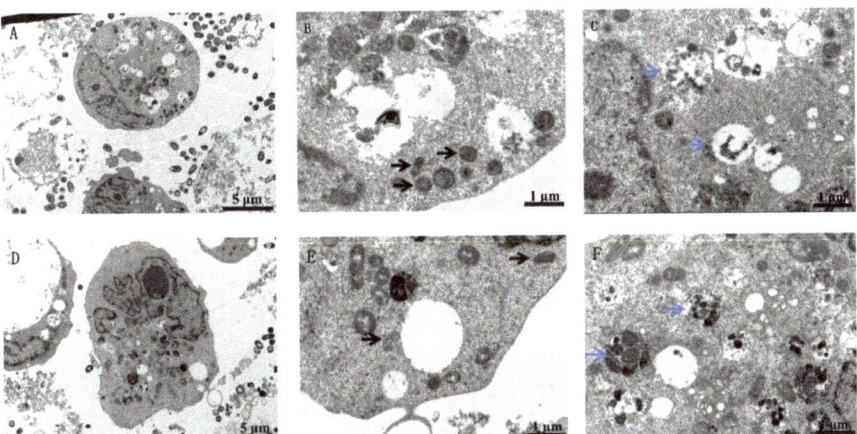

Figure 2. TEM images of U937 cells in the control group. (**A**) The overall cell structure is intact. The mitochondria ((**B**); black arrows) and lysosomes ((**C**); blue arrows) are intact. Sonicated WC solution was added to U937 cells and incubated for 24 h. TEM images of U937 cells exposed to nano-WC. (**D**) The overall cell structure is essentially intact, with an irregular nuclear membrane and a solid nucleolus. (**E**) There are large vacuoles and multiple mitochondria (black arrows) in the cytoplasm. (**F**) The lysosomes (blue arrows) are segmented internally.

3.2. Release of Tungsten Ions in Cells Exposed to Nano-WC

Studies show that the cytotoxicity of metal oxide NPs is mediated by the release of free metal ions [23,30]. Therefore, we hypothesize that the release of W^{6+} from nano-WC is the source of toxicity. To this end, lung epithelial cells and macrophages were treated with 200 µg/mL nano-WC, and the W^{6+} levels in the supernatant were measured by ICP-MS after centrifugation [31]. As shown in Figure 3A,B, at the initial time of 0 h prior to the treatment of cells, the detected W^{6+} concentration in the supernatant with only nano-WC was 0, implying that nano-WC does not spontaneously dissolve in the absence of cells. Within 12 h, the changes in the W^{6+} concentration released from nano-WC exposed to both cell types were generally consistent. After 12 h, the W^{6+} concentration decreased but remained high in the supernatant of BEAS-2B cells, while the W^{6+} concentration in the supernatant of U937 cells was relatively stable. Generally speaking, W^{6+} concentrations in the supernatants of both cell types increased significantly after 24 h of incubation.

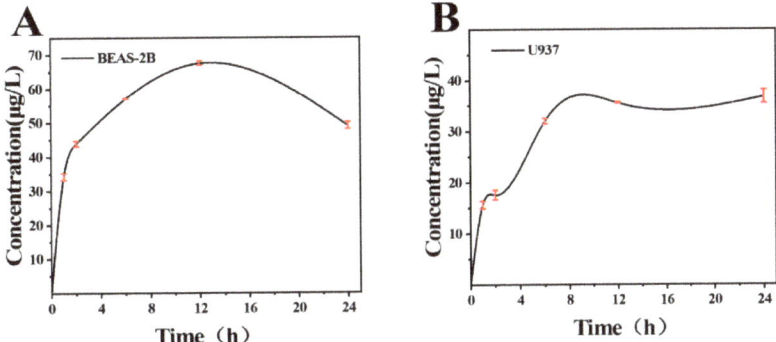

Figure 3. Temporal dissolution curves of nano-WC in BEAS-2B and U937 cells. (**A**) W^{6+} concentration in the supernatants of BEAS-2B treated with 200 µg/mL nano-WC for 0, 1, 2, 6, 12, and 24 h. (**B**) W^{6+} concentration in the supernatants of U937 treated with 200 µg/mL nano-WC for 0, 1, 2, 6, 12, and 24 h.

3.3. Mitigating the Cytotoxicity of Nano-WC by Chelation of W^{6+}

To detect the toxic effect of tungsten ion concentration in supernatant on cells, lactate dehydrogenase (LDH) levels were measured (Figure 4A,B). The cells in the nano-WC groups release significantly higher amounts of LDH compared to the control groups, and the mortality rates of BEAS-2B and U937 cells are 20% and 24%, respectively. The results showed that tungsten ions in the supernatant could also induce the release of LDH in BEAS-2B cells and U937 cells, leading to apoptosis.

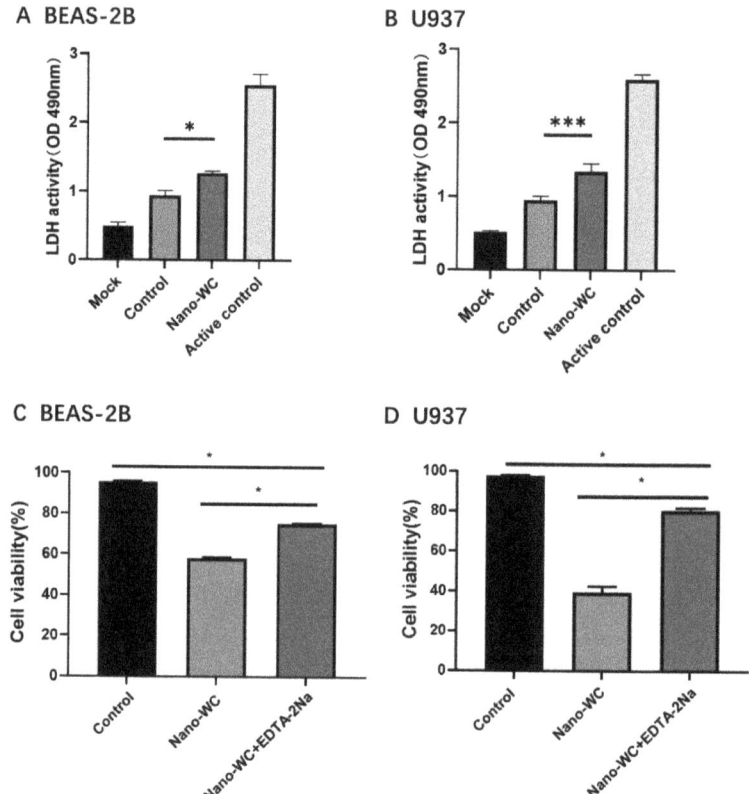

Figure 4. LDH activity of BEAS-2B cells (**A**) and U937 cells (**B**) treated with the condition medium of nano-WC-treated cells. LDH activity of BEAS-2B cells (**C**) and U937 cells (**D**) treated with the condition medium with or without EDTA-2Na. The data on the figures represent mean ± SD. * $p < 0.05$ and *** $p < 0.001$ vs. control group.

To investigate the cytotoxic impact of tungsten ions (W^{6+}) on cells, EDTA-2Na was used to chelate W^{6+} from nano-WC suspension. Subsequent to this treatment, the modified nano-WC suspension was subjected to flow cytometry analysis (Figure 5) to evaluate the rates of cellular apoptosis. The apoptosis rate of BEAS-2B cells in the nano-WC group was 36.57%; the apoptosis rate of EDTA-2Na group was 21.24%. The apoptosis rate of U937 cells in the nano-WC group was 20.58%, while that in EDTA-2Na group was 9.62%. The viability of cells treated with EDTA-2Na and nano-WC is significantly higher than that of cells treated with nano-WC alone ($p < 0.05$; Figure 4C,D). The result shows that the addition of EDTA-2Na will reduce the W^{6+} concentration, and thus toxicity will be reduced.

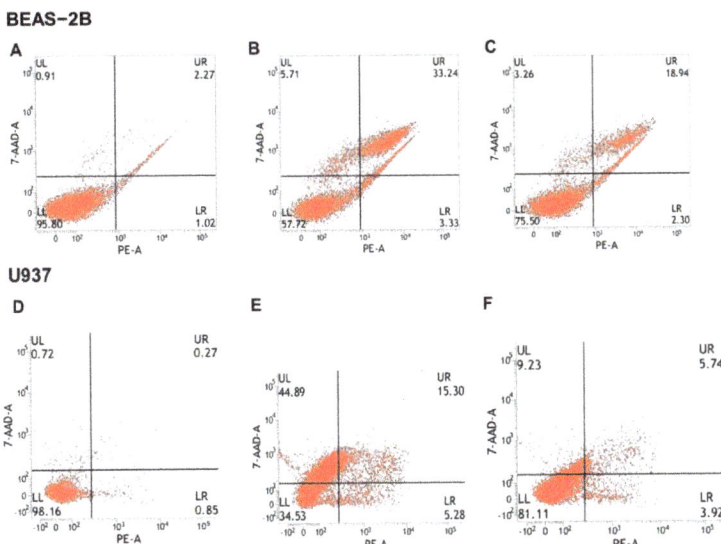

Figure 5. Flow cytometry measurements of BEAS-2B cells and U937 cells in the control (**A,D**), nano-WC (**B,E**), and nano-WC + EDTA-2Na (**C,F**) groups. Apoptosis rates were calculated based on Figure 5.

4. Discussion

The nucleus controls cellular functions and the inheritance of genetic material [32,33], and the aggregation and condensation of chromatin in the nucleus is an indicator of irreversible damage [34]. We found that nano-WC exposure led to significant chromatin condensation in human lung epithelial cells, along with loss of organelle integrity and a massive increase in the number of vesicles, which could be the cellular basis of the toxic effects of nano-WC. Recent studies have shown that lysosomal damage can trigger apoptosis [35,36]. In addition, phagocytosis of inhaled silica or asbestos dust by lung macrophages leads to lysosomal rupture, which releases hydrolytic enzymes and increases tissue fibrosis [37]. Consistent with this, the U937 cells treated with nano-WC particles showed split extracellular lysosomes.

A number of studies have proven that free metal ions released from metal oxide NPs are the primary factor for cytotoxicity [23,27,28,30]. Singh et al. [38] demonstrated that phagocytosed Ag NPs are degraded inside the cells and release Ag ions, which interfere with normal mitochondrial functions and induce apoptosis. Likewise, we detected free W^{6+} in the supernatant of the cell lines, and the release of tungsten ions is increased with increased time during the first 12 h (Figure 3A,B). Overall, tungsten ion concentrations in the supernatants of both cell types increased significantly after 24 h of incubation, and these data suggest that macrophages and epithelial cells can rapidly (within 24 h) dissolve nano-WC into W^{6+}, which are then released by dying cells into the surrounding medium.

LDH is an important cell metabolism enzyme in body tissues, which can better reflect cell proliferation and metabolism [39]. The LDH level of healthy tissue cells is generally low, and when tissue cells are damaged, the LDH level will rise. Indeed, the increase in LDH activity confirms that the tungsten ions in the supernatant could also induce the release of LDH in both cells, leading to apoptosis. This indicates that after nano-WC enters the body, BEAS-2B cells and U937 cells had similar outcomes as target cells, providing an experimental basis for subsequent animal experiments to select target organs. Furthermore, to validate the cytotoxicity derived from W^{6+} rather than nano-WC, EDTA-2Na was used to adsorb W^{6+}. EDTA-2Na can effectively prevent metal ions from acting by encapsulating metal ions into the chelating agent through its strong binding with metal ions [40–42], which effectively avoid the induction of free radicals/reactive oxygen species (ROS) causing oxidative stress by chelating the free W^{6+} [43]. These results support the hypothesis that nano-WC particles are phagocytosed by macrophages, degraded in the acidic lysosomes, and release W^{6+} that triggers apoptosis. Nanoparticle solubilization results in a local spike in ionic tungsten, which damages and permeabilizes the lysosome, causing the contents (along with the ionic tungsten) to leak out into the cytoplasm, which kills the cell [28]. Furthermore, free W^{6+} is significantly more toxic than nano-WC and can easily target neighboring macrophages or lung epithelial cells [28,44,45]. This suggests that the partial cause of cytotoxicity is W^{6+} released from nano-WC, and W^{6+} can indeed cause cell damage in the absence of nano-WC.

Moreover, apart from the toxic effect of NPs on the cell level, the effect of pulmonary surfactant on NPs should not be ignored. For different kinds of NPs, many studies have demonstrated that the pulmonary surfactant will promote or reduce the toxicity of NPs [46,47]. Therefore, the interaction of nano-WC and pulmonary surfactant needs further intensive investigation.

5. Conclusions

The mechanisms underlying lung toxicity due to nano-WC were investigated. U937 macrophages and BEAS-2B epithelial cells were cultured and then exposed to nano-WC. By TEM, it was found that human lung epithelial cells showed obvious chromatin condensation, loss of organelle integrity, and a large increase in the number of vesicles, as well as the division of extracellular lysosomes in U937 cells, confirming obvious cell damage. The cytotoxicity of nano-WC suspension was proven through a cellular LDH assay. Furthermore, a decrease in W^{6+} by the ion chelator (EDTA-2Na) reduces cytotoxicity, which indicates that the partial cause of cytotoxicity is W^{6+} released from nano-WC. Our findings provide new insights into the mechanisms underlying toxicity of nano-WC on the lung epithelium, and possible strategies for therapeutic intervention.

Supplementary Materials: The following supporting information can be downloaded at: https://www.mdpi.com/article/10.3390/toxics11060528/s1, Figure S1: Diameter distribution of nano-WC suspension; Figure S2: The distribution of zeta potential as a function of nano-WC concentration.

Author Contributions: Conceptualization, J.Y. and P.Z.; methodology, J.Y., X.Z. and B.Y.; writing—original draft preparation, J.Y. and P.Z.; validation, X.Z., B.Y. and Y.P.; writing—review and editing, X.Z., B.Y. and Y.P.; funding acquisition, Y.P.; Supervision, Y.P. and J.J. All authors have read and agreed to the published version of the manuscript.

Funding: This research was supported by the Natural Science Foundation for Distinguished Young Scholars of Jiangsu Province (No. BK20190036), and the National Natural Science Foundation of China (No. 81803274).

Institutional Review Board Statement: Not applicable.

Informed Consent Statement: Not applicable.

Data Availability Statement: The data that support the findings of this study are available from the corresponding author, (Y.P.), upon reasonable request.

Conflicts of Interest: The authors declare no conflict of interest.

References

1. Verma, S.K.; Panda, P.K.; Kumari, P.; Patel, P.; Arunima, A.; Jha, E.; Husain, S.; Prakash, R.; Hergenröder, R.; Mishra, Y.K.; et al. Determining factors for the nano-biocompatibility of cobalt oxide nanoparticles: Proximal discrepancy in intrinsic atomic interactions at differential vicinage. *Green Chem.* **2021**, *23*, 3439–3458. [CrossRef]
2. Azman, M.N.; Abualroos, N.J.; Yaacob, K.A.; Zainon, R. Feasibility of nanomaterial tungsten carbide as lead-free nanomaterial-based radiation shielding. *Radiat. Phys. Chem.* **2022**, *202*, 110492. [CrossRef]
3. Yao, Z.; Stiglich, J.J.; Sudarshan, T.S. Nanosized WC-Co holds promise for the future. *Metal Powder Rep.* **1998**, *53*, 26–33. [CrossRef]
4. Zhengui, Y.; Stiglich, J.J.; Sudarshan, T.S. Nano-grained Tungsten Carbide Cobalt (WC/Co). *Mater Modif.* **1998**, *2929*, 1–27.

5. Stefaniak, A.B.; Virji, M.A.; Day, G.A. Characterization of exposures among cemented tungsten carbide workers. Part I: Size-fractionated exposures to airborne cobalt and tungsten particles. *J. Expo. Sci. Environ. Epidemiol.* **2009**, *19*, 475–491. [CrossRef]
6. Lombaert, N.; De Boeck, M.; Decordier, I.; Cundari, E.; Lison, D.; Kirsch-Volders, M. Evaluation of the apoptogenic potential of hard metal dust (WC–Co), tungsten carbide and metallic cobalt. *Toxicol. Lett.* **2004**, *154*, 23–34. [CrossRef]
7. Rivolta, G.; Nicoli, E.; Ferretti, G.; Tomasini, M. Hard metal lung disorders: Analysis of a group of exposed workers. *Sci. Total Environ.* **1994**, *150*, 161–165. [CrossRef]
8. Forni, A. Bronchoalveolar lavage in the diagnosis of hard metal disease. *Sci. Total Environ.* **1994**, *150*, 69–76. [CrossRef]
9. Kinoshita, M.; Sueyasu, Y.; Watanabe, H.; Tanoue, S.; Okubo, Y.; Koga, T.; Kawahara, M.; Nagata, E.; Oizumi, K. Giant cell interstitial pneumonia in two hard metal workers: The role of bronchoalveolar lavage in diagnosis. *Respirology* **1999**, *4*, 263–266. [CrossRef]
10. Armstead, A.L.; Li, B. Nanotoxicity: Emerging concerns regarding nanomaterial safety and occupational hard metal (WC-Co) nanoparticle exposure. *Int. J. Nanomed.* **2016**, *2016*, 6421–6433. [CrossRef]
11. Du, X.; Liu, J.; Wang, Y.; Jin, M.; Ye, Q. Cobalt-related interstitial lung disease or hard metal lung disease: A case series of Chinese workers. *Toxicol. Ind. Health* **2021**, *37*, 280–288. [CrossRef] [PubMed]
12. Kühnel, D.; Busch, W.; Meißner, T.; Springer, A.; Potthoff, A.; Richter, V.; Gelinsky, M.; Scholz, S.; Schirmer, K. Agglomeration of tungsten carbide nanoparticles in exposure medium does not prevent uptake and toxicity toward a rainbow trout gill cell line. *Aquat. Toxicol.* **2009**, *93*, 91–99. [CrossRef] [PubMed]
13. Shan, D.; Xie, Y.; Ren, G.; Yang, Z. Attenuated effect of tungsten carbide nanoparticles on voltage-gated sodium current of hippocampal CA1 pyramidal neurons. *Toxicol. In Vitro* **2013**, *27*, 299–304. [CrossRef]
14. Huaux, F.; Lasfargues, G.; Lauwerys, R.; Lison, D. Lung toxicity of hard metal particles and production of interleukin-1, tumor necrosis factor-α, fibronectin, and cystatin-c by lung phagocytes. *Toxicol. Appl. Pharmacol.* **1995**, *132*, 53–62. [CrossRef] [PubMed]
15. Lifeng, W.; Fenghua, G.; Zhuo, Y. Effect of tungsten carbide nanoparticles on the development of zebrafish embryos. *China Environ. Sci.* **2012**, *32*, 1280–1283.
16. Afroz, T.; Hiraku, Y.; Ma, N.; Ahmed, S.; Oikawa, S.; Kawanishi, S.; Murata, M. Nitrative DNA damage in cultured macrophages exposed to indium oxide. *J. Occup. Health* **2018**, *60*, 148–155. [CrossRef]
17. Hiraku, Y.; Nishikawa, Y.; Ma, N.; Afroz, T.; Mizobuchi, K.; Ishiyama, R.; Matsunaga, Y.; Ichinose, T.; Kawanishi, S.; Murata, M. Nitrative DNA damage induced by carbon-black nanoparticles in macrophages and lung epithelial cells. *Mutat. Res./Genet. Toxicol. Environ. Mutagen.* **2017**, *818*, 7–16. [CrossRef]
18. Akiyo, T.; Miyuki, H.; Minoru, O.; Naohide, I.; Takahiro, U.; Toshiaki, H.; Kiyohisa, S. Pulmonary Toxicity of Indium-Tin Oxide and Indium Phosphide after Intratracheal Instillations into the Lung of Hamsters. *J. Occup. Health* **2002**, *44*, 99–102. [CrossRef]
19. Nagano, K.; Nishizawa, T.; Umeda, Y.; Kasai, T.; Noguchi, T.; Gotoh, K.; Ikawa, N.; Eitaki, Y.; Kawasumi, Y.; Yamauchi, T.; et al. Inhalation Carcinogenicity and Chronic Toxicity of Indium-tin Oxide in Rats and Mice. *J. Occup. Health* **2011**, *53*, 175–187. [CrossRef]
20. Oberdörster, G. Pulmonary effects of inhaled ultrafine particles. *Int. Arch. Occup. Environ. Health* **2000**, *74*, 1–8. [CrossRef]
21. Lison, D.; Lauwerys, R. Evaluation of the role of reactive oxygen species in the interactive toxicity of carbide-cobalt mixtures on macrophages in culture. *Arch. Toxicol.* **1993**, *67*, 347–351. [CrossRef] [PubMed]
22. Andersson, P.O.; Lejon, C.; Ekstrand-Hammarström, B.; Akfur, C.; Ahlinder, L.; Bucht, A.; Österlund, L. Polymorph-and size-dependent uptake and toxicity of TiO2 nanoparticles in living lung epithelial cells. *Small* **2011**, *7*, 514–523. [CrossRef] [PubMed]
23. Song, W.; Zhang, J.; Guo, J.; Zhang, J.; Ding, F.; Li, L.; Sun, Z. Role of the dissolved zinc ion and reactive oxygen species in cytotoxicity of ZnO nanoparticles. *Toxicol. Lett.* **2010**, *199*, 389–397. [CrossRef] [PubMed]
24. Tabei, Y.; Sonoda, A.; Nakajima, Y.; Biju, V.; Makita, Y.; Yoshida, Y.; Horie, M. Intracellular accumulation of indium ions released from nanoparticles induces oxidative stress, proinflammatory response and DNA damage. *J. Biochem.* **2016**, *159*, 225–237. [CrossRef]
25. Lison, D.; Laloy, J.; Corazzari, I.; Muller, J.; Rabolli, V.; Panin, N.; Huaux, F.; Fenoglio, I.; Fubini, B. Sintered indium-tin-oxide (ITO) particles: A new pneumotoxic entity. *Toxicol. Sci.* **2009**, *108*, 472–481. [CrossRef]
26. Badding, M.A.; Schwegler-Berry, D.; Park, J.-H.; Fix, N.R.; Cummings, K.J.; Leonard, S.S. Sintered indium-tin oxide particles induce pro-inflammatory responses in vitro, in part through inflammasome activation. *PLoS ONE* **2015**, *10*, e0124368. [CrossRef]
27. Gwinn, W.M.; Qu, W.; Shines, C.J.; Bousquet, R.W.; Taylor, G.J.; Waalkes, M.P.; Morgan, D.L. Macrophage Solubilization and Cytotoxicity of Indium-Containing Particles In Vitro. *Toxicol. Sci.* **2013**, *135*, 414–424. [CrossRef]
28. Gwinn, W.M.; Qu, W.; Bousquet, R.W.; Price, H.; Shines, C.J.; Taylor, G.J.; Waalkes, M.P.; Morgan, D.L. Macrophage solubilization and cytotoxicity of indium-containing particles as in vitro correlates to pulmonary toxicity in vivo. *Toxicol. Sci.* **2015**, *144*, 17–26. [CrossRef]
29. Bastian, S.; Busch, W.; Kühnel, D.; Springer, A.; Meißner, T.; Holke, R.; Scholz, S.; Iwe, M.; Pompe, W.; Gelinsky, M.; et al. Toxicity of tungsten carbide and cobalt-doped tungsten carbide nanoparticles in mammalian cells in vitro. *Environ. Health Perspect.* **2009**, *117*, 530–536. [CrossRef]
30. Roy, R.; Tripathi, A.; Das, M.; Dwivedi, P.D. Cytotoxicity and uptake of zinc oxide nanoparticles leading to enhanced inflammatory cytokines levels in murine macrophages: Comparison with bulk zinc oxide. *J. Biomed. Nanotechnol.* **2011**, *7*, 110–111. [CrossRef]

31. Böhme, S.; Baccaro, M.; Schmidt, M.; Potthoff, A.; Stärk, H.-J.; Reemtsma, T.; Kühnel, D. Metal uptake and distribution in the zebrafish (Danio rerio) embryo: Differences between nanoparticles and metal ions. *Environ. Sci. Nano* **2017**, *4*, 1005–1015. [CrossRef]
32. Fielding, J.; Hall, J. A biolchemical and cytochemical study of peroxidase activity in roots of Pisum sativum: I. a comparison of DAB-peroxidase and guaiacol-peroxidase with particular emphasis on the properties of cell wall activity. *J. Exp. Bot.* **1978**, *29*, 969–981. [CrossRef]
33. Melanie, M.; Jan, L. The Driving Force: Nuclear Mechanotransduction in Cellular Function, Fate, and Disease. *HHS Public Access* **2019**, *4*, 443–468. [CrossRef]
34. Li, L. Ginkgo Biloba Conducting Tissue Development, Transcellular Transport and Effects of Water Logging Stress. Master's Thesis, Yangzhou University, Yangzhou, China, 2007.
35. Roberg, K.; Kågedal, K.; Öllinger, K. Microinjection of cathepsin d induces caspase-dependent apoptosis in fibroblasts. *Am. J. Pathol.* **2002**, *161*, 89–96. [CrossRef]
36. Wang, F.; Gómez-Sintes, R.; Boya, P. Lysosomal membrane permeabilization and cell death. *Traffic* **2018**, *19*, 918–931. [CrossRef]
37. Leinardi, R.; Pavan, C.; Yedavally, H.; Tomatis, M.; Salvati, A.; Turci, F. Cytotoxicity of fractured quartz on THP-1 human macrophages: Role of the membranolytic activity of quartz and phagolysosome destabilization. *Arch. Toxicol.* **2020**, *94*, 2981–2995. [CrossRef]
38. Singh, R.P.; Ramarao, P. Cellular uptake, intracellular trafficking and cytotoxicity of silver nanoparticles. *Toxicol. Lett.* **2012**, *213*, 249–259. [CrossRef]
39. Bastani, A.; Asghary, A.; Karimi-Busheri, F. Evaluation of the sensitivity and specificity of serum level of prostasin, CA125, LDH, AFP, and hCG+β in epithelial ovarian cancer patients. *Eur. J. Gynaecol. Oncol.* **2017**, *38*, 418–424. [CrossRef]
40. Repo, E.; Warchol, J.K.; Kurniawan, T.A.; Sillanpää, M.E. Adsorption of Co (II) and Ni (II) by EDTA-and/or DTPA-modified chitosan: Kinetic and equilibrium modeling. *Chem. Eng. J.* **2010**, *161*, 73–82. [CrossRef]
41. Ren, Y.; Sun, M.-H.; Peng, H.; Huang, K.-X. Removal of heavy metals from extract of Angelica sinensis by EDTA-modified chitosan magnetic adsorbent. *China J. Chin. Mater. Med.* **2013**, *38*, 3709–3712. [CrossRef]
42. Monu, V.; Waseem, A.; Ju-Hyun, P.; Vinod, K.; Mikhail, S.V.; Dipti, V.; Hyunook, K. One-step functionalization of chitosan using EDTA: Kinetics and isotherms modeling for multiple heavy metals adsorption and their mechanism. *J. Water Process Eng.* **2022**, *49*, 102989. [CrossRef]
43. Chibli, H.; Carlini, L.; Park, S.; Dimitrijevic, N.M.; Nadeau, J.L. Cytotoxicity of InP/ZnS quantum dots related to reactive oxygen species generation. *Nanoscale* **2011**, *3*, 2552–2559. [CrossRef] [PubMed]
44. Oberdörster, G.; Oberdörster, E.; Oberdörster, J. Nanotoxicology: An emerging discipline evolving from studies of ultrafine particles. *Environ. Health Perspect.* **2005**, *113*, 823–839. [CrossRef] [PubMed]
45. Andersen, J.C.Ø.; Cropp, A.; Paradise, D.C. Solubility of indium-tin oxide in simulated lung and gastric fluids: Pathways for human intake. *Sci. Total Environ.* **2017**, *579*, 628–636. [CrossRef]
46. Liu, Q.; Guan, J.; Song, R.; Zhang, X.; Mao, S. Physicochemical properties of nanoparticles affecting their fate and the physiological function of pulmonary surfactants. *Acta Biomater.* **2022**, *140*, 76–87. [CrossRef]
47. Olga, B.; Manon, F.; Shirin, B.; Abdullah, K.; Jennifer, C.; Christine, D.; Antonella, B. Silica Nanoparticle-Induced Structural Reorganizations in Pulmonary Surfactant Films: What Monolayer Compression Isotherms Do Not Say. *ACS Appl. Nano Mater.* **2018**, *1*, 5268–5278. [CrossRef]

Disclaimer/Publisher's Note: The statements, opinions and data contained in all publications are solely those of the individual author(s) and contributor(s) and not of MDPI and/or the editor(s). MDPI and/or the editor(s) disclaim responsibility for any injury to people or property resulting from any ideas, methods, instructions or products referred to in the content.

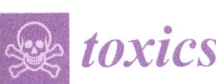

Article

Inhibitory Impact of Prenatal Exposure to Nano-Polystyrene Particles on the MAP2K6/p38 MAPK Axis Inducing Embryonic Developmental Abnormalities in Mice

Junyi Lv [1,†], Qing He [1,†], Zixiang Yan [1,†], Yuan Xie [1], Yao Wu [2], Anqi Li [1], Yuqing Zhang [3], Jing Li [1] and Zhenyao Huang [1,*]

1. Key Laboratory of Human Genetics and Environmental Medicine, School of Public Health, Xuzhou Medical University, Xuzhou 221004, China; 202005010319@stu.xzhmu.edu.cn (J.L.); 302110110929@stu.xzhmu.edu.cn (Q.H.); 202005010420@stu.xzhmu.edu.cn (Z.Y.); 202005010315@stu.xzhmu.edu.cn (Y.X.); 202105010105@stu.xzhmu.edu.cn (A.L.); 100002008046@xzhmu.edu.cn (J.L.)
2. School of Medical Imaging, Xuzhou Medical University, Xuzhou 221004, China; 202103030208@stu.xzhmu.edu.cn
3. Department of Obstetrics and Gynecology, Women's Hospital of Nanjing Medical University, Nanjing Maternity and Child Health Care Hospital, Nanjing 210004, China; yuqingzhang@njmu.edu.cn
* Correspondence: huangzhenyao@xzhmu.edu.cn
† These authors contributed equally to this work.

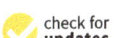

Abstract: Nanoplastics, created by the fragmentation of larger plastic debris, are a serious pollutant posing substantial environmental and health risks. Here, we developed a polystyrene nanoparticle (PS-NP) exposure model during mice pregnancy to explore their effects on embryonic development. We found that exposure to 30 nm PS-NPs during pregnancy resulted in reduced mice placental weight and abnormal embryonic development. Subsequently, our transcriptomic dissection unveiled differential expression in 102 genes under PS-NP exposure and the p38 MAPK pathway emerged as being significantly altered in KEGG pathway mapping. Our findings also included a reduction in the thickness of the trophoblastic layer in the placenta, diminished cell invasion capabilities, and an over-abundance of immature red cells in the blood vessels of the mice. In addition, we validated our findings through the human trophoblastic cell line, HTR-8/SVneo (HTR). PS-NPs induced a drop in the vitality and migration capacities of HTR cells and suppressed the p38 MAPK signaling pathway. This research highlights the embryotoxic effects of nanoplastics on mice, while the verification results from the HTR cells suggest that there could also be certain impacts on the human trophoblast layer, indicating a need for further exploration in this area.

Keywords: nanoplastics; exposure during pregnancy; placenta

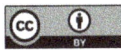

1. Introduction

Nanoplastics are formed from the degradation of larger plastic debris, initially into microplastics and eventually into nanoparticles that are less than 100 nm in size (Figure 1) [1,2]. This process is instigated by environmental factors such as ultraviolet radiation, oxygen, and mechanical abrasion from waves and sand, and can be influenced by temperature and certain microorganisms [3]. Over time, these factors gradually break down microplastics into nanoplastics. The main types of nanoplastics include polymers such as polyethylene (PE), polypropylene (PP), polystyrene (PS), and polyvinyl chloride (PVC).

The pollution caused by nanoplastics is indeed severe and poses various environmental and health issues. Due to their small size, nanoplastics have the ability to pervade different environmental compartments, including water, air, and soil. Unfortunately, as it stands currently, specific data on the global scale of nanoplastics pollution are limited. This is largely because nanoplastics are difficult to detect, measure, and isolate, given how extremely small they are. Even the most cutting-edge scientific methods have difficulty measuring nanoplastics accurately. However, to give a sense of the broader scale of plastic pollution, a study estimated that 8.3 billion tons of plastic have been produced since the 1950s, and about 60% of that plastic has ended up in either a landfill or the natural environment [4]. Meanwhile, the number of microplastic particles in our oceans is a massive 51 trillion [5]. While these figures do not provide a direct measure of nanoplastics, they underscore the seriousness of the broader plastic pollution issue, and these plastics will eventually break down into microplastics and nanoplastics in the environment, posing a greater potential hazard to the environment [6].

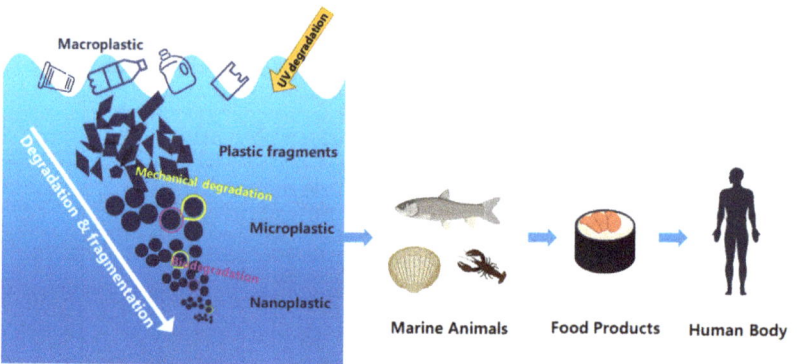

Figure 1. The sources, formation, and impact pathways of microplastics and nanoplastics on living organisms.

Microplastics and nanoplastics can easily enter the food chain as they can be ingested by small organisms and subsequently reach larger ones, potentially impacting wildlife and human health (Figure 1). A 2019 World Wildlife Fund report reveals that globally, each person ingests an average of 2000 microplastic particles weekly, weighing the same as a credit card [7]. Scientists have estimated the volume of microplastics inhaled by humans within a 24 h period to be approximately 272 particles, according to air samples taken from three apartments and a constructed human model [8]. However, nanoplastics originate from the degradation of plastic fragments, and it is estimated that the concentration of these fragments is 10^{14} times higher than that of the microplastics currently found in the aquatic environment [9]. Nanoplastics enter the human body mainly through the respiratory tract, the digestive tract, and the skin, and they can produce toxic effects on the corresponding tissues and organs through particle internalization or migration. Nanoplastics have been reported to exert toxic effects on the digestive, neurological, respiratory, immune, and reproductive endocrine systems by physically damage, causing an imbalance in intestinal flora, altering enzyme activity, activating immune cells, inducing oxidative stress, and interfering with endogenous hormones [10,11]. In animal experimental studies, it was found that exposure to nanoplastics can lead to thickening of mouse alveolar walls and pulmonary interstitial fibrosis, causing changes in lung structure [12]. Concurrently, they also cause liver damage, characterized by the infiltration of immune cells, hepatocyte vacuolization, nuclear shrinkage, and enlargement of hepatic sinusoidal spaces. The damage to the kidneys is primarily manifested in the form of renal tubule and glomerular atrophy accompanied by an inflammatory response. Exposure to nanoplastics also causes neurotoxicity in zebrafish, leading to abnormal behavior in zebrafish [13]. Nanoplastics can also disrupt the composition and function of the zebrafish gut microbiota, accompanied by immune system dysfunction [14]. This disrupts the brain–gut axis, mediated by alterations in neurotransmitter metabolites. Moreover, nanoplastics can act as carriers for other pollutants, as they have a large surface area that can adsorb harmful substances such as heavy metals and persistent organic pollutants [15–17]. When ingested by organisms, these substances can be released and cause further harm.

Embryonic development is a crucial stage in an organism's life, during which the organism undergoes rapid growth and cell division. It is agreed upon in many scientific studies that the embryo is often more sensitive to various environmental stressors, including pollution, as compared to adults. Regarding nanoplastics, little is known about their specific effects on embryonic development. However, given that nanoplastics can have harmful effects on adult organisms [10], it is reasonable to hypothesize that embryos, being in a more vulnerable and sensitive stage, might be even more adversely affected by nanoplastics exposure. A few experimental studies on aquatic organisms have indicated that exposure to nanoplastics during the embryonic stage could cause developmental abnormalities [18]. Polystyrene nanoplastic particles (PS-NPs) reduced nutrient accumulation and led to inhibition of gonadal development in juvenile river prawns [19]. PS-NPs also induce neurotoxicity (decreased spontaneous contraction frequency), cardiotoxicity (bradycardia), and morphological changes in the eyes and head of zebrafish embryos, leading to impaired embryonic development [20,21]. In addition, population studies have found higher levels of nanoplastic particles in the chorionic tissue of patients, with unexplained recurrent miscarriage (RM) relative to healthy individuals [22]. However, more research is needed to conclusively determine the risks and understand how nanoplastics could affect embryos.

In this research, our primary objective was to unravel the potential toxicological mechanisms of polystyrene nanoparticles (PS-NPs) on ICR mice during pregnancy and human trophoblast cells. We constructed a model of PS-NP (30 nm) exposure during pregnancy in mice to explore the effects and specific mechanisms of PS-NP exposure during pregnancy on dams and offspring. Through this study, we aimed to validate our argument that a certain concentration of small-sized PS-NPs is toxic to embryonic development and to probe potential mechanisms responsible for this toxicity.

2. Materials and Methods

2.1. Nanoplastics and Characterization

Polystyrene nanoplastic particles (PS-NPs) were purchased from Rigor Science (Wuxi, China), with a diameter of 30 nm and a mass percentage of 2.5 wt%. The TEM images were obtained using a JEM-2000EX microscope (JEOL, Tokyo, Japan). The size and zeta potential of PS-NPs were determined using a Zetasizer Nano (ZS90, Worcester, UK). Each measurement was made three times at a controlled temperature of $25 \pm 1\,°C$.

2.2. In Vivo Experiments

2.2.1. Modeling of PS-NP Exposure during Pregnancy in ICR Mice

The study was conducted using 8-week-old ICR mice of the Specific Pathogen Free (SPF) category, provided by the Experimental Animal Center of Xuzhou Medical University, with ethical approval granted by the Xuzhou Medical University Ethics Committee (Ethical Approval Number: 202305T002). The ICR mice were kept in an SPF-grade animal room with controlled temperature conditions ($22 \pm 2\,°C$), and subjected to alternating 12 h light and dark cycles. They had unrestricted access to food and water. One week was allocated prior to the experiment for the mice to adjust to their surroundings.

Female and male mice were co-housed in a 2:1 ratio and vaginal plug checks were carried out each morning. The identification of a vaginal plug is a conventional sign used in reproductive biology to designate that mating has occurred in mice. The day a plug is observed is defined as gestational day 0.5 (GD0.5). The study used 30 nm diameter PS-NPs and divided the pregnant mice ($n = 20$) randomly into four groups for the experiment: control group (corn oil), low-dose group (0.1 mg/kg/d), medium-dose group (1 mg/kg/d), and high-dose group (10 mg/kg/d), comprising 5 mice each. Following pregnancy confirmation, gavage of PS-NP solution was conducted based on the body weight of the pregnant mice, while also documenting their food and water intake. This continued until GD18.5, when the pregnant mice were euthanized.

2.2.2. Histopathology

Upon euthanizing the pregnant mice on GD18.5, organs such as the placenta and liver were harvested for subsequent pathological examination. Using tweezers, the placenta and fetuses were dissected, cleaned in physiological saline, weighed, and recorded. Five placentas per group (one placenta corresponding to each fetus) were then placed in a 4% paraformaldehyde solution to fix. After a process of gradient dehydration with ethanol, embedding, and sectioning, Hematoxylin and Eosin (H&E) staining was performed. Under the microscope, changes in the placental tissue pathology were observed.

2.2.3. Placental Transcriptome Sequencing

The placentas collected from both the control group and the PS-NP exposure group were used for transcriptome sequencing (3:3); the specific steps were similar to those in previous studies and are briefly described below [23,24]. The transcriptome profiling protocol commenced with the isolation and purification of the total RNA from the placental tissues using TRIzol reagent (Invitrogen, Waltham, MA, USA) in accordance with the manufacturer's instructions. Subsequently, cDNA libraries were prepared for next-generation sequencing using a NEBNext® Ultra™ RNA Library Prep Kit for Illumina® (New England Biolabs, Ipswich, MA, USA) following the manufacturer's recommendations, which subsequently generated extensive transcriptome data. The raw data were initially processed through in-house Perl scripts and clean data were obtained. Thereafter, all downstream analyses were based on clean data with high quality. Q20, Q30, and GC contents of the raw data were calculated. We utilized the Majorbio Cloud Platform (https://cloud.majorbio.com/ (accessed on 05 January 2024)) to analyze the aligned reads. When the false discovery rate (FDR) < 0.01 and Fold Change ≥ 2, differentially expressed genes (DEGs) were identified between the control and PS-NP-exposed placentas. Finally, the classification and functional enrichment of the DEGs were analyzed using Kyoto Encyclopedia of Genes and Genomes (KEGG) databases and Gene Ontology (GO) databases. Multiple testing corrections were made using FDR and only those pathways having an adjusted p-value < 0.05 were considered to be significantly enriched.

2.3. In Vitro Experiments

2.3.1. Cell Sources and Cultures

HTR-8/SVneo cells, abbreviated as HTR, were used for cell experiments (bought from HyCyte, Suzhou, China). HTR-8/SVneo cells were obtained by transfecting cells grown from human early gestation placental villous explants with a gene encoding the simian virus 40 large T antigen, and can be used to study trophoblast and placental biology [23,24]. The cells were cultured in RPMI-1640 Medium (P/S) (KeyGEN BioTECH, Nanjing, China) with added PS-NP solution and 10% fetal bovine serum (ZETA, Spring House, PA, USA). The concentrations of PS-NPs used were 0, 10, 20, 50, and 100 μg/mL.

2.3.2. Cell Proliferation Assays

Cell proliferation vitality was evaluated using a CCK8 assay. The seeding density of HTR was 2.5×10^4 mL^{-1}. After 24 h, PS-NPs were added to the culture medium for another 24 h. As per the manufacturer's instructions, a cell proliferation and cytotoxicity kit-8 (CCK8) was used (Abbkine Scientific, Wuhan, China). After incubation for 2 h, cell viability was determined under 450 nm absorbance with an enzyme-linked immunosorbent assay to assess the cell proliferation rate.

2.3.3. Cell Migration Assay

The migration ability of HTR cells was evaluated using a cell scratch test. Fully grown HTR cells were evenly inoculated into a six-well plate. After incubation for 24 h, once the cells were fully merged, a scratch was made using a 20 μL sterile pipette tip. After washing with warm PBS to remove floating cells, images were taken at the 0 h mark. The PBS was then removed from the six-well plate, and PS-NPs were added to the fetal bovine serum containing the culture medium. According to the standard of 2 mL per well, this was added to the six-well plate for further cultivation. After 24 h, scratch images were taken at the same location. The scratch area was then measured using ImageJ 1.53e software (Wayne Rasband, Bethesda, MA, USA).

2.4. RNA Extraction and Reverse Transcription-Quantitative Polymerase Chain Reaction (qRT-PCR)

Total RNA was extracted from cells and tissues using TRIzol reagent Vazyme BioTech (Nanjing, China), following the manufacturer's provided method. The total RNA was then quantitated using the nanodrop 2000c system (Thermo Fisher Scientific, Waltham, MA, USA). The RNA was then reverse transcribed into cDNA using HiScript II Q RT SuperMix for qPCR (+gDNA wiper) Vazyme BioTech (China), and amplified with ChamQ SYBR qPCR Master Mix (Applied Biosystems, Los Angeles, CA, USA) at a volume of 10 µL. Real-time fluorescence quantitative PCR was carried out based on the ChamQ SYBR qPCR Master Mix (Vazyme BioTech, China). The data were normalized using GAPDH. The primer sequences can be seen in the Supplementary Material, Table S1.

2.5. Western Blotting

After treating the cells with PS-NPs at concentrations of 0, 10, 20, 50, and 100 µg/mL for 24 h, the HTR cells were lysed with RIPA lysis buffer (Beyotime Biotechnology, Shanghai, China) containing proteinase and phosphatase inhibitors (Beyotime Biotechnology, China). Protein concentration was measured using a BCA reagent kit and proteins were denatured by adding SDS and PBS and heating at 100 °C for 5 min. After gel electrophoresis, the proteins were separated and transferred to a polyvinylidene fluoride (PVDF) membrane. QuickBlock Western Blocking Solution (Beyotime Biotechnology, China) was used for blocking for 20 min. After incubation with the primary antibody at 4 °C overnight, the membranes were washed with TBST (Servicebio, Wuhan, China), and then subjected to incubation with the secondary antibody for 1 h before being washed again with TBST. Finally, the PVDF membranes were imaged using a Bio-Rad ChemiDocXRS+ (Bio-Rad, Hercules, CA, USA). Protein band grayscale values on the images were calculated using Image J.

2.6. Statistical Analysis

The data collected from this experiment were analyzed using SPSS 21.0 statistical software. All data are represented as mean ± standard deviation. A test for homogeneity of variance was first conducted, followed by the *t*-test, Mann–Whitney U test, and Friedman test. Graph Pad Prism 5.0 was used for statistical plotting. A *p*-value below 0.05 indicates a statistically significant difference. The mechanism figure was drawn using Figdraw 2.0 (ResearchHome, Hangzhou, China).

3. Results

3.1. Characteristics of PS-NPs

The transmission electron microscope results revealed that the original particle size of PS-NPs was about 30 nm. They were in the form of spherical particles with good dispersion (Supplementary Material, Figure S1A). The hydrodynamic diameter of the PS-NPs was 167.7 ± 0.22 nm, larger than their original particle size, indicating a slight agglomeration of PS-NPs in water (Supplementary Material, Figure S1B). The zeta potential of the PS-NPs was -23.0 ± 5.0 mV (Supplementary Material, Figure S1C). At the same time, the Polymer Dispersion Index (PDI) of PS-NPs was less than 0.5, indicating good dispersion. These results demonstrate that PS-NPs possess common nanoparticle characteristics and meet the experimental requirements; thus, they could be used for subsequent experiments.

3.2. Embryonic Developmental Toxicity of PS-NPs in ICR Mice

Compared with the control group, there was no significant change in the body weight of pregnant mice fed with different doses of PS-NPs (Supplementary Material, Figure S2A). The body weight changes among all four pregnant mice groups (from GD0.5 to GD18.5) showed a steady increasing trend with no significant differences (Supplementary Material, Figure S2B). In addition, there was no difference in food and water intake during the exposure period between different dose groups and the control group (Supplementary Material, Figure S2C,D).

Compared with the control group, both the placental weight and diameter in the 10 mg/kg/d group decreased, although the placental weight and diameter in the 1 mg/kg/d group increased, and the differences were not statistically significant (Figures 2A,B and 3). Meanwhile, the number of embryos in each exposure group showed no significant differences compared to in the control group (Figure 2C). At the same time, the high-dose group showed a significantly higher rate of fetal death and absorbed fetuses compared to the control group (Figure 2D).

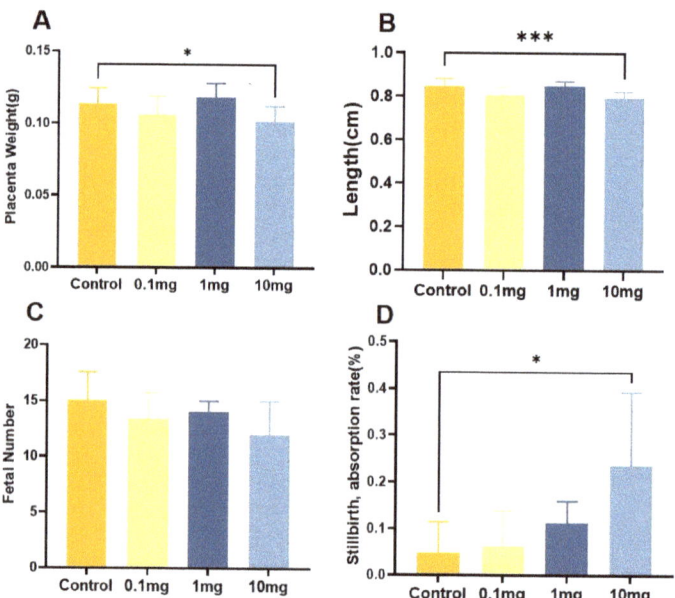

Figure 2. Biological effects of PS-NPs on fetal rats. (**A**) Placenta weight. (**B**) Placenta diameter. (**C**) Number of embryos. (**D**) Stillbirth, absorption rate. Data are represented as the mean ± SEM. * $p < 0.05$, *** $p < 0.001$.

By observing the morphological structures of the placenta via HE staining, it was found that in the PS-NP exposure group, the nourishing layer of the placenta became thinner, the invasion of nourishing cells was insufficient, and there was a large number of immature red blood cells in the blood vessels (Figure 4). All these results suggest that exposure to PS-NPs during pregnancy may lead to poor placental development, which could further cause embryonic development obstacles.

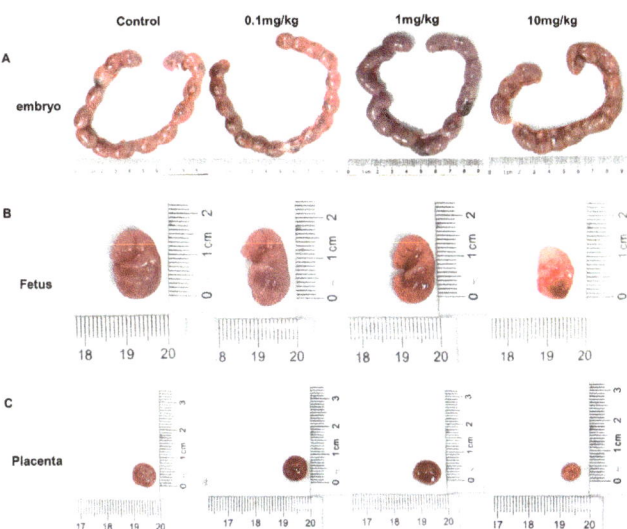

Figure 3. Exposure to PS-NPs causes placental and fetal developmental toxicity. (**A**) Representative images of maternal rat embryos. (**B**) Representative image of a fetal rat. (**C**) Representative image of placenta.

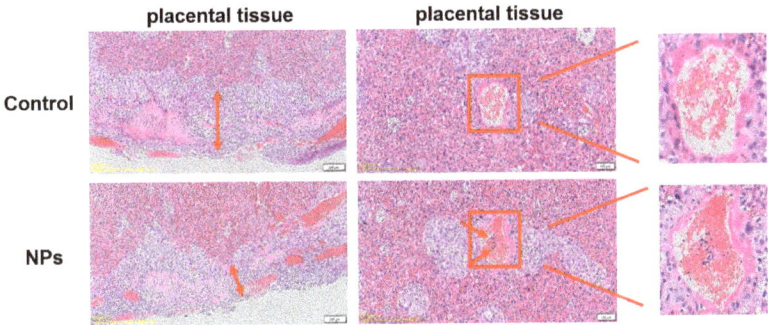

Figure 4. Exposure to PS-NPs resulted in pathological changes in the placenta at GD18.5.

3.3. Screening of Differentially Expressed Genes in Placental Tissues Exposed to PS-NPs during Pregnancy

In order to investigate the cause of placental underdevelopment due to PS-NP exposure, we employed transcriptome sequencing to identify differentially expressed genes post-PS-NP exposure in placental tissue. Gene expression differences were examined using DESeq, setting the filtering criteria for differentially expressed genes as $|\log2FoldChange| > 2$ and FDR < 0.05. The results revealed an upregulation of 39 genes and downregulation of 63 genes in the placental tissue post PS-NP exposure, giving a total of 102 differentially expressed genes. A volcano plot was used to illustrate the overall differential distribution and aid in the selection of such genes (Figure 5A). Cluster analysis suggested that genes within each sample with similar expression patterns clustered together, with distinct separation between the two groups, indicating no layered confusion (Figure 5B).

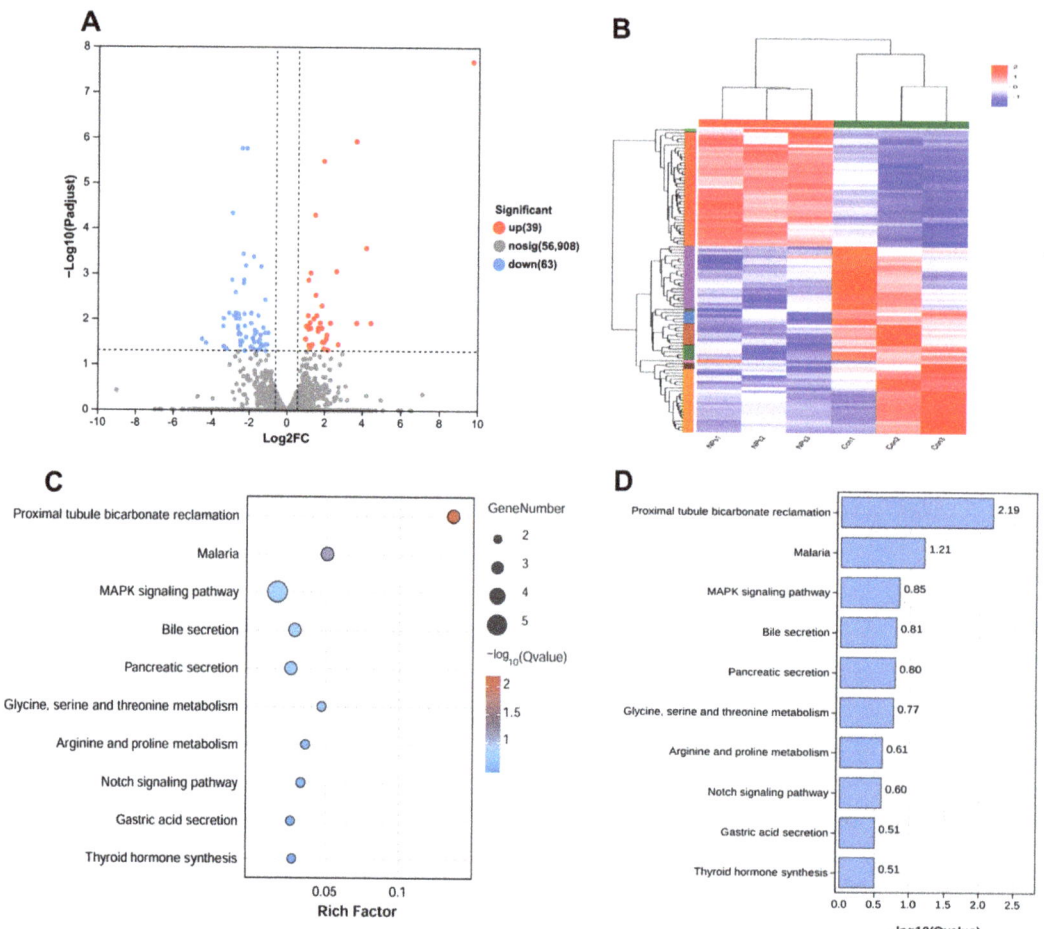

Figure 5. Transcriptomic analyses were performed on the control and 10 mg/kg/d PS-NP groups. (**A**) Volcano plots showing differential gene expression between control and PS-NP-treated groups. Red, blue, and black dots represent DEG upregulated, DEG downregulated, and no differentially expressed genes, respectively. (**B**) Cluster analysis plot of mRNA differentially expressed genes. (**C**) KEGG pathway enrichment analysis bubble plot. (**D**) KEGG pathway enrichment analysis bar graph.

We performed a KEGG pathway enrichment analysis on genes linked with PS-NP exposure using the KEGG database. Based on the results from the KEGG enrichment analysis of the differentially expressed genes, we selected the top 10 most significantly enriched pathways (those with the smallest p-value) (Figure 5C,D). The enrichment of differentially expressed genes was most significant in the MAPK signaling pathway. The downregulation of the MAPK signaling pathway is closely linked to embryonic growth and development, suggesting that regulatory factors related to this pathway may be associated with embryonic developmental delay induced by NP exposure. Further bioinformatics results are available in the Supplementary Material, Figure S3. Subsequently, we selected four genes, MAP2K6, Cacng4, Flt1, and Dtx3l, which showed differential expression in the sequencing results, for qRT-PCR validation. The results were consistent with the sequencing data (Supplementary Material, Figure S4).

3.4. Effects of PS-NPs on Trophoblast Cells

To further corroborate the correlation between the impact of PS-NPs on placental function and trophoblast cells, we exposed HTR cells to PS-NPs. The CCK8 assays demonstrated a significant reduction in HTR cells' viability, with the high-dose group experiencing an inhibition rate of up to 20% due to PS-NPs (Figure 6A). Moreover, an exposure to 100 µg/L of PS-NPs detrimentally impacted HTR cells' migration, as evidenced by the scratch tests (Figure 6B,C).

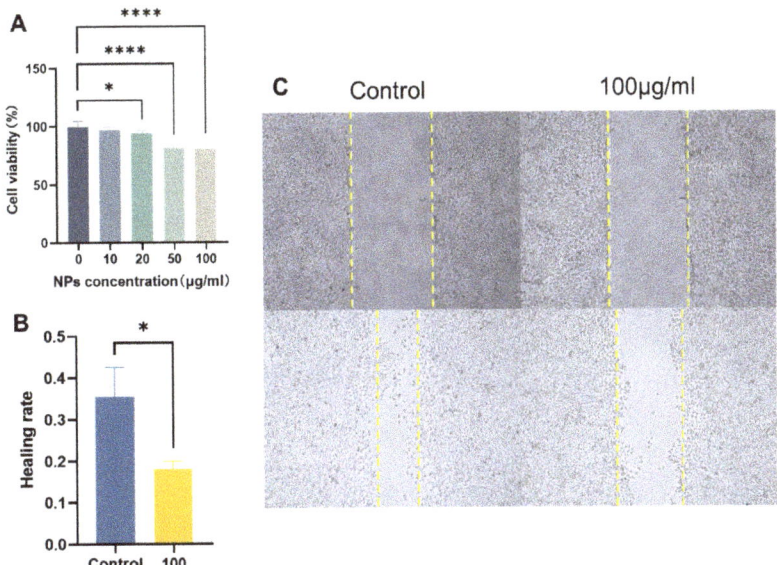

Figure 6. Exposure of PS-NPs inhibits HTR cell viability, migration, and invasion in vitro. (**A**) Twenty-four-hour cell viability of HTR cells exposed to the indicated doses was determined by Cell Counting Kit-8 assay. (**B**) Quantitative results of wound healing assay control and high-dose groups. (**C**) PS-NP exposure reduces the migration distance of HTR cells. Scale bar = 100 µm. Data are presented as the mean ± SD of three independent assays. * $p < 0.05$, **** $p < 0.0001$.

MAP2K6, a vital gene within the MAPK pathway, exhibited reduced expression levels in placental tissues upon exposure to PS-NPs, as discovered through the transcriptome sequencing and qRT-PCR results (Figure 7A). To pinpoint the mechanism underlying the impact of PS-NP exposure on trophoblast cells' proliferation and migration, we examined the expression levels of MAP2K6. We determined that NP exposure led to diminished mRNA and protein levels of MAP2K6 in the trophoblast cells (Figure 7B). In addition, MAP2K6 is involved in p38 phosphorylation. Normally, an activated MAP2K6, or MKK6, uniquely phosphorylates and activates p38 MAP kinase. The Western blot tests on HTR cells indicated that NP infection reduced the expression of phosphorylated p38 protein, but did not alter the overall p38 expression (Figure 7C).

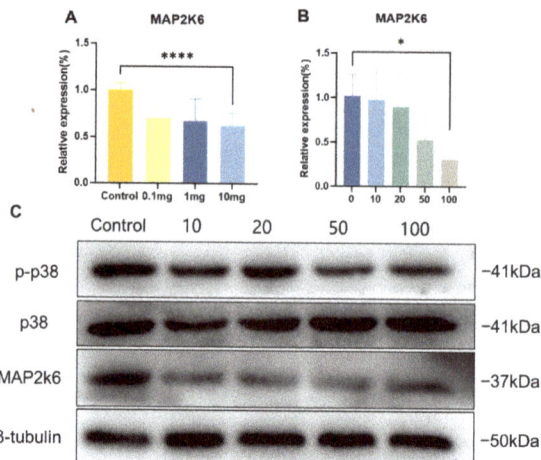

Figure 7. PS-NPs inhibit the expression of p38 MAPK-regulated genes in embryonic growth and development in vivo and in vitro by reducing MAP2K6. (**A**) mRNA levels of MAP2K6 in the placenta of GD18.5 female rats were detected by qRT-PCR. (**B**) Detection of mRNA levels of MAP2K6 by qRT-PCR in HTR cells exposed to the indicated PS-NP doses. (**C**) Protein expression of MAP2K6, p38, and p-p38 in HTR cells exposed to PS-NPs was analyzed by Western blot. Data are presented as the mean ± SD of three independent assays. * $p < 0.05$, **** $p < 0.0001$.

4. Discussion

The widespread detection of nanoplastics has raised concerns about their exposure risks to the environment and human health. In recent years, several studies have demonstrated the toxicity of nanoplastics to mammals [25–29]. Nanoplastics can accumulate in the liver, kidneys, and intestines of mice, causing disruption of energy and lipid metabolism as well as oxidative stress [25]. Exposure to PS-NPs can induce gut microbiota dysbiosis, intestinal barrier dysfunction, and metabolic disorder in mice [27]. Moreover, it has been discovered that exposure to PS-NPs during pregnancy and lactation can modify the function, structure, and cellular makeup of the offspring's neural stem cells. This leads to neurophysiological and cognitive impairments. In male mice, this exposure also triggers testicular dysgenesis, subsequently influencing their fertility [30,31]. However, studies on the potential harmful effects of nanoplastic exposure during pregnancy on placental embryos are still limited. Therefore, we established a pregnancy exposure model for PS-NPs in ICR mice and screened for differentially expressed genes in placental tissue after exposure to PS-NPs during pregnancy. In addition, we conducted corresponding verifications in the human trophoblast cell line (HTR) and further explored its possible mechanisms.

In mice experiments, exposure to PS-NPs during pregnancy had little effect on the weight, or food and water consumption, of the dams, and did not affect the survival rate or gender ratio of their offspring, which is consistent with the research results of Luo and others [32,33]. However, by weighing and measuring the diameter of the mother mouse's placenta and embryos, it was found that exposure to PS-NPs during pregnancy reduced the diameter and weight of the placenta. At the same time, pathological sections of the placenta showed that the trophoblastic layer of the treated group was thin, with insufficient invasion of trophoblastic cells, and a large number of immature red cells in the blood vessels. These results all indicate that PS-NPs may break the placental barrier and affect the growth and development of the offspring, and these adverse effects may be related to pathological changes in the placenta. Research indicates that microplastics have now infiltrated the human placenta, with a detection rate as high as 100% in samples taken after 2021 [34]. Furthermore, exposure to PS-NPs can stimulate oxidative stress in placental cells in vitro, increasing the production of ROS, inducing DNA damage, suppressing cell vitality, increasing cell apoptosis, and blocking the cell cycle, and the cytotoxicity of PS-NPs is related to particle size and whether it carries a charge [35,36]. All of these results suggest that exposure to PS-NPs during pregnancy adversely affects embryonic development.

Based on the impact of prenatal PS-NP exposure on the placenta, we further explored the gene changes in the placenta after prenatal exposure to PS-NPs using RNA-seq technology. Results showed that a total of 102 genes in the placental tissue exhibited different expression after prenatal exposure to PS-NPs, indicating that PS-NP treatment can induce significant changes in the overall gene transcription profile of the placenta. Moreover, KEGG enrichment analysis showed differences in the MAPK signaling pathway, bile secretion, pancreatic secretion, Notch signaling pathway, gastric acid secretion, and thyroid hormone synthesis, among which the MAPK signaling pathway was particularly noteworthy. Therefore, we targeted the p38 MAPK signaling pathway to explore the molecular mechanism of PS-NPs' toxicity.

In the p38 MAPK signaling pathway, MAP2K6 serves as a crucial regulatory switch in the cellular response to cytokines and growth factors [37–39]. Once activated, MAP2K6 phosphorylates p38 MAPK, thereby activating p38. The active form of p38 can then transfer these signals to the downstream targets, which then modulate various cellular activities such as inflammation, cell proliferation, differentiation, and apoptosis. In essence, MAP2K6 serves as a molecular switch to relay the signals to the appropriate response points in the cell when it receives a stimulus from cytokines and growth factors. It is this precise regulation by MAP2K6 that ensures the cells react correctly to these external stimuli [37]. The potential mechanism of the MAP2K6/p38 MAPK axis in cell growth, differentiation, apoptosis, movement, and inflammation has garnered widespread attention. Multiple studies show that a decline in the expression level of MAP2K6 can inhibit the phosphorylation of p38, leading to a reduction in the level of phospho-p38 (p-p38), which in turn causes a reduction in cell proliferation and migratory invasion capabilities. By using transfection to decrease the level of MAP2K6 in human gastric cancer cells, the phosphorylation of p38 can be inhibited, affecting autophagy in GC cells, inducing a G2 phase cell cycle block, and suppressing cell proliferation and migration [40]. The use of MAP2K6 inhibitors can suppress the growth of esophageal cancer cells both in vitro and in vivo [41]. Moreover, the p38 protein plays a pivotal role in embryonic development by regulating the initial differentiation of trophoblast cells and participating in the formation of the placental blood vessels, to the extent that a significant deficiency in p38 phosphorylation can result in fetal death within the uterus [42–44]. After exposure to PS-NPs, we found a decrease in the expression of MAP2K6 in the placentas of pregnant ICR mice and a decrease in cell vitality and migration ability in HTR cells. These results suggest that exposure to PS-NPs induces a decrease in the expression of MAP2K6 in the placenta and trophoblastic cells, thus inhibiting the phosphorylation of p38, and affecting the proliferation and migration of trophoblastic cells, leading to inhibition of placental and embryonic growth. Therefore, PS-NPs may affect placental embryonic growth and development by regulating the MAP2K6/p38 MAPK axis.

5. Conclusions

In conclusion, this study investigated the biological effects of PS-NPs on the embryos in the placenta of pregnant mice and HTR cells. The findings suggest that exposure to PS-NPs during pregnancy may not significantly affect the biological responses of the dams, but can notably impact the growth and development of the mice placenta and embryo. The harm inflicted on the placenta by PS-NPs mainly manifests as an inhibition of trophoblast cell proliferation and migration, potentially achieved through the impediment of p38 phosphorylation, regulated by MAP2K6 (Figure 8). This study provides a possible molecular mechanism for understanding the potential embryonic developmental toxicity induced by PS-NPs. The verification results from the HTR cells suggest that there could also be certain impacts on the human trophoblast layer, indicating a need for further exploration in this area.

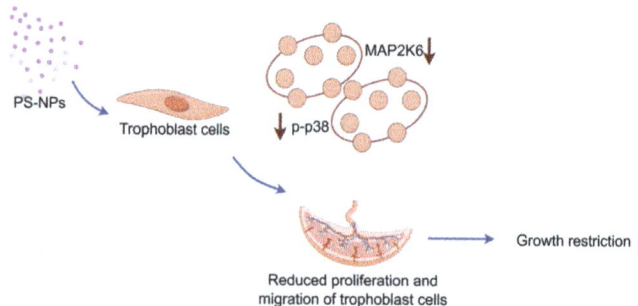

Figure 8. Possible mechanism. PS-NPs may inhibit placental embryo growth and development by decreasing MAP2K6 expression and targeting inhibition of the p38 MAPK pathway, causing embryonic developmental toxicity.

Supplementary Materials: The following supporting information can be downloaded at: https://www.mdpi.com/article/10.3390/toxics12050370/s1, Figure S1: Polystyrene nanoparticle characterization, Figure S2: Biological effects of PS-NP particles on pregnant rats, Figure S3: Differential analysis of placental expression and pathway analysis in PS-NP-exposed pregnant female rats, Figure S4: Validation of qRT-PCR of differentially expressed genes in the placenta of female mice, Table S1: Primers for real time qRT-PCR, Table S2: Antibodies for Western blot.

Author Contributions: Conceptualization, J.L. (Junyi Lv) and Z.H.; Data curation, Y.X., Y.W. and A.L.; Formal analysis, J.L. (Junyi Lv) and Q.H.; Funding acquisition, Y.Z., J.L. (Jing Li) and Z.H.; Investigation, Z.Y., Y.X. and Y.W.; Methodology, Q.H. and Z.H.; Project administration, J.L. (Jing Li) and Z.H.; Resources, Y.Z., J.L. (Jing Li) and Z.H.; Software, J.L. (Junyi Lv), Z.Y. and A.L.; Supervision, Y.Z., J.L. (Jing Li) and Z.H.; Validation, J.L. (Junyi Lv); Visualization, J.L. (Junyi Lv); Writing—original draft, Y.X., Y.W. and A.L.; Writing—review and editing, J.L. (Junyi Lv), Z.Y., Q.H. and Z.H. All authors have read and agreed to the published version of the manuscript.

Funding: This work was supported by the National Natural Science Foundation of China (82103880, 82103793), Natural Science Foundation of Jiangsu Province of China (BK20210905) and Natural Science Foundation for Colleges Universities in Jiangsu Province (21KJB330003), Jiangsu Training Program of Innovation and Entrepreneurship for Undergraduates (202310313035Z) and Xuzhou Medical University Start-up Grant (D2020021). Funders had no roles in study design, data collection, data analysis, interpretation, or report writing.

Institutional Review Board Statement: The study was conducted using 8-week-old ICR mice of the Specific Pathogen Free (SPF) category, provided by the Experimental Animal Center of Xuzhou Medical University, with ethical approval granted by the Xuzhou Medical University Ethics Committee (Ethical Approval Number: 202305T002).

Informed Consent Statement: Not applicable.

Data Availability Statement: Data are contained within the article or Supplementary Material.

Conflicts of Interest: The authors declare no conflicts of interest.

Abbreviations

PS-NPs, Polystyrene nanoplastics; TEM images, Transmission Electron Microscope; ICR mice, Institute of Cancer Research mice; HTR, HTR-8/SVneo cells; KEGG, Kyoto Encyclopedia of Genes and Genomes; GO, Gene Ontology; DEGs, Differentially Expressed Genes; PE, polyethylene; PP, polypropylene; PS, polystyrene; PVC, polyvinyl chloride; BCA, Bicinchoninic Acid Assay; SDS, Sodium dodecyl sulfate; PBS, phosphate buffered saline; PVDF, polyvinylidene difluoride; TBST, Tris-buffered saline with Tween 20; qRT-PCR, quantitative reverse transcription polymerase chain reaction; GAPDH, glyceraldehyde-3-phosphate dehydrogenase; MAP2K6, Recombinant Mitogen Activated Protein Kinase Kinase 6; p38, p38 mitogen-activated protein kinase; p-p38, Phospho-p38 mitogen-activated protein kinase; MAPK, mitogen-activated protein kinase; CCK8, Cell Counting Kit-8.

References

1. Thompson, R.C.; Olsen, Y.; Mitchell, R.P.; Davis, A.; Rowland, S.J.; John, A.W.; McGonigle, D.; Russell, A.E. Lost at sea: Where is all the plastic? *Science* **2004**, *304*, 838. [CrossRef]
2. Jambeck, J.R.; Geyer, R.; Wilcox, C.; Siegler, T.R.; Perryman, M.; Andrady, A.; Narayan, R.; Law, K.L. Marine pollution. Plastic waste inputs from land into the ocean. *Science* **2015**, *347*, 768–771. [CrossRef]
3. Lin, Z.; Jin, T.; Zou, T.; Xu, L.; Xi, B.; Xu, D.; He, J.; Xiong, L.; Tang, C.; Peng, J.; et al. Current progress on plastic/microplastic degradation: Fact influences and mechanism. *Environ. Pollut.* **2022**, *304*, 119159. [CrossRef]
4. Mossman, S. Plastics and social responsibility. In *Provocative Plastics: Their Value in Design and Material Culture*; Palgrave Macmillan: Cham, Switzerland, 2020; pp. 275–295.
5. Burgess, R.M.; Ho, K.T. Microplastics in the aquatic environment-Perspectives on the scope of the problem. *Environ. Toxicol. Chem.* **2017**, *36*, 2259–2265. [CrossRef]
6. Zaki, M.R.M.; Aris, A.Z. An overview of the effects of nanoplastics on marine organisms. *Sci. Total Environ.* **2022**, *831*, 154757. [CrossRef]
7. Aliko, V.; Beqiraj, E.G.; Qirjo, M.; Cani, M.; Rama, A.; Bego, K.; Reka, A.; Faggio, C. Plastic invasion tolling: First evaluation of microplastics in water and two crab species from the nature reserve lagoonary complex of Kune-Vain, Albania. *Sci. Total Environ.* **2022**, *849*, 157799. [CrossRef] [PubMed]
8. Vianello, A.; Jensen, R.L.; Liu, L.; Vollertsen, J. Simulating human exposure to indoor airborne microplastics using a Breathing Thermal Manikin. *Sci. Rep.* **2019**, *9*, 8670. [CrossRef] [PubMed]
9. Zhao, J.; Lan, R.; Wang, Z.; Su, W.; Song, D.; Xue, R.; Liu, Z.; Liu, X.; Dai, Y.; Yue, T.; et al. Microplastic fragmentation by rotifers in aquatic ecosystems contributes to global nanoplastic pollution. *Nat. Nanotechnol.* **2024**, *19*, 406–414. [CrossRef] [PubMed]
10. Yong, C.Q.Y.; Valiyaveettil, S.; Tang, B.L. Toxicity of Microplastics and Nanoplastics in Mammalian Systems. *Int. J. Environ. Res. Public Health* **2020**, *17*, 1509. [CrossRef]
11. Liu, Z.; You, X.Y. Recent progress of microplastic toxicity on human exposure base on in vitro and in vivo studies. *Sci. Total Environ.* **2023**, *903*, 166766. [CrossRef]
12. Xu, D.; Ma, Y.; Han, X.; Chen, Y. Systematic toxicity evaluation of polystyrene nanoplastics on mice and molecular mechanism investigation about their internalization into Caco-2 cells. *J. Hazard. Mater.* **2021**, *417*, 126092. [CrossRef] [PubMed]
13. Sarasamma, S.; Audira, G.; Siregar, P.; Malhotra, N.; Lai, Y.H.; Liang, S.T.; Chen, J.R.; Chen, K.H.; Hsiao, C.D. Nanoplastics Cause Neurobehavioral Impairments, Reproductive and Oxidative Damages, and Biomarker Responses in Zebrafish: Throwing up Alarms of Wide Spread Health Risk of Exposure. *Int. J. Mol. Sci.* **2020**, *21*, 1410. [CrossRef]
14. Teng, M.; Zhao, X.; Wang, C.; Wang, C.; White, J.C.; Zhao, W.; Zhou, L.; Duan, M.; Wu, F. Polystyrene Nanoplastics Toxicity to Zebrafish: Dysregulation of the Brain-Intestine-Microbiota Axis. *ACS Nano* **2022**, *16*, 8190–8204. [CrossRef] [PubMed]
15. Hartmann, N.B.; Rist, S.; Bodin, J.; Jensen, L.H.; Schmidt, S.N.; Mayer, P.; Meibom, A.; Baun, A. Microplastics as vectors for environmental contaminants: Exploring sorption, desorption, and transfer to biota. *Integr. Environ. Assess. Manag.* **2017**, *13*, 488–493. [CrossRef] [PubMed]
16. Liu, J.; Ma, Y.; Zhu, D.; Xia, T.; Qi, Y.; Yao, Y.; Guo, X.; Ji, R.; Chen, W. Polystyrene Nanoplastics-Enhanced Contaminant Transport: Role of Irreversible Adsorption in Glassy Polymeric Domain. *Environ. Sci. Technol.* **2018**, *52*, 2677–2685. [CrossRef]
17. Caruso, G. Microplastics as vectors of contaminants. *Mar. Pollut. Bull.* **2019**, *146*, 921–924. [CrossRef] [PubMed]
18. Torres-Ruiz, M.; De la Vieja, A.; de Alba Gonzalez, M.; Esteban Lopez, M.; Castaño Calvo, A.; Cañas Portilla, A.I. Toxicity of nanoplastics for zebrafish embryos, what we know and where to go next. *Sci. Total Environ.* **2021**, *797*, 149125. [CrossRef] [PubMed]
19. Li, Y.; Ye, Y.; Rihan, N.; Jiang, Q.; Liu, X.; Zhao, Y.; Che, X. Polystyrene nanoplastics decrease nutrient accumulation, disturb sex hormones, and inhibit reproductive development in juvenile Macrobrachium nipponense. *Sci. Total Environ.* **2023**, *891*, 164481. [CrossRef]
20. Santos, A.L.; Rodrigues, L.C.; Rodrigues, C.C.; Cirqueira, F.; Malafaia, G.; Rocha, T.L. Polystyrene nanoplastics induce developmental impairments and vasotoxicity in zebrafish (Danio rerio). *J. Hazard. Mater.* **2024**, *464*, 132880. [CrossRef]
21. Chen, J.; Liang, Q.; Zheng, Y.; Lei, Y.; Gan, X.; Mei, H.; Bai, C.; Wang, H.; Ju, J.; Dong, Q.; et al. Polystyrene nanoplastics induced size-dependent developmental and neurobehavioral toxicities in embryonic and juvenile zebrafish. *Aquat. Toxicol.* **2024**, *267*, 106842. [CrossRef]
22. Wan, S.; Wang, X.; Chen, W.; Wang, M.; Zhao, J.; Xu, Z.; Wang, R.; Mi, C.; Zheng, Z.; Zhang, H. Exposure to high dose of polystyrene nanoplastics causes trophoblast cell apoptosis and induces miscarriage. *Part. Fibre Toxicol.* **2024**, *21*, 13. [CrossRef] [PubMed]
23. Huang, Z.; Yu, H.; Du, G.; Han, L.; Huang, X.; Wu, D.; Han, X.; Xia, Y.; Wang, X.; Lu, C. Enhancer RNA lnc-CES1-1 inhibits decidual cell migration by interacting with RNA-binding protein FUS and activating PPARγ in URPL. *Mol. Ther. Nucleic Acids* **2021**, *24*, 104–112. [CrossRef] [PubMed]

24. Huang, Z.; Du, G.; Huang, X.; Han, L.; Han, X.; Xu, B.; Zhang, Y.; Yu, M.; Qin, Y.; Xia, Y.; et al. The enhancer RNA lnc-SLC4A1-1 epigenetically regulates unexplained recurrent pregnancy loss (URPL) by activating CXCL8 and NF-kB pathway. *EBioMedicine* **2018**, *38*, 162–170. [CrossRef] [PubMed]
25. Deng, Y.; Zhang, Y.; Lemos, B.; Ren, H. Tissue accumulation of microplastics in mice and biomarker responses suggest widespread health risks of exposure. *Sci. Rep.* **2017**, *7*, 46687. [CrossRef]
26. Deng, Y.; Zhang, Y.; Qiao, R.; Bonilla, M.M.; Yang, X.; Ren, H.; Lemos, B. Evidence that microplastics aggravate the toxicity of organophosphorus flame retardants in mice (Mus musculus). *J. Hazard. Mater.* **2018**, *357*, 348–354. [CrossRef] [PubMed]
27. Jin, Y.; Lu, L.; Tu, W.; Luo, T.; Fu, Z. Impacts of polystyrene microplastic on the gut barrier, microbiota and metabolism of mice. *Sci. Total Environ.* **2019**, *649*, 308–317. [CrossRef] [PubMed]
28. Li, B.; Ding, Y.; Cheng, X.; Sheng, D.; Xu, Z.; Rong, Q.; Wu, Y.; Zhao, H.; Ji, X.; Zhang, Y. Polyethylene microplastics affect the distribution of gut microbiota and inflammation development in mice. *Chemosphere* **2020**, *244*, 125492. [CrossRef] [PubMed]
29. Hu, Q.; Wang, H.; He, C.; Jin, Y.; Fu, Z. Polystyrene nanoparticles trigger the activation of p38 MAPK and apoptosis via inducing oxidative stress in zebrafish and macrophage cells. *Environ. Pollut.* **2021**, *269*, 116075. [CrossRef]
30. Jeong, B.; Baek, J.Y.; Koo, J.; Park, S.; Ryu, Y.K.; Kim, K.S.; Zhang, S.; Chung, C.; Dogan, R.; Choi, H.S.; et al. Maternal exposure to polystyrene nanoplastics causes brain abnormalities in progeny. *J. Hazard. Mater.* **2022**, *426*, 127815. [CrossRef]
31. Zhao, T.; Shen, L.; Ye, X.; Bai, G.; Liao, C.; Chen, Z.; Peng, T.; Li, X.; Kang, X.; An, G. Prenatal and postnatal exposure to polystyrene microplastics induces testis developmental disorder and affects male fertility in mice. *J. Hazard. Mater.* **2023**, *445*, 130544. [CrossRef]
32. Luo, T.; Zhang, Y.; Wang, C.; Wang, X.; Zhou, J.; Shen, M.; Zhao, Y.; Fu, Z.; Jin, Y. Maternal exposure to different sizes of polystyrene microplastics during gestation causes metabolic disorders in their offspring. *Environ. Pollut.* **2019**, *255*, 113122. [CrossRef] [PubMed]
33. Luo, T.; Wang, C.; Pan, Z.; Jin, C.; Fu, Z.; Jin, Y. Maternal Polystyrene Microplastic Exposure during Gestation and Lactation Altered Metabolic Homeostasis in the Dams and Their F1 and F2 Offspring. *Environ. Sci. Technol.* **2019**, *53*, 10978–10992. [CrossRef] [PubMed]
34. Weingrill, R.B.; Lee, M.J.; Benny, P.; Riel, J.; Saiki, K.; Garcia, J.; Oliveira, L.; Fonseca, E.; Souza, S.T.; D'Amato, F.O.S.; et al. Temporal trends in microplastic accumulation in placentas from pregnancies in Hawai'i. *Environ. Int.* **2023**, *180*, 108220. [CrossRef] [PubMed]
35. Shen, F.; Li, D.; Guo, J.; Chen, J. Mechanistic toxicity assessment of differently sized and charged polystyrene nanoparticles based on human placental cells. *Water Res.* **2022**, *223*, 118960. [CrossRef] [PubMed]
36. Hu, J.; Zhu, Y.; Zhang, J.; Xu, Y.; Wu, J.; Zeng, W.; Lin, Y.; Liu, X. The potential toxicity of polystyrene nanoplastics to human trophoblasts in vitro. *Environ. Pollut.* **2022**, *311*, 119924. [CrossRef] [PubMed]
37. Stramucci, L.; Pranteda, A.; Bossi, G. Insights of Crosstalk between p53 Protein and the MKK3/MKK6/p38 MAPK Signaling Pathway in Cancer. *Cancers* **2018**, *10*, 131. [CrossRef] [PubMed]
38. Martínez-Limón, A.; Joaquin, M.; Caballero, M.; Posas, F.; de Nadal, E. The p38 Pathway: From Biology to Cancer Therapy. *Int. J. Mol. Sci.* **2020**, *21*, 1913. [CrossRef] [PubMed]
39. New, L.; Han, J. The p38 MAP kinase pathway and its biological function. *Trends Cardiovasc. Med.* **1998**, *8*, 220–228. [CrossRef] [PubMed]
40. Li, X.; Zhu, M.; Zhao, G.; Zhou, A.; Min, L.; Liu, S.; Zhang, N.; Zhu, S.; Guo, Q.; Zhang, S.; et al. MiR-1298-5p level downregulation induced by Helicobacter pylori infection inhibits autophagy and promotes gastric cancer development by targeting MAP2K6. *Cell. Signal.* **2022**, *93*, 110286. [CrossRef]
41. Xie, X.; Liu, K.; Liu, F.; Chen, H.; Wang, X.; Zu, X.; Ma, X.; Wang, T.; Wu, Q.; Zheng, Y.; et al. Gossypetin is a novel MKK3 and MKK6 inhibitor that suppresses esophageal cancer growth in vitro and in vivo. *Cancer Lett.* **2019**, *442*, 126–136. [CrossRef]
42. Daoud, G.; Amyot, M.; Rassart, E.; Masse, A.; Simoneau, L.; Lafond, J. ERK1/2 and p38 regulate trophoblasts differentiation in human term placenta. *J. Physiol.* **2005**, *566*, 409–423. [CrossRef] [PubMed]
43. Mudgett, J.S.; Ding, J.; Guh-Siesel, L.; Chartrain, N.A.; Yang, L.; Gopal, S.; Shen, M.M. Essential role for p38alpha mitogen-activated protein kinase in placental angiogenesis. *Proc. Natl. Acad. Sci. USA* **2000**, *97*, 10454–10459. [CrossRef] [PubMed]
44. Adams, R.H.; Porras, A.; Alonso, G.; Jones, M.; Vintersten, K.; Panelli, S.; Valladares, A.; Perez, L.; Klein, R.; Nebreda, A.R. Essential role of p38alpha MAP kinase in placental but not embryonic cardiovascular development. *Mol. Cell* **2000**, *6*, 109–116. [CrossRef] [PubMed]

Disclaimer/Publisher's Note: The statements, opinions and data contained in all publications are solely those of the individual author(s) and contributor(s) and not of MDPI and/or the editor(s). MDPI and/or the editor(s) disclaim responsibility for any injury to people or property resulting from any ideas, methods, instructions or products referred to in the content.

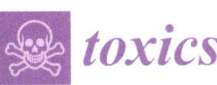

Article

Titanium Dioxide Nanoparticles Induce Maternal Preeclampsia-like Syndrome and Adverse Birth Outcomes via Disrupting Placental Function in SD Rats

Haixin Li [1,†], Dandan Miao [2,†], Haiting Hu [1], Pingping Xue [1], Kun Zhou [3,4,5,*] and Zhilei Mao [1,3,4,*]

1. Changzhou Maternity and Child Health Care Hospital, Changzhou Medical Center, Nanjing Medical University, Changzhou 213003, China; sungirllhx@163.com (H.L.); hht1173@126.com (H.H.); 13616118039@163.com (P.X.)
2. Huai'an Center for Disease Control and Prevention, Huai'an 223001, China; amiaodandan@126.com
3. State Key Laboratory of Reproductive Medicine, Center for Global Health, Nanjing Medical University, Nanjing 211100, China
4. Key Laboratory of Modern Toxicology of Ministry of Education, School of Public Health, Nanjing Medical University, Nanjing 211100, China
5. Department of Epidemiology, Center for Global Health, School of Public Health, Nanjing Medical University, Nanjing 211166, China
* Correspondence: mao598808386@126.com (Z.M.); zk@njmu.edu.cn (K.Z.); Tel.: +86-25-86868425 (Z.M.); Fax: +86-25-86868427 (Z.M.)
† These authors contributed equally to this work.

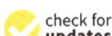

Citation: Li, H.; Miao, D.; Hu, H.; Xue, P.; Zhou, K.; Mao, Z. Titanium Dioxide Nanoparticles Induce Maternal Preeclampsia-like Syndrome and Adverse Birth Outcomes via Disrupting Placental Function in SD Rats. *Toxics* 2024, 12, 367. https://doi.org/10.3390/toxics12050367

Academic Editor: Gunnar Toft

Received: 21 April 2024
Revised: 8 May 2024
Accepted: 13 May 2024
Published: 16 May 2024

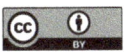

Copyright: © 2024 by the authors. Licensee MDPI, Basel, Switzerland. This article is an open access article distributed under the terms and conditions of the Creative Commons Attribution (CC BY) license (https://creativecommons.org/licenses/by/4.0/).

Abstract: The escalating utilization of titanium dioxide nanoparticles (TiO_2 NPs) in everyday products has sparked concerns regarding their potential hazards to pregnant females and their offspring. To address these concerns and shed light on their undetermined adverse effects and mechanisms, we established a pregnant rat model to investigate the impacts of TiO_2 NPs on both maternal and offspring health and to explore the underlying mechanisms of those impacts. Pregnant rats were orally administered TiO_2 NPs at a dose of 5 mg/kg body weight per day from GD5 to GD18 during pregnancy. Maternal body weight, organ weight, and birth outcomes were monitored and recorded. Maternal pathological changes were examined by HE staining and TEM observation. Maternal blood pressure was assessed using a non-invasive blood analyzer, and the urinary protein level was determined using spot urine samples. Our findings revealed that TiO_2 NPs triggered various pathological alterations in maternal liver, kidney, and spleen, and induced maternal preeclampsia-like syndrome, as well as leading to growth restriction in the offspring. Further examination unveiled that TiO_2 NPs hindered trophoblastic cell invasion into the endometrium via the promotion of autophagy. Consistent hypertension and proteinuria resulted from the destroyed kidney GBM. In total, an exposure to TiO_2 NPs during pregnancy might increase the risk of human preeclampsia through increased maternal arterial pressure and urinary albumin levels, as well as causing fetal growth restriction in the offspring.

Keywords: titanium dioxide nanoparticles; pregnant model; preeclampsia-like syndrome; autophagy; placenta development; trophoblastic cell function

1. Introduction

Titanium dioxide nanoparticles (TiO_2 NPs) were among the first nanoparticles produced and used worldwide, mainly finding applications in sunscreen, paint, ink, and as a food additive [1–3]. TiO_2 NPs are present in various environmental media, with the primary route of human exposure being through the digestive tract via food [4]. Pregnant women, therefore, cannot avoid exposure to them. Studies have shown that fetuses are more sensitive to toxins than adults, and prenatal exposure can lead to developmental toxicity in offspring [5]. To date, limited human epidemiological evidence regarding the hazards of TiO$_2$ NPs to pregnant women and birth outcomes has been reported. Existing studies about the toxicity of TiO$_2$ NPs mainly focus on animal models [6,7], making related studies urgently necessary.

Previous research has indicated that TiO$_2$ NPs can reach and accumulate in the placenta, leading to a smaller feto-placental unit [8]. They can even penetrate the placental barrier, reach fetal brains, and ultimately affect the offspring's neurodevelopment [9]. These findings underscore that the placenta is one of the target organs of TiO$_2$ NPs. The placenta plays a vital role in embryo development, facilitating substrate exchange, hormone secretion, and immune defense [10]. Trophoblastic cells are a type of cell that plays a crucial role in the development of the placenta during pregnancy, and their migration and invasion ability are crucial for placental development [11]. The impaired function of trophoblastic cells can result in inadequate infiltration of the placenta into the endometrium and a failure to complete spiral artery (SA) remodeling. Placental dysfunction can lead to abortion, fetal growth restriction, intrauterine anoxia, and even fetal death [12–14]. Other pregnancy-related diseases, such as preeclampsia and uteroplacental apoplexy, have also been linked to placental dysfunction [15]. However, whether TiO$_2$ NPs affect placental development and induce maternal pregnancy diseases and adverse birth outcomes remains unclear and requires further study.

The placental development and trophoblastic cell invasion pattern in rats closely resemble those in humans. Thus, we utilized pregnant rats as an in vivo model to investigate the potential effects of TiO$_2$ NPs on placental development and to uncover the potential underlying mechanisms. Rats have a gestation period of 21 days, with embryos being implanted around 4–5 days after fertilization. Therefore, we selected the 5th day of pregnancy as the starting point for exposure. Throughout this study, we closely monitored maternal changes and recorded pregnancy outcomes after TiO$_2$ NPs exposures, with a particular emphasis on observing placental development to elucidate the potential mechanisms at play.

2. Materials and Methods

2.1. Animals

The animal study was conducted in compliance with the ethical guidelines set forth by the Nanjing Medical University Ethics Committee (Approved No: IACUC-24040115) and followed the principles outlined in the ARRIVE Guidelines for reporting in vivo experiments. Titanium dioxide nanoparticles (TiO$_2$ NPs, CAS number: 13463-67-7) were purchased from Sigma-Aldrich(Sigma Chemical Co., St. Louis, MO, USA). Adult male and female SD rats (8 weeks, 280–300 g) were obtained from Beijing Vital River Laboratory Animal Technology Co., Ltd. All rats were housed separately, by gender, and acclimatized in a controlled environment maintained at a temperature of 22 ± 2 °C and humidity of 40–60%, with a 12 h light/dark cycle, for one week of rest prior to the commencement of the experiments. Female rats were paired with males in a 1:1 ratio following random grouping, with 10 rats in each group. Male rats were separated from females after confirming the presence of a vaginal plug every morning, and this was recorded as gestational day 0.5 (GD 0.5).

2.2. Cell Culture

Trophoblastic cells (HTR8-Svneo) were purchased from American Type Culture Collection (ATCC® CRL-3271™) and cultured in Roswell Park Memorial Institute 1640 (RPMI-1640) medium supplemented with 10% fetal bovine serum (FBS), 100 U/mL penicillin, and 100 µg/mL streptomycin. The culture dishes were incubated in a 37 °C, 5% CO$_2$ atmosphere, and the medium was replaced every day.

2.3. TiO$_2$ NPs Preparation and Exposure Design

The TiO$_2$ NPs were dispersed in a 5% methylcellulose solution at a concentration of 5 mg/mL. Their characteristics were assessed following sonication at 100 W for 30 min.

A morphological analysis was conducted using transmission electron microscopy (TEM), while their hydrodynamic diameter was determined using dynamic light scattering (DLS). To mimic human exposure routes and doses, pregnant rats were orally administered TiO$_2$ NPs at a dose of 5 mg/kg body weight per day from GD5 to GD18 during pregnancy. Control rats received treatment with a 0.5% methylcellulose solution [16]. The dose of 5 mg/kg/day was selected based on the average daily human consumption of TiO$_2$ [17]. Following delivery, except for those euthanized for further analysis, the remaining female rats ceased their TiO$_2$ NP exposure. Throughout the study, all pregnant rats were monitored for weight changes before supplying food.

2.4. Tissue Collection and Preparation

The pregnant rats were euthanized using 10% chloral hydrate on gestational day 18 (GD 18). Subsequently, maternal organs including the liver, spleen, kidney, and placenta were carefully dissected, counted, and weighed to calculate the organ coefficients (weight of the organ/total body weight) and then preserved in 4% polyformaldehyde for subsequent analysis. Pregnancy outcomes including fetal numbers and fetal growth conditions were documented simultaneously. To prevent the separation of the placenta from the uterus, the placenta–uterus units were carefully kept intact, ensuring the preservation of the placental invasion ability for subsequent analyses.

2.5. Histopathological Analysis and Immunohistochemical Analysis

The tissues were fixed and dehydrated before being embedded in paraffin. Subsequently, tissue blocks were sectioned into slices. These slices underwent dewaxing with xylene, followed by rehydration with graded alcohol. Hematoxylin and eosin (HE) staining and periodic acid-Schiff (PAS) staining were performed using a commercial kit and antibody (Beyotime, C0105, Shanghai, China; Abcam, ab150680, Cambridge, UK), following the manufacturer's instructions. PAS staining was employed to highlight the elastic fibers, collagen, and other components in the kidney. The immunohistochemical analysis was conducted using an anti-LC3B antibody (Abcam, ab48394) in conjunction with an HRP-conjugated secondary antibody. All sections were examined under a light microscope, and images were semi-quantified using ImageJ Software 1.8.0 (National Institute of Health, USA).

2.6. Placenta Invasion Ability Assessment

The placental invasion ability assessment was conducted following the methodology outlined in a previous study [18]. The percentage of interstitial trophoblast invasion into the mesometrial triangle (MT) was utilized to quantify the invasion ability, with infiltrated trophoblast cells identified using a cytokeratin-7 (CK-7) antibody (Abcam, ab181598). Evidence of spiral artery (SA) remodeling was also identified through the presence of CK-7-positive cells arranged on a fibrinoid layer, alongside the absence of α-actin-positive smooth muscle cells. Additionally, the cross-sectional area, as reported by Cotechini et al., was included as an informative indicator [19]. Both the ratio of the cytokeratin-7-positive trophoblast cell area to the MT area and the cross-sectional areas were measured using image J analysis software.

2.7. Immunofluorescence Analysis

A trophoblastic cell (HTR8-Svneo) model was employed for in vitro mechanism verification. Cellular autophagy levels were assessed using an anti-LC3B antibody in conjunction with a confocal microscope. Cells were seeded onto specialized dishes and incubated with 10 μg/mL TiO$_2$ NPs. After exposure for 24 h, cells were fixed and treated with the primary antibody overnight, followed by a CY3-labeled secondary antibody. Images were captured using a confocal microscope system.

2.8. Cell Invasion and Migration Ability Analysis

Cell invasion and migration ability were evaluated using a transwell assay. In brief, HTR cells were exposed to 10 μg/mL TiO$_2$ NPs and suspended in serum-free medium. These cells were then seeded onto matrigel-coated upper chambers, while a serum-containing medium was added to the lower chambers. After a 24 h incubation period, the cells were fixed and stained with crystal violet, and the number of penetrated cells was counted using a light microscope.

2.9. Maternal Blood Pressure Monitoring

Maternal mean arterial pressure (MAP) was assessed using a non-invasive blood pressure analyzer on GD0 (before mating), GD18, and the third day after delivery (AD3) in both experimental groups. The research was conducted in a controlled environment to minimize noise, with room temperature maintained between 25 and 26 °C. Female rats were gently restrained, and the pressure detector was securely positioned on their tails. Once the animals had calmed for approximately 3 min, the measurements were initiated. Each rat underwent 6 consecutive series of measurements, and any aberrant data points were excluded from the analysis.

2.10. Determination of Proteinuria

Spot urine samples from female rats in both experimental groups were collected at the corresponding time points to assess the occurrence of proteinuria, as previously described [20]. Urinary albumin and urine creatinine concentrations were quantified using commercial assay kits (TRFIA) (Lumigenx, Suzhou, China) following the manufacturer's instructions. The albumin to creatinine ratio (ACR) was utilized as an indicator of proteinuria.

2.11. Statistical Analysis

Statistical analyses were performed using SPSS software(IBM, Armonk, NY, USA). The normality and homogeneity of variance for all data were assessed using the Kolmogorov–Smirnov test. Quantitative data were presented as mean ± SD. The comparison of differences between two groups or among multiple groups was conducted using the *t*-test and a one-way ANOVA, respectively. The difference between the two ratios was assessed using the Chi-square test. A *p*-value of less than 0.05 was considered statistically significant.

3. Results

3.1. Main Characteristics of TiO$_2$ NPs

The main characteristics of TiO$_2$ NPs in 0.5% methylcellulose and in cell culture medium were determined and are presented in Figure 1A. The transmission electron microscopy (TEM) results (Figure 1B) revealed that the morphology of TiO$_2$ NPs was nearly spherical, with a primary size of approximately 21 nm. The purity of the TiO$_2$ NPs was reported to be $\geq$99.5% in terms of trace metals, with a BET surface area ranging from 35 to 65 m^2/g, and their crystal form was determined to be 80% anatase and 20% rutile according to the manufacturer's reports. Additionally, the results of dynamic light scattering (DLS) indicated that the average hydrodynamic diameter of the TiO$_2$ NPs was approximately 190 nm in 0.5% methylcellulose and about 80 nm in complete cell culture medium containing serum, which is consistent with our previous study.

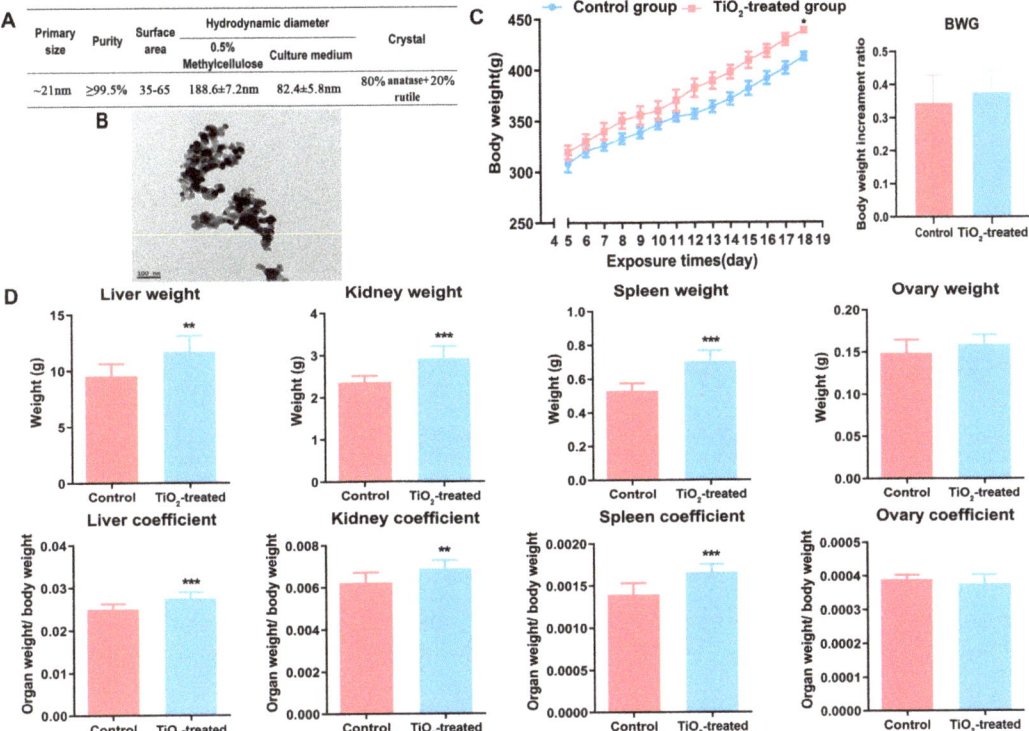

Figure 1. (**A**,**B**) The characteristics of TiO$_2$ NPs determined by a transmission electronic microscope (TEM), dynamic light scattering (DLS), and by the manufacturer's report. (**C**) Maternal body weights were determined before the female rats were fed every morning. Body weight gain (BWG) = (mf − mi)/mi. "mf" represents the final body weight and "mi" represents the initial body weight. (**D**) The main organs (liver, kidney, spleen, and ovary) were weighed and the organ coefficients were calculated after the pregnant rats were executed on GD18. * $p < 0.05$, ** $p < 0.01$, *** $p < 0.001$. There were 7 rats in the control group and 8 rats in the exposure group.

3.2. Effects of TiO$_2$ NPs on Maternal Conditions

The results revealed that the conception rate, with both groups showing 7 or 8 out of 9 successful conceptions, exhibited no difference after the observation of vaginal plugs. Maternal body weight and organ weights were recorded before and after the TiO$_2$ NPs exposure. The monitoring of body weight indicated that the maternal body weight did not differ at the beginning of the study but increased throughout the entire pregnancy period in both groups, with a significant difference observed at the end stage of pregnancy, while the body weight gain (BWG) showed no significant change (Figure 1C). Additionally, compared to control rats, the weight of the maternal liver, kidney, spleen, and their corresponding organ coefficients, all increased on GD18 following exposure. Conversely, the weight of the ovary and the ovarian coefficient showed no significant change between the two groups on GD18 (Figure 1D).

3.3. Pathological Changes of Maternal Organs after TiO$_2$ NPs Exposure

The maternal liver, kidney, spleen and ovary were examined by hematoxylin–eosin (HE) staining. Compared with the control group, hyperemia occurred in the liver after exposure, resulting in an edema and the degeneration of liver cells in the hyperemic areas, with degenerative particles appearing in the cytoplasm. This occurred partly, rather than diffusing throughout the entire organ. After the TiO$_2$ NPs exposure, we observed that the volume of glomeruli increased and the renal tubular cells exhibited edema. The maternal splenic corpuscles either disappeared or were demolished, with splenic sinusoids exhibiting hyperemia. The area of white pulp decreased, indicating atrophy of the white pulp. Additionally, the splenic marginal zone widened. In comparison to the control group, the maternal ovary showed no pathological changes after exposure (Figure 2).

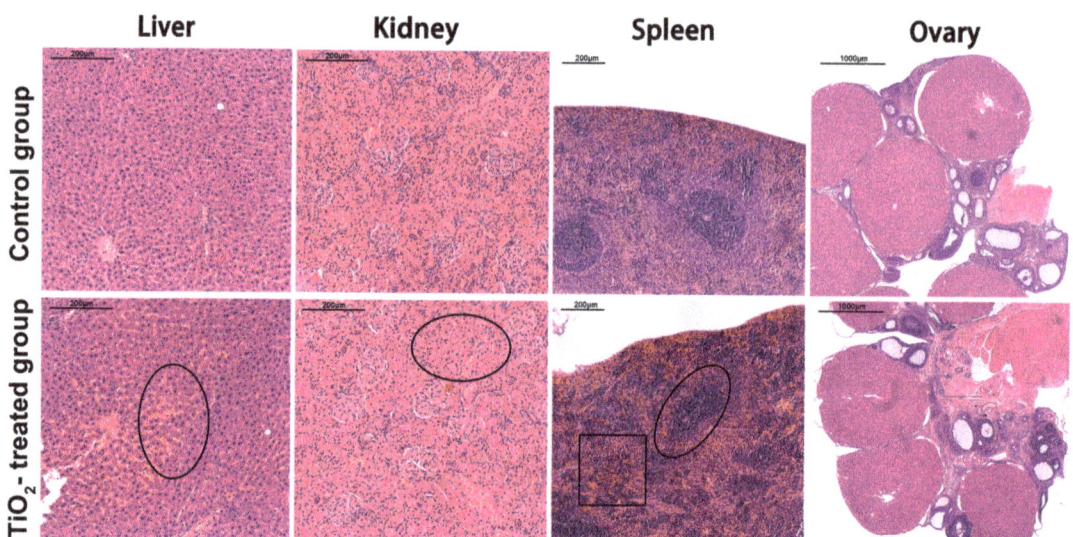

Figure 2. The pathological changes in the maternal liver, kidney, spleen, and ovary after exposure were examined by light microscope after hematoxylin and eosin (HE) staining. Scale bar = 200 μm in the liver, kidney, and spleen. Scale bar = 1000 μm in the ovary. Pathological changes in the liver, kidney, and spleen were indicated with black circles, and hyperemia region was indicated with black square. There were 7 rats in the control group and 8 rats in the exposure group.

3.4. Effects of TiO$_2$ NPs on Fetal Birth Outcomes

Compared with the control group, the early embryo resorption rate significantly increased after an exposure to TiO$_2$ NPs, with a ratio of 0.019 (2/105) in the control group and 0.0737 (7/95) in the exposure group. Moreover, the number of pregnant rats experiencing embryo loss significantly increased (2/7 in the control group and 5/8 in the exposure group). Even a monocyesis was observed after exposure, which barely happens during normal pregnancy (Figure S1). Although there was a decreasing trend, the total number and total weight of the fetuses (including the fetus, placenta, and uterus) did not show a significant difference after their exposure to TiO$_2$ NPs (Figure 3A,B). However, the average body weight (Figure 3C) and body length (Figure 3D,E) of the fetal rats decreased significantly ($p < 0.05$). The average placental diameters showed no difference (Figure 3G,H), while their corresponding weights exhibited a slight but significant increase (0.05 g) in the exposure group (Figure 3F).

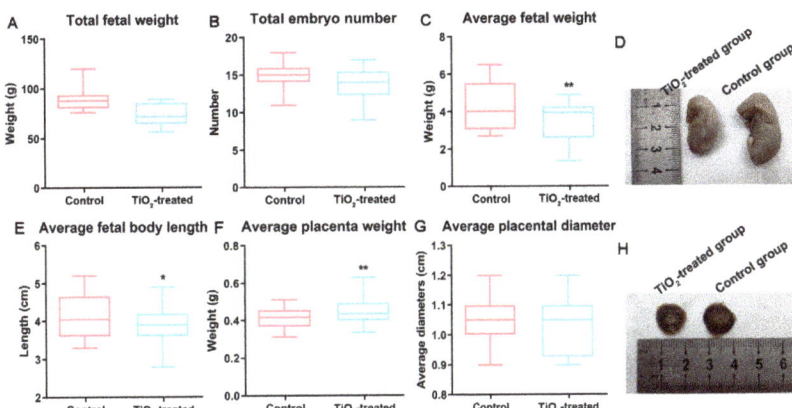

Figure 3. The main birth outcomes were recorded on GD18 after the mothers were executed. The total fetal weight (**A**), total embryo number (**B**), average fetal weight (**C**), average fetal body length (**E**), average placental weight (**F**), and placental diameter (**G**) were obtained from the control and TiO$_2$-treated group. (**D,H**) show images of the fetuses and placenta. * $p < 0.05$, ** $p < 0.01$. There were 105 fetal rats in the control group and 95 fetal rats in the exposure group.

3.5. TiO$_2$ NPs Increased Maternal Mean Arterial Pressure (MAP)

Maternal mean arterial pressures (MAPs) were measured on GD0 (before mating), GD18, and on the third day after delivery (AD3). The blood pressure monitoring results indicated no significant difference between the two groups on GD0. However, the MAP significantly increased in the exposure group on GD18 (Figure 4A). Furthermore, even after delivery, their maternal MAPs remained significantly higher than those of the control rats, indicating irreversible damage to the mothers.

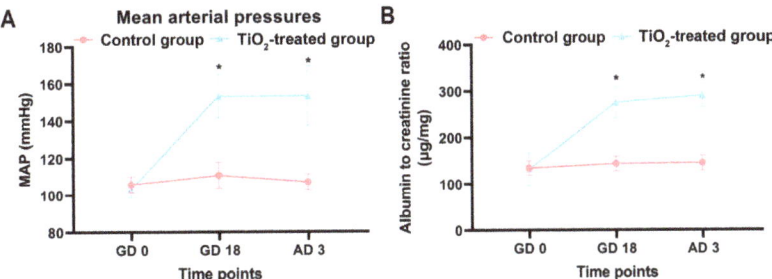

Figure 4. (**A**) The average maternal arterial pressures were measured using a non-invasive blood pressure analyzer before pregnancy (GD0), on the 18th day of gestation (GD18), and on the third day after delivery (AD3). (**B**) The maternal urinary protein levels were determined using spot urine samples, and the urinary albumin to creatinine ratio (ACR) was utilized to normalize the proteinuria. The data were indicated as mean ± SD. * $p < 0.05$. There were 7 rats in the control group and 8 rats in the exposure group.

3.6. TiO$_2$ NPs Induced Maternal Proteinuria

Maternal proteinuria was assessed on GD0, GD18, and AD3. The findings revealed that, after adjusting for the effects of creatinine, the albumin-to-creatinine ratio (ACR) significantly increased in the TiO$_2$ NPs exposure group on GD18, indicating the occurrence of proteinuria (Figure 4B). Moreover, the proteinuria persisted on the third day after delivery, showing no signs of diminishing.

3.7. Effects of TiO₂ NPs on Placental Infiltration into Uterus

Placental infiltration and spiral artery (SA) remodeling were assessed using image analysis software after revealing interstitial trophoblastic cells and smooth muscle cells. The immunohistochemistry results indicated a decreased ratio of cytokeratin-positive and an increased ratio of actin-positive cells in SA (Figure 5A,B). The area percentage of interstitial trophoblast invasion into the maternal tissue (MT) significantly decreased after the maternal exposure to TiO₂ NPs (Figure 5C). Additionally, a reduction in both the number and cross-section areas of the spiral arteries (SAs) in the placental triangle was observed in the TiO₂ NPs group compared to the control group (Figure 5D).

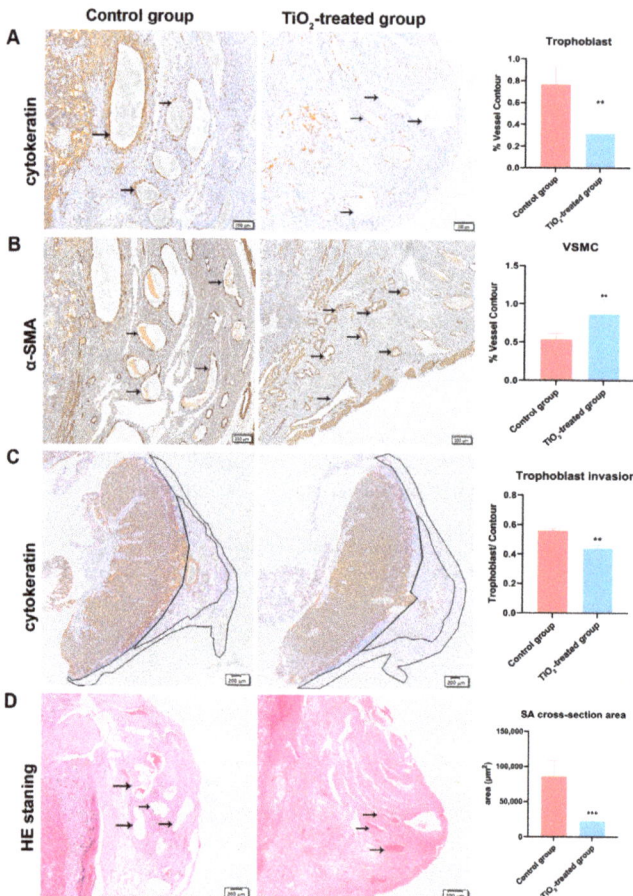

Figure 5. (**A**) A placental invasion ability assessment was conducted using the percentage of interstitial trophoblast invasion into the mesometrial triangle (MT). The infiltrated trophoblast cells were identified using a cytokeratin-7 (CK-7) antibody. (**B**) Evidence of spiral artery (SA) remodeling was also identified through the α-actin-positive smooth muscle cells. (**C**) The ratio of the cytokeratin-7-positive trophoblast cell area to the MT area. (**D**) The cross-sectional areas and SA numbers were measured by HE staining. A quantitative analysis was carried out with the Olympus OlyVIA software. The data were indicated as mean ± SD. ** $p < 0.01$, *** $p < 0.001$. The obvious pathological changes were indicated with black arrows, and the trophoblast invasion areas were outlined. There were 7 rats in the control group and 8 rats in the exposure group.

3.8. Effects of TiO₂ NPs on Maternal Glomerular Basement Membrane (GBM)

This glomerulus was stained with PAS to reveal the basement membranes. As shown in Figure 6A, after the TiO_2 NPs exposure, the capillary loops of the glomerulus were thin and well defined, while the loops were blurred and the normal structures had disappeared, indicating that the GBM was destroyed. A fibrinous deposition was easily observed in the glomerulus. Figure 6B showed the ultra-microstructure observed by TEM; as shown, the control tissue showed a clear and consecutive GBM, while the GBM in the exposure group was fuzzy and became thin, fractures even occurred in certain areas.

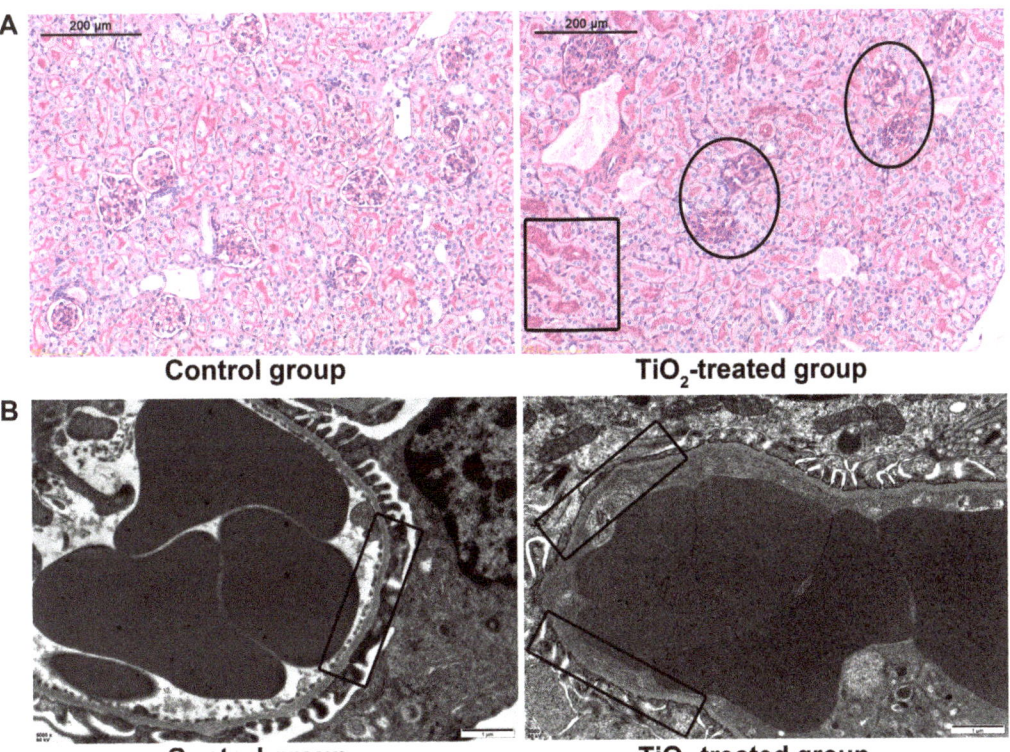

Figure 6. (**A**) The glomerular basement membrane (GBM) and deposit of fibrin were revealed by periodic acid-Schiff (PAS) staining. (**B**) The ultra microstructure of the GBM was revealed by TEM after a series of sample preparations, bar = 1 µm. The glomerular lesions were indicated with black circles, and the fibrin deposition region was indicated with a black square. The normal and impaired GBM were highlighted with black squares in TEM images. There were 7 rats in the control group and 8 rats in the exposure group.

3.9. Effects of TiO₂ NPs on the Migration and Invasion Ability of Human Trophoblastic Cells

The migration and invasion abilities of human trophoblastic cells were assessed using a transwell assay. The results (Figure 7A) revealed that, after an exposure to 10 µg/mL TiO_2 NPs, the number of penetrated cells significantly decreased when observed under a light microscope.

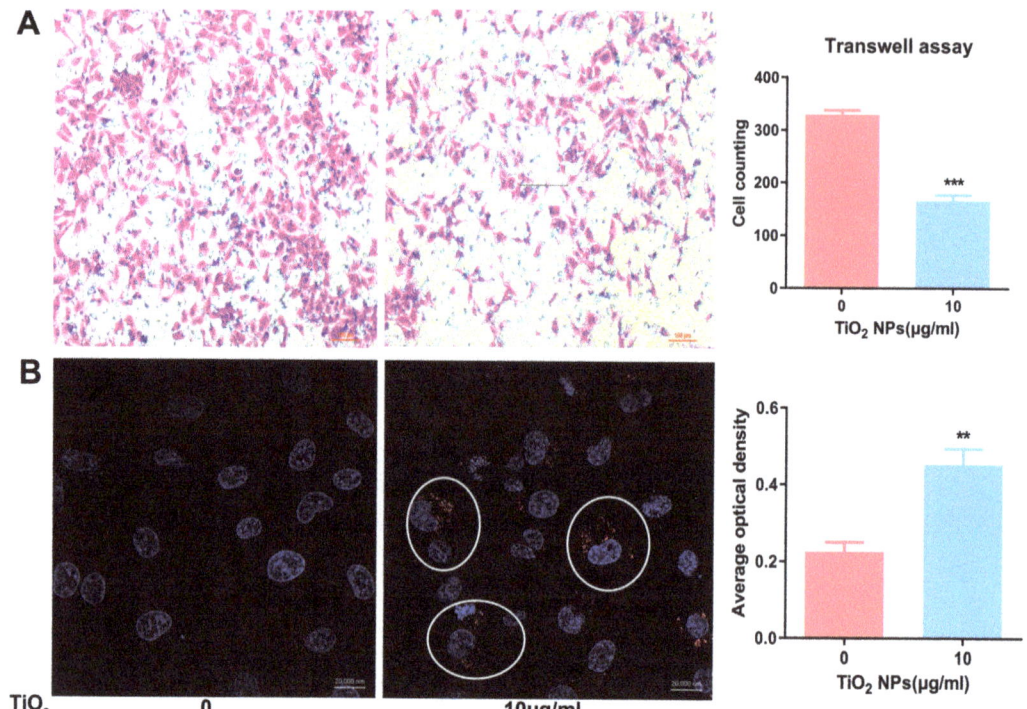

Figure 7. (**A**) The cellular migration and invasion ability of trophoblastic cell lines (HTR) were determined by a transwell assay; cell counting was obtained from five independent fields of the light microscope, and the data were presented as mean ± SD, scale bar = 100 µm. (**B**) The autophagy levels of HTR cells exposed to TiO_2 NPs were examined by immunofluorescence; the nuclei were stained blued with DAPI and the autophagosomes were stained red with CY3. Their fluorescence density was measured with the Zeiss software (https://www.zeiss.com/microscopy/en/products/software/zeiss-zen.html accessed on 9 May 2024) within the laser confocal microscope software package. Scale bar = 20,000 nm. *** $p < 0.001$, ** $p < 0.01$. The autophagsomes are indicated by the white circles in the image.

3.10. Effects of TiO_2 NPs on the Autophagy of Human Trophoblastic Cells

The autophagy levels of HTR cells were assessed through immunofluorescence combined with a confocal microscope examination following their exposure to 10 µg/mL TiO_2 NPs. Figure 7B showed that, after the exposure of TiO_2 NPs, there was an observed increase in the autophagy level of HTR cells. Specifically, in the control cells, there were few LC3-positive dots, whereas, in the treated group, numerous autophagosomes formed and accumulated in the cytoplasm.

4. Discussion

Due to the widespread use of TiO_2 NPs in everyday products and the indications of their toxicity to humans from numerous animal studies [21,22], concerns regarding their safety for human beings, particularly pregnant women, have been raised. However, to date, there is limited epidemiological evidence proving the risks of TiO_2 NPs to pregnant women and their fetuses. Therefore, establishing pregnant animal models is essential to explore the potential effects following from TiO_2 NPs exposures. In a previous study, Yamashita et al. established a pregnant mice model to investigate the adverse effects of TiO_2 NPs on maternal and fetal health. They found that the placenta played a significant role as a target organ in mediating toxicity during pregnancy [23]. However, it has been suggested that the rat placenta may be more suitable for studying human placental function, considering the similarities in its trophoblastic cell invasion and spiral arterial remodeling [24]. In this study, we opted for a pregnant rat model as it represents a suitable model and we primarily focused on placental development after TiO_2 NPs exposures.

To our knowledge, pregnant females are sensitive to their surroundings and to different manipulations, which can sometimes lead to abortion during the early stages of pregnancy [25]. However, our results indicated that the conception rate did not differ between the two groups, suggesting that the effects of manual manipulation could be disregarded. We observed that the maternal body weight across the two groups significantly increased from the 12th day. We attribute this finding to the complex changes involving organ weights and fetal weights, as well as the enhanced maternal blood glucose level reported in our previous study [26]. Specifically, major maternal organs such as the liver, kidney, and spleen exhibited hyperemia, with both organ weight and organ coefficient showing significant increases. Meanwhile, the total fetal weight decreased, a phenomenon also reported in Hong's study [27].

Previous studies evaluating TiO_2 NPs' toxicity have shown similar pathological changes in the liver, with researchers attributing these changes to inflammatory responses or disturbances in the antioxidant system [28]. The kidney, which is the main organ for TiO_2 NPs' excretion [29], exhibited glomerular swelling and an accumulation of red blood cells after exposure, consistent with previous findings [30]. This alteration may result from inflammation, as similar results have been reported in other studies [31]. The spleen, an important immune organ, contains numerous macrophages at its edges, which play a crucial role in responding to foreign substances [32]. In our study, we observed a widening of the spleen edge after exposure, indicating a vigorous immune response, consistent with previous findings that TiO_2 NPs prime a specific activation state of macrophages [33]. Additionally, a previous study demonstrated that TiO_2 NPs exert immune toxicity by inducing apoptosis and Toll-like receptor signaling [34], a finding supported by the observed atrophy of the white pulp in our study.

Researchers have found that TiO_2 NPs can induce premature ovarian failure, follicle disorders, and ovarian dysfunction in female mice [35–37], indicating reproductive toxicity in this species. However, no obvious pathological changes were observed in the present study. This might be explained by the fact that, during pregnancy, follicle development halts and its blood supply decreases compared to that in non-pregnant females, potentially reducing the impact on the ovary, similar to the kidney responses.

Following the exposure to TiO_2 NPs, there was a significant increase in embryo loss, consistent with a previous finding [38]. Our results, along with those of previous reports, suggest that TiO_2 NPs may increase the abortion rate in humans after maternal exposure. Decreases in average body weight and length suggest inhibited fetal development, raising concerns about the potential associations between TiO_2 NPs exposure and low fetal birth weight or fetal growth restriction (FGR) in humans. As far as our knowledge extends, the placenta plays a crucial role in embryo development, and the failure of proper placental invasion can lead to abnormal fetal development. Therefore, placental infiltration was further evaluated in our study.

The migration and invasion of trophoblast cells are known to be associated with the maternal vascular network [39], and the invasion of trophoblast cells into the spiral arteries is a critical process for vascular remodeling during pregnancy. Therefore, we evaluated indicators closely related to placental development, including the percentage of the area invaded by trophoblast cells in the mesometrial triangles, the presence of trophoblast cells resting on a fibrinoid layer [18], and the cross-sectional area of the spiral arteries [19]. Our results suggested an insufficient invasion of the placenta into the endometrium and a failure to complete spiral artery remodeling. This restricted fetal blood supply and affected fetal development, resulting in decreased fetal weight and length in the exposure group, resembling the progression of preeclampsia.

Inflammatory responses, cell apoptosis, and reactive oxygen species (ROS) were observed in a placenta model after a maternal exposure to TiO_2 NPs [40,41]. The authors suggested these as possible mechanisms for placental vascular dysfunction. Recent studies have shown that autophagy is an important mechanism contributing to placental dysplasia [42]. Additionally, TiO_2 NPs have been reported to induce autophagy in various cell lines [43], potentially inhibiting the normal development of the rat placenta by inducing autophagy in trophoblastic cells. Therefore, we investigated whether autophagy plays a crucial role in TiO_2 NPs-induced placental dysfunction. Our results showed a significant increase in autophagy levels in the labyrinthine placenta after exposure. The evidence indicates that TiO_2 NPs can accumulate in the placenta and reach relatively high levels even after exposure during pregnancy [27]. To verify whether TiO_2 NPs could induce autophagy at relatively low doses, we administered 10 µg/mL of TiO_2 NPs to HTR, a human-derived cell line, for further study. The results confirmed that TiO_2 NPs could induce cell autophagy and inhibit the migration and invasion ability of human trophoblastic cells, validating the results observed in animal studies and raising concerns about the risks to pregnant women.

Considering that TiO_2 NPs induced significant pathological and functional changes in both the kidney and placenta, resembling those seen in preeclampsia, our study observed increased blood pressure and the appearance of proteinuria after exposure, on GD18. Previous animal studies suggested that TiO_2 NPs may deposit on the glomerular basement membrane, inducing kidney inflammation, although the total urine protein levels did not significantly change [44]. In our study, proteinuria was detected, potentially indicating an increased kidney burden during pregnancy and protein leakage. It has been reported that nanoparticles can induce kidney injury and elevate urinary retinol-binding proteins, supporting our findings [45]. The kidney plays a crucial role in blood pressure regulation [46], and TiO_2 has been shown to activate ROS [47] or induce fibrosis via the Wnt pathway [48], thus contributing to increased blood pressure through renal impairment via reported or undetermined pathways after a TiO_2 NPs exposure. An important characteristic of preeclampsia is the resolution of hypertension and proteinuria after delivery. However, in our study, hypertension and proteinuria did not revert to pre-pregnancy levels. It is important to note that the disease induced by TiO_2 NPs is not traditional preeclampsia, and treatments for preeclampsia may not be effective and could potentially exacerbate these related clinical symptoms during pregnancy. In our previous work, we identified targets for reversing autophagy to mitigate the adverse effects of TiO_2 NPs during human placental development [49]. However, considering that microRNAs are species-specific and the candidate microRNAs identified in human trophoblastic cells may not be suitable for use in rats, we were unable to observe birth outcomes and placental development after reversing placental autophagy. Nonetheless, targeting autophagy reversal may be a useful approach to alleviating TiO_2 NPs-related symptoms in pregnant women.

5. Conclusions

In this study, we demonstrated that pregnant rats exposed to TiO_2 NPs via their digestive tract from GD5 to GD18 exhibited significant alterations in maternal physiology, organ pathology, fetal growth restriction, and a maternal preeclampsia-like syndrome. The adverse effects on the fetus and mother may be associated with placental dysplasia, which may be related to deficiencies in autophagy-related cell migration and invasion. Overall, TiO_2 NPs induced symptoms resembling those of preeclampsia in pregnant rats.

Supplementary Materials: The following supporting information can be downloaded at https://www.mdpi.com/article/10.3390/toxics12050367/s1, Figure S1: The image of the maternal uterus that carried single pregnancy.

Author Contributions: H.L. carried out the animal study and wrote the manuscript, H.H. was responsible for the cell study, D.M. was responsible for the data analysis, P.X. guided the placenta function assessment, Z.M. and K.Z. designed the study and provided the funding support, K.Z.

also helped to revise the draft. All authors have read and agreed to the published version of the manuscript.

Funding: The study was founded by Social Developmental Project of Changzhou Science and Technology Bureau (CE20215037); Top Talent of Changzhou "The 14th Five Year Plan" High-Level Health Talents Training Project (2022CZLJ088).

Institutional Review Board Statement: The animal study protocol was approved by the Ethics Committee of Nanjing Medical University (IACUC-24040115).

Informed Consent Statement: Not applicable.

Data Availability Statement: The data presented in this study are available on request from the corresponding author.

Conflicts of Interest: The authors declare no conflicts of interest.

References

1. Baranowska-Wojcik, E.; Szwajgier, D.; Oleszczuk, P.; Winiarska-Mieczan, A. Effects of Titanium Dioxide Nanoparticles Exposure on Human Health—A Review. *Biol. Trace Elem. Res.* **2019**, *193*, 118–129. [CrossRef]
2. Warheit, D.B.; Donner, E.M. Risk assessment strategies for nanoscale and fine-sized titanium dioxide particles: Recognizing hazard and exposure issues. *Food Chem. Toxicol.* **2015**, *85*, 138–147. [CrossRef] [PubMed]
3. Gulson, B.; McCall, M.J.; Bowman, D.M.; Pinheiro, T. A review of critical factors for assessing the dermal absorption of metal oxide nanoparticles from sunscreens applied to humans, and a research strategy to address current deficiencies. *Arch. Toxicol.* **2015**, *89*, 1909–1930. [CrossRef] [PubMed]
4. Shi, H.; Magaye, R.; Castranova, V.; Zhao, J. Titanium dioxide nanoparticles: A review of current toxicological data. *Part. Fibre Toxicol.* **2013**, *10*, 15. [CrossRef]
5. Takeda, K.; Shinkai, Y.; Suzuki, K.; Yanagita, S.; Umezawa, M.; Yokota, S.; Tainaka, H.; Oshio, S.; Ihara, T.; Sugamata, M. Health effects of nanomaterials on next generation. *Yakugaku Zasshi* **2011**, *131*, 229–236. [CrossRef]
6. Warheit, D.B. Hazard and risk assessment strategies for nanoparticle exposures: How far have we come in the past 10 years? *F1000Research* **2018**, *7*, 376. [CrossRef]
7. Grande, F.; Tucci, P. Titanium Dioxide Nanoparticles: A Risk for Human Health? *Mini Rev. Med. Chem.* **2016**, *16*, 762–769. [CrossRef] [PubMed]
8. Naserzadeh, P.; Ghanbary, F.; Ashtari, P.; Seydi, E.; Ashtari, K.; Akbari, M. Biocompatibility assessment of titanium dioxide nanoparticles in mice fetoplacental unit. *J. Biomed. Mater. Res. A* **2018**, *106*, 580–589. [CrossRef]
9. Hong, F.; Zhou, Y.; Ji, J.; Zhuang, J.; Sheng, L.; Wang, L. Nano-TiO$_2$ Inhibits Development of the Central Nervous System and Its Mechanism in Offspring Mice. *J. Agric. Food Chem.* **2018**, *66*, 11767–11774. [CrossRef]
10. Burton, G.J.; Fowden, A.L. The placenta: A multifaceted, transient organ. *Philos. Trans. R. Soc. Lond. B Biol. Sci.* **2015**, *370*, 20140066. [CrossRef]
11. Silva, J.F.; Serakides, R. Intrauterine trophoblast migration: A comparative view of humans and rodents. *Cell Adh. Migr.* **2016**, *10*, 88–110. [CrossRef]
12. Salavati, N.; Smies, M.; Ganzevoort, W.; Charles, A.K.; Erwich, J.J.; Plosch, T.; Gordijn, S.J. The Possible Role of Placental Morphometry in the Detection of Fetal Growth Restriction. *Front. Physiol.* **2018**, *9*, 1884. [CrossRef]
13. Zong, S.; Li, C.; Luo, C.; Zhao, X.; Liu, C.; Wang, K.; Jia, W.; Bai, M.; Yin, M.; Bao, S.; et al. Dysregulated expression of IDO may cause unexplained recurrent spontaneous abortion through suppression of trophoblast cell proliferation and migration. *Sci. Rep.* **2016**, *6*, 19916. [CrossRef]
14. Lyall, F.; Robson, S.C.; Bulmer, J.N. Spiral artery remodeling and trophoblast invasion in preeclampsia and fetal growth restriction: Relationship to clinical outcome. *Hypertension* **2013**, *62*, 1046–1054. [CrossRef] [PubMed]
15. Gutierrez, J.A.; Gomez, I.; Chiarello, D.I.; Salsoso, R.; Klein, A.D.; Guzman-Gutierrez, E.; Toledo, F.; Sobrevia, L. Role of proteases in dysfunctional placental vascular remodelling in preeclampsia. *Biochim. Biophys. Acta Mol. Basis Dis.* **2019**, *1866*, 165448. [CrossRef]
16. Auttachoat, W.; McLoughlin, C.E.; White, K.L., Jr.; Smith, M.J. Route-dependent systemic and local immune effects following exposure to solutions prepared from titanium dioxide nanoparticles. *J. Immunotoxicol.* **2014**, *11*, 273–282. [CrossRef]
17. Jovanović, B. Critical review of public health regulations of titanium dioxide, a human food additive. *Integr. Environ. Assess. Manag.* **2015**, *11*, 10–20. [CrossRef] [PubMed]
18. Vercruysse, L.; Caluwaerts, S.; Luyten, C.; Pijnenborg, R. Interstitial trophoblast invasion in the decidua and mesometrial triangle during the last third of pregnancy in the rat. *Placenta* **2006**, *27*, 22–33. [CrossRef]
19. Cotechini, T.; Komisarenko, M.; Sperou, A.; Macdonald-Goodfellow, S.; Adams, M.A.; Graham, C.H. Inflammation in rat pregnancy inhibits spiral artery remodeling leading to fetal growth restriction and features of preeclampsia. *J. Exp. Med.* **2014**, *211*, 165–179. [CrossRef]

20. Aziz, K.M.A. Association of High Levels of Spot Urine Protein with High Blood Pressure, Mean Arterial Pressure and Pulse Pressure with Development of Diabetic Chronic Kidney Dysfunction or Failure among Diabetic Patients. Statistical Regression Modeling to Predict Diabetic Proteinuria. *Curr. Diabetes Rev.* **2018**, *15*, 486–496.
21. Asare, N.; Duale, N.; Slagsvold, H.H.; Lindeman, B.; Olsen, A.K.; Gromadzka-Ostrowska, J.; Meczynska-Wielgosz, S.; Kruszewski, M.; Brunborg, G.; Instanes, C. Genotoxicity and gene expression modulation of silver and titanium dioxide nanoparticles in mice. *Nanotoxicology* **2016**, *10*, 312–321. [CrossRef] [PubMed]
22. Ebrahimzadeh Bideskan, A.; Mohammadipour, A.; Fazel, A.; Haghir, H.; Rafatpanah, H.; Hosseini, M.; Rajabzadeh, A. Maternal exposure to titanium dioxide nanoparticles during pregnancy and lactation alters offspring hippocampal mRNA BAX and Bcl-2 levels, induces apoptosis and decreases neurogenesis. *Exp. Toxicol. Pathol.* **2017**, *69*, 329–337. [CrossRef] [PubMed]
23. Yamashita, K.; Yoshioka, Y.; Higashisaka, K.; Mimura, K.; Morishita, Y.; Nozaki, M.; Yoshida, T.; Ogura, T.; Nabeshi, H.; Nagano, K.; et al. Silica and titanium dioxide nanoparticles cause pregnancy complications in mice. *Nat. Nanotechnol.* **2011**, *6*, 321–328. [CrossRef] [PubMed]
24. Grigsby, P.L. Animal Models to Study Placental Development and Function throughout Normal and Dysfunctional Human Pregnancy. *Semin. Reprod. Med.* **2016**, *34*, 11–16. [CrossRef] [PubMed]
25. Bettahar, K.; Pinton, A.; Boisrame, T.; Cavillon, V.; Wylomanski, S.; Nisand, I.; Hassoun, D. Medical induced abortion. *J. Gynecol. Obstet. Biol. Reprod.* **2016**, *45*, 1490–1514. [CrossRef]
26. Mao, Z.; Li, Y.; Dong, T.; Zhang, L.; Zhang, Y.; Li, S.; Hu, H.; Sun, C.; Xia, Y. Exposure to Titanium Dioxide Nanoparticles During Pregnancy Changed Maternal Gut Microbiota and Increased Blood Glucose of Rat. *Nanoscale Res. Lett.* **2019**, *14*, 26. [CrossRef]
27. Hong, F.; Zhou, Y.; Zhao, X.; Sheng, L.; Wang, L. Maternal exposure to nanosized titanium dioxide suppresses embryonic development in mice. *Int. J. Nanomed.* **2017**, *12*, 6197–6204. [CrossRef] [PubMed]
28. Shakeel, M.; Jabeen, F.; Iqbal, R.; Chaudhry, A.S.; Zafar, S.; Ali, M.; Khan, M.S.; Khalid, A.; Shabbir, S.; Asghar, M.S. Assessment of Titanium Dioxide Nanoparticles (TiO$_2$-NPs) Induced Hepatotoxicity and Ameliorative Effects of Cinnamomum cassia in Sprague-Dawley Rats. *Biol. Trace Elem. Res.* **2018**, *182*, 57–69. [CrossRef]
29. Cho, W.S.; Kang, B.C.; Lee, J.K.; Jeong, J.; Che, J.H.; Seok, S.H. Comparative absorption, distribution, and excretion of titanium dioxide and zinc oxide nanoparticles after repeated oral administration. *Part. Fibre Toxicol.* **2013**, *10*, 9. [CrossRef]
30. Alidadi, H.; Khorsandi, L.; Shirani, M. Effects of Quercetin on Tubular Cell Apoptosis and Kidney Damage in Rats Induced by Titanium Dioxide Nanoparticles. *Malays. J. Med. Sci.* **2018**, *25*, 72–81. [CrossRef]
31. Hong, F.; Wu, N.; Ge, Y.; Zhou, Y.; Shen, T.; Qiang, Q.; Zhang, Q.; Chen, M.; Wang, Y.; Wang, L.; et al. Nanosized titanium dioxide resulted in the activation of TGF-beta/Smads/p38MAPK pathway in renal inflammation and fibration of mice. *J. Biomed. Mater. Res. A* **2016**, *104*, 1452–1461. [CrossRef]
32. Mebius, R.E.; Kraal, G. Structure and function of the spleen, Nature reviews. *Immunology* **2005**, *5*, 606–616.
33. Huang, C.; Sun, M.; Yang, Y.; Wang, F.; Ma, X.; Li, J.; Wang, Y.; Ding, Q.; Ying, H.; Song, H.; et al. Titanium dioxide nanoparticles prime a specific activation state of macrophages. *Nanotoxicology* **2017**, *11*, 737–750. [CrossRef]
34. Dhupal, M.; Oh, J.M.; Tripathy, D.R.; Kim, S.K.; Koh, S.B.; Park, K.S. Immunotoxicity of titanium dioxide nanoparticles via simultaneous induction of apoptosis and multiple toll-like receptors signaling through ROS-dependent SAPK/JNK and p38 MAPK activation. *Int. J. Nanomed.* **2018**, *13*, 6735–6750. [CrossRef]
35. Hong, F.; Wang, L. Nanosized titanium dioxide-induced premature ovarian failure is associated with abnormalities in serum parameters in female mice. *Int. J. Nanomed.* **2018**, *13*, 2543–2549. [CrossRef]
36. Zhao, X.; Ze, Y.; Gao, G.; Sang, X.; Li, B.; Gui, S.; Sheng, L.; Sun, Q.; Cheng, J.; Cheng, Z.; et al. Nanosized TiO$_2$-induced reproductive system dysfunction and its mechanism in female mice. *PLoS ONE* **2013**, *8*, e59378. [CrossRef]
37. Gao, G.; Ze, Y.; Li, B.; Zhao, X.; Zhang, T.; Sheng, L.; Hu, R.; Gui, S.; Sang, X.; Sun, Q.; et al. Ovarian dysfunction and gene-expressed characteristics of female mice caused by long-term exposure to titanium dioxide nanoparticles. *J. Hazard. Mater.* **2012**, *243*, 19–27. [CrossRef]
38. Philbrook, N.A.; Winn, L.M.; Afrooz, A.R.; Saleh, N.B.; Walker, V.K. The effect of TiO$_{(2)}$ and Ag nanoparticles on reproduction and development of Drosophila melanogaster and CD-1 mice. *Toxicol. Appl. Pharmacol.* **2011**, *257*, 429–436. [CrossRef] [PubMed]
39. Pijnenborg, R.; Vercruysse, L.; Hanssens, M. The uterine spiral arteries in human pregnancy: Facts and controversies. *Placenta* **2006**, *27*, 939–958. [CrossRef]
40. Yin, F.; Zhu, Y.; Zhang, M.; Yu, H.; Chen, W.; Qin, J. A 3D human placenta-on-a-chip model to probe nanoparticle exposure at the placental barrier. *Toxicol. In Vitro* **2019**, *54*, 105–113. [CrossRef]
41. Zhang, L.; Xie, X.; Zhou, Y.; Yu, D.; Deng, Y.; Ouyang, J.; Yang, B.; Luo, D.; Zhang, D.; Kuang, H. Gestational exposure to titanium dioxide nanoparticles impairs the placentation through dysregulation of vascularization, proliferation and apoptosis in mice. *Int. J. Nanomed.* **2018**, *13*, 777–789. [CrossRef]
42. Huang, X.; Han, X.; Huang, Z.; Yu, M.; Zhang, Y.; Fan, Y.; Xu, B.; Zhou, K.; Song, L.; Wang, X.; et al. Maternal pentachlorophenol exposure induces developmental toxicity mediated by autophagy on pregnancy mice. *Ecotoxicol. Environ. Saf.* **2019**, *169*, 829–836. [CrossRef]
43. Dai, X.; Liu, R.; Li, N.; Yi, J. Titanium dioxide nanoparticles induce in vitro autophagy. *Hum. Exp. Toxicol.* **2019**, *38*, 56–64. [CrossRef] [PubMed]
44. Valentini, X.; Rugira, P.; Frau, A.; Tagliatti, V.; Conotte, R.; Laurent, S.; Colet, J.M.; Nonclercq, D. Hepatic and Renal Toxicity Induced by TiO$_2$ Nanoparticles in Rats: A Morphological and Metabonomic Study. *J. Toxicol.* **2019**, *2019*, 5767012. [CrossRef]

45. Fontana, L.; Leso, V.; Marinaccio, A.; Cenacchi, G.; Papa, V.; Leopold, K.; Schindl, R.; Bocca, B.; Alimonti, A.; Iavicoli, I. The effects of palladium nanoparticles on the renal function of female Wistar rats. *Nanotoxicology* **2015**, *9*, 843–851. [CrossRef] [PubMed]
46. Sato, R.; Luthe, S.K.; Nasu, M. Blood pressure and acute kidney injury. *Crit. Care* **2017**, *21*, 28. [CrossRef]
47. Niu, L.; Shao, M.; Liu, Y.; Hu, J.; Li, R.; Xie, H.; Zhou, L.; Shi, L.; Zhang, R.; Niu, Y. Reduction of oxidative damages induced by titanium dioxide nanoparticles correlates with induction of the Nrf2 pathway by GSPE supplementation in mice. *Chem.-Biol. Interact.* **2017**, *275*, 133–144. [CrossRef]
48. Hong, F.; Hong, J.; Wang, L.; Zhou, Y.; Liu, D.; Xu, B.; Yu, X.; Sheng, L. Chronic exposure to nanoparticulate TiO_2 causes renal fibrosis involving activation of the Wnt pathway in mouse kidney. *J. Agric. Food Chem.* **2015**, *63*, 1639–1647. [CrossRef]
49. Mao, Z.; Yao, M.; Li, Y.; Fu, Z.; Li, S.; Zhang, L.; Zhou, Z.; Tang, Q.; Han, X.; Xia, Y. miR-96-5p and miR-101-3p as potential intervention targets to rescue TiO_2 NP-induced autophagy and migration impairment of human trophoblastic cells. *Biomater. Sci.* **2018**, *6*, 3273–3283. [CrossRef]

Disclaimer/Publisher's Note: The statements, opinions and data contained in all publications are solely those of the individual author(s) and contributor(s) and not of MDPI and/or the editor(s). MDPI and/or the editor(s) disclaim responsibility for any injury to people or property resulting from any ideas, methods, instructions or products referred to in the content.

Cigarette Smoke-Induced Gastric Cancer Cell Exosomes Affected the Fate of Surrounding Normal Cells via the Circ0000670/Wnt/β-Catenin Axis

Zhaofeng Liang [1,*,†], Shikun Fang [1,2,†], Yue Zhang [1], Xinyi Zhang [1], Yumeng Xu [1], Hui Qian [1] and Hao Geng [3,*]

[1] Jiangsu Key Laboratory of Medical Science and Laboratory Medicine, School of Medicine, Jiangsu University, Zhenjiang 212013, China
[2] Department of Clinical Laboratory, The Affiliated Taizhou People's Hospital of Nanjing Medical University, Taizhou 225300, China
[3] Department of Urology, Hospital of Anhui Medical University, Hefei 230032, China
* Correspondence: liangzhaofeng@ujs.edu.cn (Z.L.); 13739296089@163.com (H.G.)
† These authors contributed equally to this work.

Abstract: Cigarette smoke is a major risk factor for gastric cancer. Exosomes are an important part of intercellular and intra-organ communication systems and can carry circRNA and other components to play a regulatory role in the occurrence and development of gastric cancer. However, it is unclear whether cigarette smoke can affect exosomes and exosomal circRNA to promote the development of gastric cancer. Exosomes secreted by cancer cells promote cancer development by affecting surrounding normal cells. Herein, we aimed to clarify whether the exosomes secreted by cigarette smoke-induced gastric cancer cells can promote the development of gastric cancer by affecting the surrounding gastric mucosal epithelial cells (GES-1). In the present study, we treated gastric cancer cells with cigarette smoke extract for 4 days and demonstrated that cigarette smoke promotes the stemness and EMT of gastric cancer cells and cigarette smoke-induced exosomes promote stemness gene expression, EMT processes and the proliferation of GES-1 cells. We further found that circ0000670 was up-regulated in tissues of gastric cancer patients with smoking history, cigarette smoke-induced gastric cancer cells and their exosomes. Functional assays showed that circ0000670 knockdown inhibited the promoting effects of cigarette smoke-induced exosomes on the stemness and EMT characteristic of GES-1 cells, whereas its overexpression had the opposite effect. In addition, exosomal circ0000670 was found to promote the development of gastric cancer by regulating the Wnt/β-catenin pathway. Our findings indicated that exosomal circ0000670 promotes cigarette smoke-induced gastric cancer development, which might provide a new basis for the treatment of cigarette smoke-related gastric cancer.

Keywords: gastric cancer; cigarette smoke; circRNA; exosomes; Wnt/β-catenin

1. Introduction

Gastric cancer is the fourth most common malignant cancer and the third most common cause of cancer-related death worldwide, with more than 1 million new cases and 769,000 deaths annually [1]. Many factors are related to the occurrence and development of gastric cancer, including gene mutations, infection, dietary factors, environmental factors and cigarette smoke, among other [2,3]. Increasing evidence has shown that cigarette smoke is closely related to the initiation and progression of gastric cancer [2]. Our previous studies also found that cigarette smoke exposure induced malignant transformation and epithelial–mesenchymal transition (EMT) in mouse gastric tissues [4,5]. Although progress has been made in understanding the relationship between cigarette smoke and gastric cancer, the underlying mechanisms are still unclear. Whether cigarette smoke-induced gastric cancer cells can somehow affect surrounding normal cells and promote the development of gastric cancer is also not clear.

Exosomes are an important component of extracellular vesicles, with a size of 30–150 nm, and they are secreted by almost all cell types. Exosomes are an important part of the communication system between cells and within organs, and they can transfer active molecules and biological signals from one cell type or tissue to another [6,7]. Many studies have indicated that exosomes play a decisive role in the occurrence and development of gastric cancer [8,9]. The results of Yoon et al. identified that gastric cancer exosomes induce the transformation and field cancerization of the surrounding gastric epithelial cells [10]. Another study showed that cancer-associated fibroblasts secrete exosomal miR-522 to inhibit ferroptosis in gastric cancer cells by targeting ALOX15 and blocking lipid reactive oxygen species (ROS) accumulation [11]. Cao et al. demonstrated that linc00852 from cisplatin-resistant gastric cancer cell-derived exosomes regulates the COMM domain protein 7 to promote the resistance of recipient cells [12]. It was further reported that exosomes inhibit HSP90 degradation and promote gastric cancer progression by regulating the circSHKBP1/miR-582-3p/HUR axis [13]. Zhang et al. found that circNRIP1 affects metabolic changes in gastric cancer cells and promotes the occurrence and development of gastric cancer through exosome transport and the regulation of the miR-149-5p-AKT1/mTOR axis [14]. Previous studies by our research team also found that exosomes transport active molecules and play a regulatory role in the occurrence and development of gastric cancer [15–17]. However, it is unclear whether cigarette smoke can affect exosomes and their transport molecules, such as circular RNAs (circRNAs), to promote the occurrence and development of gastric cancer.

CircRNAs are covalently closed noncoding RNA with obvious tissue specificity and cell specificity [18,19]. The abnormal expression of circRNAs is closely related to the occurrence and development of gastric cancer. Previous results have shown that METTL14-mediated circORC5 mA modification inhibited the progression of gastric cancer by regulating the miR-30c-2-3p/AKT1S1 axis [20]. Furthermore, a study by Peng et al. revealed that circAXIN1 encodes protein AXIN1-295aa, which activates the Wnt/β-catenin pathway to promote gastric cancer progression [21]. Moreover, as the protein decoy of IGF2BP3, circTNPO3 regulates the Myc/Snail axis to inhibit gastric cancer cell proliferation and metastasis [22]. A previous study by our team found that circDIDO1 encodes DIDO1-529aa and inhibits gastric cancer development by regulating PRDX2 stability [15].

CircRNA transport through exosomes has an important role in the occurrence and development of gastric cancer [23]. Exosomal cirHKBP1 promotes the progression of gastric cancer by regulating the miR-582-3p/HuR/VEGF axis and inhibiting Hsp90 degradation [13]. Exosomal circNEK9 accelerates the progression of gastric cancer by regulating the miR-409-3p/MAP7 axis [24]. Li et al. reported that the exosome-mediated transport of circ29 promotes angiogenesis and gastric cancer progression by targeting the miR-29a/VEGF pathway [25]. Studies have also found that cigarette smoke promotes the occurrence and development of diseases by affecting the secretion or transport of active components of exosomes [26–29]. In addition, cigarette smoke can regulate the expression of circRNAs [30–33]. However, it is unclear whether cigarette smoke can regulate the expression of exosomal circRNA derived from gastric cancer cells, ultimately affecting the surrounding normal cells to promote the development of gastric cancer.

In summary, we speculated that circRNAs derived from cigarette smoke-induced gastric cancer cell exosomes might affect surrounding normal cells to promote gastric cancer development. As expected, we present in vitro evidence to demonstrate that cigarette smoke-induced gastric cancer cell exosomes can enter surrounding normal cells to promote the development of gastric cancer. Moreover, we found that circ0000670 is a key exosomal component that promotes the development of cigarette smoke-related gastric cancer via the Wnt/β-catenin pathway.

2. Materials and Methods

2.1. Cell and Cell Culture

The human gastric cancer cell lines HGC-27 and AGS were purchased from Shanghai EK-Bioscience Biotechnology (Shanghai, China). Human gastric epithelial cells (GES-1) were purchased from Shanghai GEFAN Biotechnology (Shanghai, China). HGC-27 cells were cultured in RPMI-1640 medium (BioInd biological industries, Israel, catalog number: 01-100-1A). GES-1 and AGS cells were cultured in RPMI-1640 medium (BioInd biological industries, Kibbutz Beit Haemek, Israel). All cells were cultured in medium supplemented with 10% FBS (Bovogen Biologicals, Keilor East, Australia, catalog number: SFBS) at 37 °C and 5% CO_2.

2.2. Preparation of Cigarette Smoke Extract

Cigarette smoke extract was prepared daily before use according to the reported method [34]. Briefly, one filterless 3R4F reference cigarette (9.4 mg tar and 0.73 mg nicotine/cigarette) was lit and the smoke was continuously drawn through a glass syringe containing 10 mL of fetal bovine serum-free medium pre-warmed to 37 °C at a rate of 5 min/cigarette to generate a cigarette smoke extract solution. A control solution was prepared with the same protocol, except that the cigarette was unlit. The resulting solution was adjusted to pH 7.4 and then filtered through a 0.22 μm pore filter. The obtained suspension was referred to as a 100% cigarette smoke extract solution.

2.3. Cell Counting Kit-8 Assay

For the cell counting kit-8 (CCK8) assay, which can be used to detect changes in cell viability, cells were digested, resuspended, counted and planted in 96-well plates (1×10^3 cells/well) [34] (Corning, New York, NY, USA, catalog number: 3599). Next, 110 μL medium containing 10 μL CCK-8 reagent (Vazyme, Nanjing, China, catalog number: A311-02) was added to each well and then incubated for 2 h at 37 °C. The absorbance of each well at 450 nm was measured using a microplate reader (Themo, Waltham, MA, USA). The experiment was repeated at least three times in each group.

2.4. Colony Formation Assay

Cells were digested, resuspended, counted and seeded into 6-well plates (1000 cells/well) for the indicated time [35]. The culture medium of cells in each group was changed every 3 days. At the end of the incubation period, the cells were fixed with 4% paraformaldehyde and stained with crystal violet.

2.5. Cell Migration Assays

The exponential growth period cells (4×10^4) were seeded into the upper chamber in 24-well plates. The lower chamber was filled with 500 μL medium with 10% FBS. After 12–24 h of culture, these migrated cells at the bottom of the transwells (8 μm) were fixed with 4% paraformaldehyde, stained with crystal violet and then photographed under a microscope [15].

2.6. Lentiviral Transfection

The circ0000670 overexpression, knockdown and control lentivectors were purchased from Hanbio Biotechnology (Shanghai, China). Cells in good condition at the logarithmic growth stage were seeded in 6-well plates (8×10^4 cells/well). After 24 h, lentivirus particles at an appropriate MOI (when overexpressed, the MOI of HGC-27 cells is 125, while that of AGS cells is 60. For knockdown, the MOI of HGC-27 cells is 100, while that of AGS cells is 60) were then added to the medium and incubated for 24–48 h. An appropriate concentration of puromycin and 10% FBS medium were used to select the stably transfected cell lines [35].

2.7. RNA Extraction and Real-Time PCR

Total RNA was isolated from cells using Trizol (Gibco, New York, USA, catalog number: 15596018) and other reagents according to the experimental protocol. Reverse transcription was performed according to the protocol of the reverse transcription kit manufacturer (Vazyme, Nanjing, China, catalog number: R111-02) using 1 μg RNA [36].

A real-time PCR experiment was carried out on a Step One Plus Real Time PCR System (ABI, Shrewsbury, MA, USA) by using AceQ qpcr Sybr green master mix (Vazyme, Nanjing, China, catalog number: Q111). β-actin served as the loading control. Fold changes in genes expression were evaluated using the $2^{-\Delta\Delta Ct}$ method. The primers were synthesized by biological companies (Invitrogen, Waltham, MA, USA) and the primer sequences are listed in Table 1.

Table 1. Primer sequences.

Gene Name	Primer Sequences (5'-3')
OCT4	F:5'-TGGAGAAGGTGGAACCAACT-3' R:5'-AGATGGTGGTCTGGCTGAAC-3'
NANOG	F:5'-GGAACGCCTCATCAATGC-3' R:5'-TGTCAGCCTCAGGACTTGAGA-3'
SOX2	F:5'-ACACCAATCCCATCCACACT-3' R:5'-GCAAACTTCCTGCAAAGCTC-3'
N-cadherin	F:5'-CTCCACTTCCACCTCCACAT-3' R:5'-GGACTCGCACCAGGAGTAAT-3'
E-cadherin	F:5'-GGACTCGCACCAGGAGTAAT-3' R:5'-TTGGCTGAGGATGGTGTAAG-3'
Vimentin	F:5'-GAGCTGCAGGAGCTGAATG-3' R:5'-AGGTCAAGACGTGCCAGAG-3'
circ0000670	F:5'-GGTTCATACCTCTAATTCATGTGG-3' R:5'-CATTTTCTTCCTAGACAAAGCCTTA-3'
β-catenin	F:5'-TGACACCTCCCAAGTCCTTT-3' R:5'-TTGCATACTGCCCGTCAAT-3'
GAPDH	F:5'-GCTGCCCAACGCACCGAATA-3' R:5'-GAGTCAACGGATTTGGTCGT-3'

2.8. Agarose Gel Electrophoresis

We laced the agarose gel (2.0%) in the electrophoresis tank, mixed 10 μL of PCR product, buffer solution and marker, then added this into the sample well. We performed electrophoresis for 40 min at 110 V then EB staining for 10 min, and the results were observed with a gel imaging system [37].

2.9. Western Blotting

Total proteins from cells were harvested and lysed in radioimmunoprecipitation buffer supplemented with 1% protease inhibitors (Pierce, Dorchester, MA, USA, catalog number: 88668). Equal amounts of the total protein were separated on 7.5%–10% SDS-polyacrylamide gel and transferred to 0.45 μm PVDF membranes [38] (Millipore, Burlington, MA, USA, catalog number: IPVH00010). After being blocked with 5% skimmed milk for 1 h, the membranes were incubated with the primary antibodies for GAPDH (1:5000, Bioworld, Minneapolis, MN, USA, catalog number: AP0063), Vimentin, SOX2 (1:1000, Bioworld, Minneapolis, MN, USA, catalog number: BS1491, MB0064), E-cadherin, N-cadherin (1:1000, CST, USA, catalog number: 3195T, 13116P), NANOG, LIN28 and CD44 (1:500, SAB, Los Angeles, CA, USA, catalog number: 21423, 21626) at 4 °C overnight. After being washed three times with tris-buffered saline and Tween, the membrane was incubated with horseradish peroxidase-conjugated secondary antibody (1:5000, Bioworld, Minneapolis, MN, USA) for 1 h. Then, the protein bands were visualized using an enhanced chemiluminescent substrate detection system (Millipore, Burlington, MA, USA, catalog number: WBKLS0500).

2.10. Extraction and Identification of Exosomes

We inoculated the same number of cells into the culture dishes, and then each group of cells received different treatments. We collected cell culture supernatant and extracted exosomes from each group of cells using the ultracentrifugation method as reported previously [39]. Transmission electron microscopy was used to detect the morphology of exosomes, a NanoSight nanoparticle tracking analyzer was used to detect the particle size of exosomes and Western blotting was used to detect the expression of markers such as CD9, CD63, CD81, Albumin, Calnexin, HSP70, etc.

2.11. NanoSight Nanoparticle Tracking

Exosomes of gastric cancer cells were diluted to the appropriate proportion with PBS (1:1000–1:5000); then, 1 mL of the suspension was analyzed with a NanoSight nanoparticle analyzer [40] (Particle Metrix, Dusseldorf, Germany). Changes in the particle size and concentration of exosomes were analyzed using NanoSight nanoparticle tracking.

2.12. Transmission Electron Microscope Scanning

The gastric cancer cell exosome suspensions, with an appropriate dilution of PBS, were transferred to copper mesh and allowed to stand at room temperature for 2–5 min, and then counterstained with 3% phosphotungstic acid for 1–3 min. The morphology of gastric cancer cell exosomes was observed with a transmission electron microscope [41] (Philips, Amsterdam, The Netherlands).

2.13. Immunofluorescence Assay

Exosomes were added to DIL cell tracer at a ratio of 1:1000, mixed well and placed in a 37 °C constant-temperature incubator for 30 min. Cells were centrifuged at 4 °C at $1500 \times g$ for 30 min and resuspended in PBS. Cells were fixed with 4% paraformaldehyde for 20 min and washed with PBS. They were then treated with 0.2% triton X-100 for 10 min and washed with PBS. Serum was used for blocking for 30 min, and samples were washed three times with PBS. A β-actin antibody was incubated with the cells overnight at 4 °C, and they were then washed three times with PBS. The secondary antibody was incubated with the sample at room temperature for 2 h. DAPI staining and PBS washing were then performed three times. Cells were observed under a fluorescence microscope.

2.14. Ethics Statement

The gastric cancer tissues and adjacent noncancerous tissues were collected from advanced gastric cancer patients with a history of smoking for more than 5 years who had not received chemotherapy at the affiliated hospital of Jiangsu University. This study was approved by the institutional ethical committee of Jiangsu University (2012258) and written informed consent was obtained from all patients prior to tissue collection.

2.15. Statistical Analysis

All the statistical data are presented as mean ± standard deviation and were analyzed by using SPSS software 22.0 (SPSS, Chicago, IL, USA). Unpaired Student's t-test and one-way analysis were used according to actual conditions. Values of $p < 0.05$ were considered significant.

3. Results

Cigarette smoke extract promotes EMT and stemness gene expression in gastric cancer cells.

To investigate the effect of cigarette smoke on gastric cancer cells, gastric cancer cells (HGC-27 and AGS) were treated with various concentrations of cigarette smoke extract for 4 days, and 0.5% cigarette smoke extract was selected for the following experiments (Figure 1A). We found that cigarette smoke extract promoted the expression of OCT4, Lin28, Nanog, Vimentin and N-cadherin (Figure 1B,C). At the same time, the expression of E-cadherin was inhibited (Figure 1B,C). These results suggested that cigarette smoke could promote the EMT and stemness of gastric cancer cells.

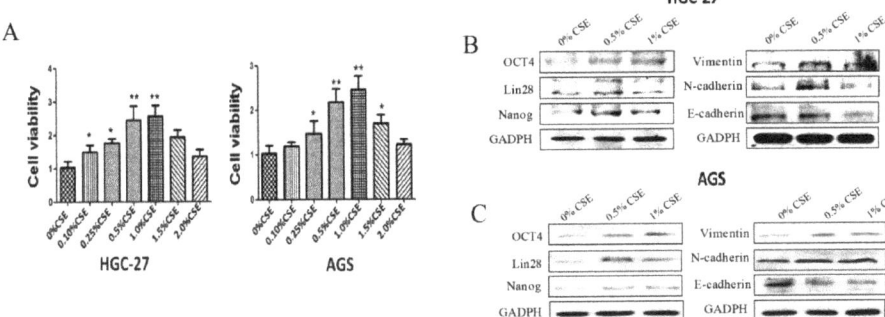

Figure 1. Cigarette smoke promotes EMT and stemness of gastric cancer cells. Gastric cancer cells (HGC-27 and AGS) were treated with cigarette smoke extract for 4 days. (**A**) Effects of different concentrations of cigarette smoke extract on the activity of gastric cancer cells. (**B,C**) Protein expression of stemness and EMT markers in gastric cancer cells after cigarette smoke extract exposure. * $p < 0.05$, ** $p < 0.01$.

3.1. Effect of Cigarette Smoke on Exosomes of Gastric Cancer Cells

We next extracted the exosomes secreted by gastric cancer cells before and after cigarette smoke extract exposure and analyzed the effect of cigarette smoke on the exosomes of gastric cancer cells. We found that compared with the group without cigarette smoke extract exposure, cigarette smoke extract did not significantly affect the particle size or average secretion level of exosomes (Figure 2A). We identified the extracted exosomes using surface marker proteins (Figure 2B). Transmission electron microscopy showed that exosomes were spherical or oval vesicles, and there were no significant changes in the morphology before and after cigarette smoke extract exposure (Figure 2C). These results suggest that cigarette smoke had no significant effect on the particle size, secretion or surface markers of exosomes secreted by gastric cancer cells.

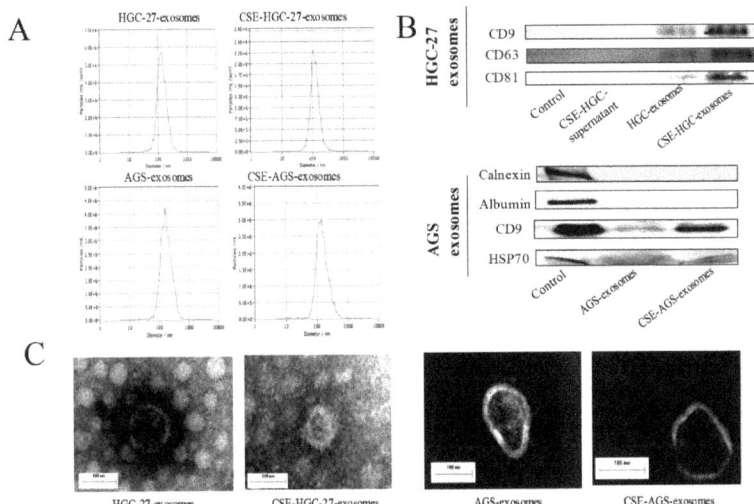

Figure 2. Effect of cigarette smoke on exosomes of gastric cancer cells. Gastric cancer cell exosomes were extracted before and after cigarette smoke exposure. (**A**) Detection of exosomes with a nanoparticle tracking analyzer. (**B**) Exosome-labeled proteins such as CD9, CD63, CD81, Calnexin, Albumin and HSP70 were detected using Western blotting. (**C**) The morphology of exosomes before and after cigarette smoke extract treatment were observed using transmission electron microscopy.

3.2. Cigarette Smoke-Induced Exosomes Promote the Stemness and EMT of GES-1 Cells

The enhancement of the stemness and EMT characteristic of cells plays an important role in the occurrence and development of gastric cancer. To clarify whether cigarette smoke-induced gastric cancer cell exosomes could affect surrounding normal cells to promote the development of gastric cancer, 300 μg of gastric cancer cell exosomes treated with cigarette smoke extract was cocultured with GES-1 cells. An immunofluorescence assay showed that the exosomes treated with cigarette smoke extract were absorbed by GES-1 cells (Figure 3A). Changes in the protein and mRNA levels of stemness and EMT makers in GES-1 cells before and after treatment with cigarette smoke-induced exosomes were detected (Figure 3B–E). The results showed that cigarette smoke-treated exosomes from gastric cancer cells promoted the expression of Vimentin and N-cadherin and inhibited the expression of E-cadherin. Furthermore, the migration ability of GES-1 cells was significantly enhanced (Figure 3F,G). In addition, cigarette smoke-treated exosomes increased the expression of stemness genes (Nanog, OCT4, Lin28). These data revealed that cigarette smoke-treated exosomes of gastric cancer cells promote the stemness and EMT of GES-1 cells, and might play an important role in gastric cancer progression.

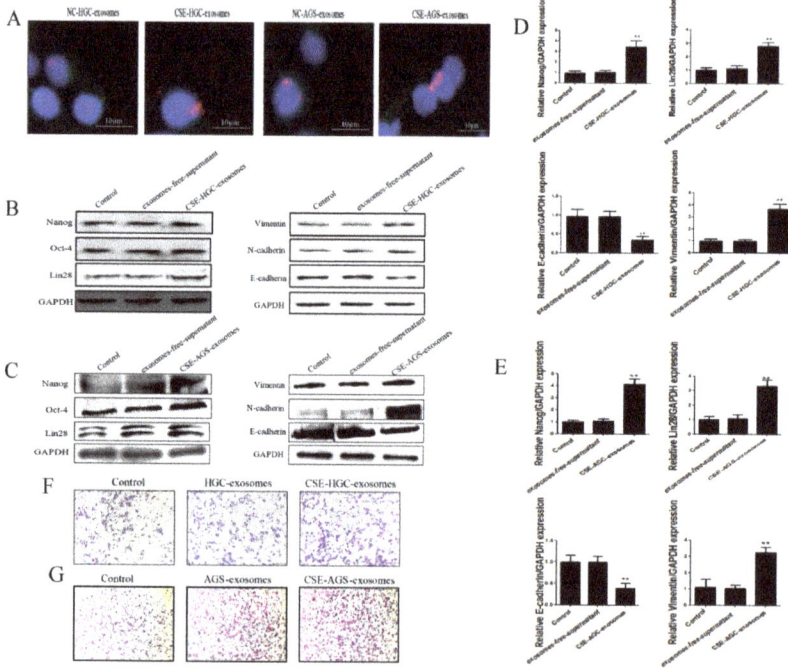

Figure 3. Cigarette smoke-induced exosomes promote the stemness and EMT of GES-1 cells. Cigarette smoke-induced GC cell exosomes were administered to GES-1 cells for 4 days. (**A**) Exosomes of gastric cancer cells were taken up by GES-1 cells. (**B,C**) Effect of cigarette smoke-induced exosomes on the protein levels of stemness and EMT markers. (**D,E**) Effect of cigarette smoke-induced exosomes on stemness and EMT marker mRNA expression. (**F,G**) Cigarette smoke-induced exosomes promoted GES-1 cell migration. ** $p < 0.01$.

3.3. Circ0000670 Was Highly Expressed in Cigarette Smoke-Exposed Gastric Cancer Cells and Exosomes

Emerging evidence indicates that circRNA plays an important role in the progression of gastric cancer. To determine whether circRNA is involved in the process through which cigarette smoke-induced exosomes promote gastric cancer progression, we analyzed circRNA microarray data (GSE83521 and GSE93541) from the Gene Expression Omnibus database (GEO, https://www.ncbi.nlm.nih.gov/geo/, accessed on 31 December 2021) to obtain circRNA expression profiles, which were verified in the tissues of gastric cancer patients with a smoking history (Figure 4A,B). The results of agarose gel electrophoresis (Figure 4D) and Sanger sequencing (Figure 4E) showed that the circ0000670 primer design was successful. The results showed that circ0000670 expression was significantly up-regulated in gastric cancer tissues. We also found that cigarette smoke could up-regulate the expression of circ0000670 in gastric cancer cells and the exosomes secreted by gastric cancer cells (Figure 4G). In addition, we found that the expression of circ0000670 showed an increasing trend in gastric cancer patients with a smoking history ($n = 40, 34/40$) (Figure 4H). These results determined that circ0000670 was highly expressed in cigarette smoke-exposed gastric cancer cells and exosomes.

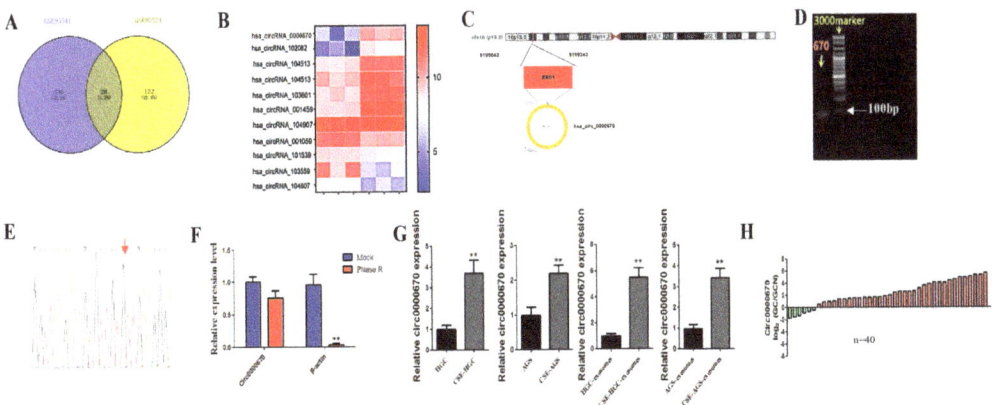

Figure 4. Circ0000670 is highly expressed in cigarette smoke-exposed gastric cancer cells and exosomes. The differentially expressed circRNAs were screened and verified in gastric cancer tissues, gastric cancer cells and exosomes. (**A**) Screening of differentially expressed circRNAs from the GEO database. (**B**) Major circRNAs with obvious differential expression. (**C**) Schematic diagram of mode of circ0000670 formation. (**D**) The results of agarose gel electrophoresis. (**E**) Sanger sequencing results of PCR products of circ0000670. (**F**) The level of circ0000670 in GSE-1 cells after RNase R treatment compared with the level of β-actin. (**G**) Expression of circ0000670 in gastric cancer cells and their exosomes exposed to cigarette smoke. (**H**) Expression of circ0000670 in the tissues of 40 gastric cancer patients with a smoking history. ** $p < 0.01$, compared with control.

3.4. Role of Circ0000670 in Cigarette Smoke-Induced Exosomes Promoted GES-1 Cell Stemness and EMT

To study the mechanism through which circ0000670 from CS-treated exosomes promotes the stemness and EMT of GES-1 cells, we constructed circ0000670 knockdown and overexpression lentivirus vectors. Cigarette smoke-induced gastric cancer cells were transfected with the circ0000670 knockdown and overexpression lentivirus vectors, and the expression of circ0000670 in exosomes was detected. The knockdown lentivirus had no significant effect on the particle size and morphology of exosomes (Figure 5C). Our results further showed that the circ0000670 knockdown lentivirus vector could significantly inhibit the high expression of circ0000670 in cigarette smoke-treated exosomes (Figure 5D). The promoting effect of cigarette smoke-treated exosomes on the protein and mRNA expression of stemness and EMT markers of GES-1 cells was significantly inhibited by the low expression of circ0000670 (Figure 5E,G). The migration ability of GES-1 cells was significantly weakened (Figure 5F). Moreover, the circ0000670 overexpression lentivirus vector increased the expression of circ0000670 in gastric cancer cell exosomes (Figure 5I). The results suggested that the overexpression of circ0000670 in exosomes significantly promotes the protein and mRNA levels of stemness and EMT markers of GES-1 cells (Figure 5J,L). The migration ability of GES-1 cells was also enhanced (Figure 5K). These results indicated that circ0000670 plays a crucial role in the development of cigarette smoke-induced gastric cancer.

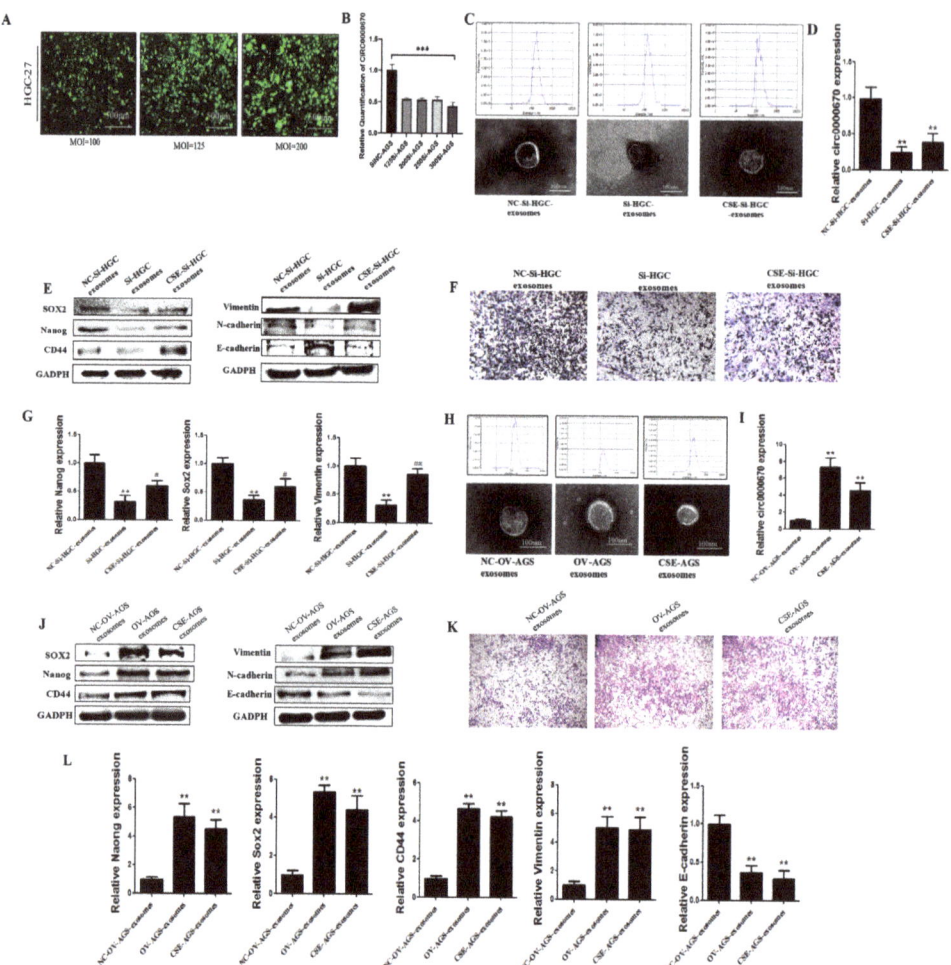

Figure 5. Role of circ0000670 in the promotion of GES-1 cell stemness and EMT by cigarette smoke-induced exosomes. A circ0000670 knockdown lentivirus vector was transferred into the cigarette smoke-induced gastric cancer cells, and exosomes were extracted to treat GES-1 cells. (**A**) Cell infection after treatment with circ0000670 knockdown lentivirus vector. (**B**) Expression of circ0000670 in gastric cancer cells after knockdown. (**C**) Effects of circ0000670 knockdown on the morphology and particle size of HGC-27 exosomes. (**D**) Expression of circ0000670 in exosomes after circ0000670 knockdown. (**E**) Protein expression of stemness and EMT markers after knockdown. (**F**) Changes in migration ability of GES-1 cells after knockdown of circ0000670. (**G**) mRNA expression of stemness and EMT markers after knockdown. (**H**) Effects of overexpression of circ0000670 on the morphology and particle size of AGC exosomes. (**I**) Expression of circ0000670 in exosomes after circ0000670 overexpression. (**J**) Protein expression of stemness and EMT markers after circ0000670 overexpression. (**K**) Changes in migration ability of GES-1 cells after overexpression of circ0000670. (**L**) mRNA expression of stemness and EMT markers after overexpression. ** $p < 0.01$, *** $p < 0.001$, compared with control, # $p < 0.05$, ## $p < 0.01$ compared with si-HGC-exosomes.

The Wnt/β-catenin pathway might be a downstream effector of the cigarette smoke-induced exosomal circ0000670-mediated promotion of gastric cancer progression.

To further explore the mechanism through which cigarette smoke-induced exosomal circ0000670 promotes the development of gastric cancer, we performed bioinformatics analysis and found that circ0000670 was associated with the Wnt/β-catenin signaling pathway. Gastric cancer cells were treated with the β-catenin-targeting inhibitor jw55, cigarette smoke and lentivirus, alone or in combination, and then the exosomes were extracted.

The results showed that the high expression of β-catenin and c-Myc induced by cigarette smoke was inhibited by jw55 in gastric cancer cells. Moreover, circ0000670 overexpression significantly up-regulated the expression of β-catenin and c-Myc in gastric cancer cells, whereas jw55 inhibited this (Figure 6A). The expression of β-catenin, c-Myc and stemness genes as well as EMT, which was promoted by gastric cancer cell exosomes treated with cigarette smoke, was blocked in the jw55 group (Figure 6A–C). Gastric cancer cell exosomes of the circ0000670overexpression group up-regulated the expression of β-catenin, c-Myc and stemness genes and promoted EMT in GES-1 cells. Exosomes from GC cells of the combined jw55-treated and circ0000670 overexpression group inhibited the enhanced expression of stemness genes, β-catenin, c-Myc and EMT caused by circ0000670 overexpression.

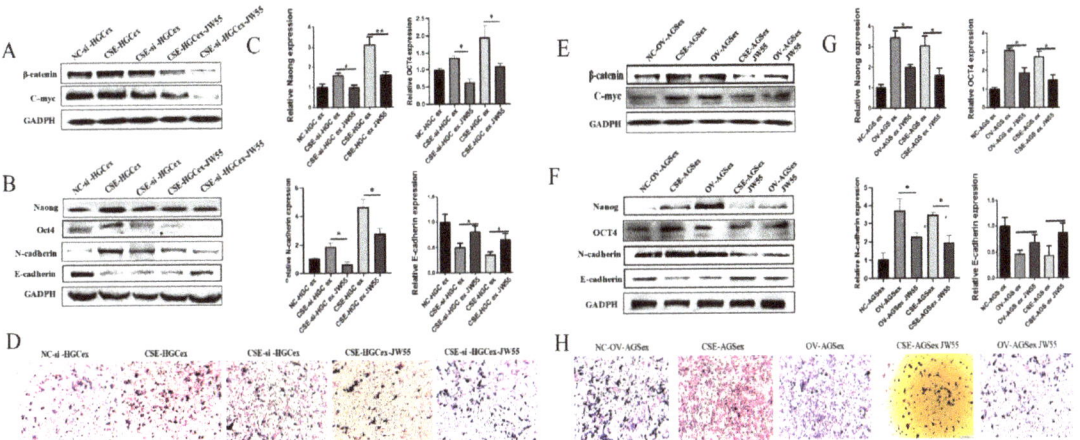

Figure 6. Wnt/β-catenin pathway regulates the gastric cancer-promoting effect of cigarette smoke-induced exosomes. A circ0000670 overexpression lentivirus and the β-catenin-targeting inhibitor jw55 were used to treat cigarette smoke-induced GC cells alone or in combination, and exosomes were extracted to treat GES-1 cells. (**A**) Changes in the protein levels of β-catenin and c-Myc. (**B**) Changes in the protein levels of stemness and EMT markers in GES-1 cells. (**C**) Changes in the mRNA levels of stemness and EMT markers in GES-1 cells. (**D**) Changes in the migration ability of GES-1 cells. (**E**) Changes in the protein levels of β-catenin and c-Myc. (**F**) Changes in the protein levels of stemness and EMT markers in GES-1 cells. (**G**) Changes in the mRNA levels of stemness and EMT markers in GES-1 cells. (**H**) Changes in the migration ability of GES-1 cells. * $p < 0.05$, ** $p < 0.01$, compared with control.

It was also found that inhibition of the Wnt/β-catenin pathway could inhibit the expression of stemness genes and EMT in gastric cancer cells (Figure 6E–H). Furthermore, the circ0000670 knockdown lentivirus vector inhibited the up-regulation of β-catenin and c-Myc expression induced by cigarette smoke (Figure 6E). The circ0000670 knockdown virus combined with jw55 treatment significantly inhibited the cigarette smoke-induced up-regulation of β-catenin and c-Myc expression compared to that with the jw55 treatment alone. Further study found that the exosomes of the jw55 treatment group of gastric cancer cells inhibited the expression of stemness genes and EMT in GES-1 cells. Meanwhile, exosomes of gastric cancer cells in the circ0000670 knockdown group inhibited the upregulation of β-catenin and c-Myc expression induced by cigarette smoke. Exosomes of gastric cancer cells treated with the circ0000670 knockdown vector and jw55 significantly inhibited the cigarette smoke-induced up-regulation of β-catenin, c-Myc, stemness gene expression and EMT compared to those with treatment alone (Figure 6E–H). Based on these results, we speculated that the Wnt/β-catenin pathway might be downstream of cigarette smoke-induced exosomal circ0000670 with respect to the promotion of gastric cancer progression.

4. Discussion

There is substantive evidence demonstrating that cigarette smoke is one of the primary causes of gastric cancer. However, the molecular mechanisms by which cigarette smoke promotes gastric cancer are not well established. Exosomes transmit active substances and signals to surrounding cells, which promote the development of gastric cancer. In this study, we found that cigarette smoke enhances the proliferation, stemness and EMT of gastric cancer cells. Furthermore, exosomes derived from cigarette smoke-treated gastric cancer cells promoted the stemness and EMT process of GES-1 cells. In addition, our data indicated that exosomal circ0000670 plays a regulatory role in the mechanism through which cigarette smoke enhances the stemness and EMT of GES-1 cells. Furthermore, the Wnt/β-catenin pathway might be downstream of cigarette smoke-induced exosomal circ0000670 with respect to the promotion of gastric cancer progression. In conclusion, circ0000670 transported by gastric cancer cell exosomes regulates the Wnt/β-catenin pathway, affecting the biological characteristics of surrounding GES-1 cells and ultimately promoting the development of gastric cancer.

Cigarette smoke plays an important role in the occurrence and development of gastric cancer [42,43], but it is unclear whether cigarette smoke can promote the development of gastric cancer via exosomes. Exosomes are an important part of the communication system between cells and within organs, and they can transfer active molecules and biological signals from one cell type or tissue to another [6,7]. Many studies have indicated that exosomes play a decisive role in the occurrence and development of gastric cancer [8,9]. Cigarette smoke is involved in the occurrence and development of a variety of diseases by affecting exosomes [28,44,45]. In this study, we mainly clarified that cigarette smoke could affect the fate of surrounding GES-1 cells through gastric cancer cell exosomes and then promote the development of gastric cancer. Gastric cancer cell-derived exosomes were extracted before and after cigarette smoke exposure, and we examined the effects of cigarette smoke on exosomes. The results identified that there were no significant changes in exosome size and average secretion after cigarette smoke exposure. EMT is a common cellular process. Cells lose epithelial properties and acquire mesenchymal properties. Normal cells can acquire EMT properties, which may be an important feature in the carcinogenic process. Meanwhile, EMT participates in pro-cancerous tissue remodeling of gastric cancer and other tumors. Many cancers, including gastric cancer, arise from cancer stem cells. Therefore, the enhancement of stem cell characteristics plays an important indicator role in the occurrence and development of gastric cancer. We also observed the effects of cigarette smoke-treated gastric cancer cell exosomes on the stemness and EMT of GES-1 cells. We found that cigarette smoke-induced exosomes could promote the expression of Nanog, OCT4, Lin28 and vimentin and inhibit the expression of E-cadherin. In addition, the migration of GES-1 cells was also significantly enhanced (Figure 3). These results suggested that cigarette smoke-induced exosomes of gastric cancer cells promote the proliferation, stemness and EMT of GES-1 cells, and play an important role in gastric cancer progression.

Exosomes carry noncoding RNA, protein and other molecules to participate in cell communication and have a critical role in gastric cancer and other cancers [46,47]. The abnormal expression of circRNAs is closely related to the occurrence and development of gastric cancer [20,48,49]. It was found that cigarette smoke affects circRNAs and other noncoding RNAs transported by exosomes and plays a role in the occurrence and development of diseases [27,28,32]. In the current study, we investigated whether cigarette smoke promotes gastric cancer by affecting the components carried by exosomes, such as circRNA. We first screened and verified abnormally expressed circRNAs from the GEO database (GSE83521 and GSE93541) and tissues of gastric cancer patients with a smoking history. The results indicated that circ0000670 is highly expressed in the tissues of gastric cancer patients with a smoking history. Liu et al. also reported that circ0000670 plays an important role in the development of gastric cancer [50], but its role in cigarette smoke-induced gastric cancer and the effects of cigarette smoke-induced gastric cancer cell exosomes on the fate of surrounding normal cells was not clear. Our results showed an increasing trend in 40 gastric cancer patients with a smoking history (85%). We also found that cigarette smoke promoted the expression of circ0000670 in gastric cancer cells (HGC-27 and AGS) and associated exosomes (Figure 4). To study the role of exosomal circ0000670 in promoting the stemness and EMT of GES-1 cells, we commissioned a biological company to construct circ0000670 knockdown and overexpression lentivirus vectors. In further experiments, circ0000670 knockdown and overexpression lentivirus vectors were transferred into cigarette smoke-treated gastric cancer cells, and the expression of circ0000670 in gastric cancer cell exosomes was detected. We found that the augmenting effect of gastric cancer cell exosomes on the stemness and EMT of GES-1 cells was inhibited by the knockdown of circ0000670 (Figure 5C–G). In contrast, the results showed that gastric cancer cell exosomes of the circ0000670-overexpressing group could promote the stemness and EMT of GES-1 cells (Figure 5H–L).

In order to further explore the mechanism through which cigarette smoke-induced exosomal circ0000670 promotes the development of gastric cancer, we performed bioinformatic analysis and found that circ0000670 was associated with the Wnt/β-catenin signaling pathway. A previous study revealed that the activation of the Wnt/β-catenin pathway promotes the occurrence and development of cancers, including gastric cancer [51–53]. CircRNA also affects the occurrence and development of gastric cancer by regulating the activity of the Wnt/β-catenin pathway [21,54]. In this study, gastric cancer cells were treated with the β-catenin-targeting inhibitor jw55, cigarette smoke and lentivirus, alone or in combination, and then the exosomes were extracted. The results suggested that the Wnt/β-catenin pathway might be downstream of cigarette smoke-induced exosomal circ0000670 with respect to the effects on the surrounding normal cells and the promotion of gastric cancer progression.

5. Conclusions

In summary, cigarette smoke-induced gastric cancer cell exosomal circ0000670 acts as a promoter of gastric cancer by affecting the fate of surrounding normal cells and might be a potential target for the prevention and treatment of gastric cancer. These findings provide new insights into the mechanism of cigarette smoke-related gastric cancer.

Author Contributions: Writing—original draft preparation, Z.L.; writing—review and editing, Z.L., H.Q. and H.G.; investigation, Z.L. and S.F.; data curation, S.F. and Y.Z.; formal analysis, X.Z. and Y.X. analyzed data. funding acquisition, Z.L., H.Q. and H.G. All authors have read and agreed to the published version of the manuscript.

Funding: This study was supported by a project of social development in Zhenjiang (No. SH2021045), the Foundation for excellent young teachers of Jiangsu University and the Zhenjiang key laboratory of high technology research on exosome foundation and transformation application (Grant SS2018003) and Technology Development Project of Jiangsu University (20220516), Anhui Institute of Translational Medicine (2022zhyx-C82).

Institutional Review Board Statement: All of the mouse experiments were approved by the Animal Care and Use Committee of Jiangsu University (Approval code: 2020040205) and efforts were made to minimize suffering and distress.

Informed Consent Statement: Not applicable.

Data Availability Statement: All data generated or analyzed in this study are included in thispublished article.

Conflicts of Interest: The authors declare no conflict of interest.

References

1. Sung, H.; Ferlay, J.; Siegel, R.L.; Laversanne, M.; Soerjomataram, I.; Jemal, A.; Bray, F. Global Cancer Statistics 2020: GLOBOCAN Estimates of Incidence and Mortality Worldwide for 36 Cancers in 185 Countries. *CA A Cancer J. Clin.* **2021**, *71*, 209–249. [CrossRef]
2. Lu, L.; Chen, J.; Li, M.; Tang, L.; Wu, R.; Jin, L.; Liang, Z. β-carotene reverses tobacco smoke induced gastric EMT via Notch pathway in vivo. *Oncol. Rep.* **2018**, *39*, 1867–1873. [CrossRef] [PubMed]
3. Song, M.; Camargo, M.C.; Katki, H.A.; Weinstein, S.J.; Mannisto, S.; Albanes, D.; Surcel, H.-M.; Rabkin, C.S. Association of Antiparietal Cell and Anti-Intrinsic Factor Antibodies with Risk of Gastric Cancer. *JAMA Oncol.* **2022**, *8*, 268–274. [CrossRef] [PubMed]
4. Lu, L.; Chen, J.; Tang, H.; Bai, L.; Lu, C.; Wang, K.; Li, M.; Yan, Y.; Tang, L.; Wu, R.; et al. EGCG Suppresses ERK5 Activation to Reverse Tobacco Smoke-Triggered Gastric Epithelial-Mesenchymal Transition in BALB/c Mice. *Nutrients* **2016**, *8*, 380. [CrossRef] [PubMed]
5. Liang, Z.; Wu, R.; Xie, W.; Geng, H.; Zhao, L.; Xie, C.; Wu, J.; Geng, S.; Li, X.; Zhu, M.; et al. Curcumin Suppresses MAPK Pathways to Reverse Tobacco Smoke-induced Gastric Epithelial-Mesenchymal Transition in Mice. *Phytother. Res. PTR* **2015**, *29*, 1665–1671. [CrossRef] [PubMed]
6. Isaac, R.; Reis, F.C.G.; Ying, W.; Olefsky, J.M. Exosomes as mediators of intercellular crosstalk in metabolism. *Cell Metab.* **2021**, *33*, 1744–1762. [CrossRef]
7. Morrissey, S.M.; Zhang, F.; Ding, C.; Montoya-Durango, D.E.; Hu, X.; Yang, C.; Wang, Z.; Yuan, F.; Fox, M.; Zhang, H.-G.; et al. Tumor-derived exosomes drive immunosuppressive macrophages in a pre-metastatic niche through glycolytic dominant metabolic reprogramming. *Cell Metab.* **2021**, *33*, 2040–2058.e10. [CrossRef] [PubMed]
8. Tang, X.H.; Guo, T.; Gao, X.Y.; Wu, X.L.; Xing, X.F.; Ji, J.F.; Li, Z.-Y. Exosome-derived noncoding RNAs in gastric cancer: Functions and clinical applications. *Mol. Cancer* **2021**, *20*, 99. [CrossRef]
9. Wu, H.; Fu, M.; Liu, J.; Chong, W.; Fang, Z.; Du, F.; Liu, Y.; Shang, L.; Li, L. The role and application of small extracellular vesicles in gastric cancer. *Mol. Cancer* **2021**, *20*, 71. [CrossRef]
10. Yoon, J.H.; Choi, B.J.; Nam, S.W.; Park, W.S. Gastric cancer exosomes contribute to the field cancerization of gastric epithelial cells surrounding gastric cancer. *Gastric Cancer* **2022**, *25*, 490–502. [CrossRef]
11. Zhang, H.; Deng, T.; Liu, R.; Ning, T.; Yang, H.; Liu, D.; Zhang, Q.; Lin, D.; Ge, S.; Bai, M.; et al. CAF secreted miR-522 suppresses ferroptosis and promotes acquired chemo-resistance in gastric cancer. *Mol. Cancer* **2020**, *19*, 43. [CrossRef] [PubMed]
12. Cao, S.; Fu, B.; Cai, J.; Zhang, D.; Wang, C.; Wu, H. Linc00852 from cisplatin-resistant gastric cancer cell-derived exosomes regulates COMMD7 to promote cisplatin resistance of recipient cells through microRNA-514a-5p. *Cell Biol. Toxicol.* **2022**. [CrossRef] [PubMed]
13. Xie, M.; Yu, T.; Jing, X.; Ma, L.; Fan, Y.; Yang, F.; Ma, P.; Jiang, H.; Wu, X.; Shu, Y.; et al. Exosomal circSHKBP1 promotes gastric cancer progression via regulating the miR-582-3p/HUR/VEGF axis and suppressing HSP90 degradation. *Mol. Cancer* **2020**, *19*, 112. [CrossRef] [PubMed]
14. Zhang, X.; Wang, S.; Wang, H.; Cao, J.; Huang, X.; Chen, Z.; Xu, P.; Sun, G.; Xu, J.; Lv, J.; et al. Circular RNA circNRIP1 acts as a microRNA-149-5p sponge to promote gastric cancer progression via the AKT1/mTOR pathway. *Mol. Cancer* **2019**, *18*, 20. [CrossRef] [PubMed]
15. Zhang, Y.; Jiang, J.; Zhang, J.; Shen, H.; Wang, M.; Guo, Z.; Zang, X.; Shi, H.; Gao, J.; Cai, H.; et al. CircDIDO1 inhibits gastric cancer progression by encoding a novel DIDO1-529aa protein and regulating PRDX2 protein stability. *Mol. Cancer* **2021**, *20*, 101. [CrossRef] [PubMed]
16. Wang, M.; Zhao, X.; Qiu, R.; Gong, Z.; Huang, F.; Yu, W.; Shen, B.; Sha, X.; Dong, H.; Huang, J.; et al. Lymph node metastasis-derived gastric cancer cells educate bone marrow-derived mesenchymal stem cells via YAP signaling activation by exosomal Wnt5a. *Oncogene* **2021**, *40*, 2296–2308. [CrossRef]
17. Lu, L.; Fang, S.; Zhang, Y.; Jin, L.; Xu, W.; Liang, Z. Exosomes and Exosomal circRNAs: The Rising Stars in the Progression, Diagnosis and Prognosis of Gastric Cancer. *Cancer Manag. Res.* **2021**, *13*, 8121–8129. [CrossRef]
18. Kristensen, L.S.; Andersen, M.S.; Stagsted, L.V.W.; Ebbesen, K.K.; Hansen, T.B.; Kjems, J. The biogenesis, biology and characterization of circular RNAs. *Nat. Rev. Genet.* **2019**, *20*, 675–691. [CrossRef]
19. Mostafazadeh, M.; Kahroba, H.; Haiaty, S.; TazeKand, A.P.; Samadi, N.; Rahbarghazi, R.; Nouri, M. In vitro exosomal transfer of Nrf2 led to the oxaliplatin resistance in human colorectal cancer LS174T cells. *Cell Biochem. Funct.* **2022**, *40*, 391–402. [CrossRef]
20. Fan, H.N.; Chen, Z.Y.; Chen, X.Y.; Chen, M.; Yi, Y.C.; Zhu, J.S.; Zhang, J. METTL14-mediated m(6)A modification of circORC5 suppresses gastric cancer progression by regulating miR-30c-2-3p/AKT1S1 axis. *Mol. Cancer* **2022**, *21*, 51. [CrossRef]
21. Peng, Y.; Xu, Y.; Zhang, X.; Deng, S.; Yuan, Y.; Luo, X.; Hossain, M.T.; Zhu, X.; Du, K.; Hu, F.; et al. A novel protein AXIN1-295aa encoded by circAXIN1 activates the Wnt/beta-catenin signaling pathway to promote gastric cancer progression. *Mol. Cancer* **2021**, *20*, 158. [CrossRef] [PubMed]

22. Yu, T.; Ran, L.; Zhao, H.; Yin, P.; Li, W.; Lin, J.; Mao, H.; Cai, D.; Ma, Q.; Pan, X.; et al. Circular RNA circ-TNPO3 suppresses metastasis of GC by acting as a protein decoy for IGF2BP3 to regulate the expression of MYC and SNAIL. *Mol. Ther. Nucleic Acids* **2021**, *26*, 649–664. [CrossRef] [PubMed]
23. Wang, H.; Zeng, X.; Zheng, Y.; Wang, Y.; Zhou, Y. Exosomal circRNA in Digestive System Tumors: The Main Player or Coadjuvants? *Front. Oncol.* **2021**, *11*, 614462. [CrossRef] [PubMed]
24. Yu, L.; Xie, J.; Liu, X.; Yu, Y.; Wang, S. Plasma Exosomal CircNEK9 Accelerates the Progression of Gastric Cancer via miR-409-3p/MAP7 Axis. *Dig. Dis. Sci.* **2021**, *66*, 4274–4289. [CrossRef] [PubMed]
25. Li, S.; Li, J.; Zhang, H.; Zhang, Y.; Wang, X.; Yang, H.; Zhou, Z.; Hao, X.; Ying, G.; Ba, Y. Gastric cancer derived exosomes mediate the delivery of circRNA to promote angiogenesis by targeting miR-29a/VEGF axis in endothelial cells. *Biochem. Biophys. Res. Commun.* **2021**, *560*, 37–44. [CrossRef] [PubMed]
26. Zhu, Z.; Lian, X.; Su, X.; Wu, W.; Zeng, Y.; Chen, X. Exosomes derived from adipose-derived stem cells alleviate cigarette smoke-induced lung inflammation and injury by inhibiting alveolar macrophages pyroptosis. *Respir. Res.* **2022**, *23*, 5. [CrossRef] [PubMed]
27. Chen, Z.; Wu, H.; Shi, R.; Fan, W.; Zhang, J.; Su, W.; Wang, Y.; Li, P. miRNAomics analysis reveals the promoting effects of cigarette smoke extract-treated Beas-2B-derived exosomes on macrophage polarization. *Biochem. Biophys. Res. Commun.* **2021**, *572*, 157–163. [CrossRef]
28. Wang, L.; Chen, Q.; Yu, Q.; Xiao, J.; Zhao, H. Cigarette smoke extract-treated airway epithelial cells-derived exosomes promote M1 macrophage polarization in chronic obstructive pulmonary disease. *Int. Immunopharmacol.* **2021**, *96*, 107700. [CrossRef]
29. Xu, B.; Gan, C.X.; Chen, S.S.; Li, J.Q.; Liu, M.Z.; Guo, G.H. BMSC-derived exosomes alleviate smoke inhalation lung injury through blockade of the HMGB1/NF-kappaB pathway. *Life Sci.* **2020**, *257*, 118042. [CrossRef]
30. Zhao, J.; Xia, H.; Wu, Y.; Lu, L.; Cheng, C.; Sun, J.; Xiang, Q.; Bian, T.; Liu, Q. CircRNA_0026344 via miR-21 is involved in cigarette smoke-induced autophagy and apoptosis of alveolar epithelial cells in emphysema. *Cell Biol. Toxicol.* **2021**. [CrossRef]
31. Qiao, D.; Hu, C.; Li, Q.; Fan, J. Circ-RBMS1 Knockdown Alleviates CSE-Induced Apoptosis, Inflammation and Oxidative Stress via Up-Regulating FBXO11 Through miR-197-3p in 16HBE Cells. *Int. J. Chronic Obstr. Pulm. Dis.* **2021**, *16*, 2105–2118. [CrossRef] [PubMed]
32. Chen, J.; Rong, N.; Liu, M.; Xu, C.; Guo, J. The exosome-circ_0001359 derived from cigarette smoke exposed-prostate stromal cells promotes epithelial cells collagen deposition and primary ciliogenesis. *Toxicol. Appl. Pharmacol.* **2022**, *435*, 115850. [CrossRef] [PubMed]
33. Bai, J.; Deng, J.; Han, Z.; Cui, Y.; He, R.; Gu, Y.; Zhang, Q. CircRNA_0026344 via exosomal miR-21 regulation of Smad7 is involved in aberrant cross-talk of epithelium-fibroblasts during cigarette smoke-induced pulmonary fibrosis. *Toxicol. Lett.* **2021**, *347*, 58–66. [CrossRef]
34. Gal, K.; Cseh, A.; Szalay, B.; Rusai, K.; Vannay, A.; Lukacsovits, J.; Heemann, U.; Szabó, A.J.; Losonczy, G.; Tamási, L.; et al. Effect of cigarette smoke and dexamethasone on Hsp72 system of alveolar epithelial cells. *Cell Stress Chaperones* **2011**, *16*, 369–378. [CrossRef]
35. Wang, Y.; Wang, H.; Zheng, R.; Wu, P.; Sun, Z.; Chen, J.; Zhang, L.; Zhang, C.; Qian, H.; Jiang, J.; et al. Circular RNA ITCH suppresses metastasis of gastric cancer via regulating miR-199a-5p/Klotho axis. *Cell Cycle* **2021**, *20*, 522–536. [CrossRef] [PubMed]
36. Liang, J.H.; Xu, Q.D.; Gu, S.G. LncRNA RSU1P2-microRNA let-7a-Testis-Expressed Protein 10 axis modulates tumorigenesis and cancer stem cell-like properties in liver cancer. *Bioengineered* **2022**, *13*, 4285–4300. [CrossRef]
37. Gong, X.; Lu, X.; Cao, J.; Liu, H.; Chen, H.; Bao, F.; Shi, X.; Cong, H. Serum hsa_circ_0087776 as a new oncologic marker for the joint diagnosis of multiple myeloma. *Bioengineered* **2021**, *12*, 12447–12459. [CrossRef]
38. Jiang, K.; Zou, H. microRNA-20b-5p overexpression combing Pembrolizumab potentiates cancer cells to radiation therapy via repressing programmed death-ligand 1. *Bioengineered* **2022**, *13*, 917–929. [CrossRef]
39. Tan, Y.; Huang, Y.; Mei, R.; Mao, F.; Yang, D.; Liu, J.; Xu, W.; Qian, H.; Yan, Y. HucMSC-derived exosomes delivered BECN1 induces ferroptosis of hepatic stellate cells via regulating the xCT/GPX4 axis. *Cell Death Dis.* **2022**, *13*, 319. [CrossRef]
40. Han, X.; Wu, P.; Li, L.; Sahal, H.M.; Ji, C.; Zhang, J.; Wang, Y.; Wang, Q.; Qian, H.; Shi, H.; et al. Exosomes derived from autologous dermal fibroblasts promote diabetic cutaneous wound healing through the Akt/beta-catenin pathway. *Cell Cycle* **2021**, *20*, 616–629. [CrossRef]
41. Shou, Y.; Wang, X.; Liang, Y.; Liu, X.; Chen, K. Exosomes-derived miR-154-5p attenuates esophageal squamous cell carcinoma progression and angiogenesis by targeting kinesin family member 14. *Bioengineered* **2022**, *13*, 4610–4620. [CrossRef] [PubMed]
42. Ghosh, P.; Mandal, S.; Mitra Mustafi, S.; Murmu, N. Clinicopathological Characteristics and Incidence of Gastric Cancer in Eastern India: A Retrospective Study. *J. Gastrointest. Cancer* **2021**, *52*, 863–871. [CrossRef] [PubMed]
43. Li, J.; Xu, H.L.; Yao, B.D.; Li, W.X.; Fang, H.; Xu, D.L.; Zhang, Z.-F. Environmental tobacco smoke and cancer risk, a prospective cohort study in a Chinese population. *Environ. Res.* **2020**, *191*, 110015. [CrossRef] [PubMed]
44. Benedikter, B.J.; Volgers, C.; van Eijck, P.H.; Wouters, E.F.M.; Savelkoul, P.H.M.; Reynaert, N.L.; Haenen, G.R.; Rohde, G.G.; Weseler, A.R.; Stassen, F.R. Cigarette smoke extract induced exosome release is mediated by depletion of exofacial thiols and can be inhibited by thiol-antioxidants. *Free Radic. Biol. Med.* **2017**, *108*, 334–344. [CrossRef] [PubMed]
45. He, S.; Chen, D.; Hu, M.; Zhang, L.; Liu, C.; Traini, D.; Grau, G.E.; Zeng, Z.; Lu, J.; Zhou, G.; et al. Bronchial epithelial cell extracellular vesicles ameliorate epithelial-mesenchymal transition in COPD pathogenesis by alleviating M2 macrophage polarization. *Nanomed. Nanotechnol. Biol. Med.* **2019**, *18*, 259–271. [CrossRef]

46. Gao, J.; Li, S.; Xu, Q.; Zhang, X.; Huang, M.; Dai, X.; Liu, L. Exosomes Promote Pre-Metastatic Niche Formation in Gastric Cancer. *Front. Oncol.* **2021**, *11*, 652378. [CrossRef]
47. Fu, M.; Gu, J.; Jiang, P.; Qian, H.; Xu, W.; Zhang, X. Exosomes in gastric cancer: Roles, mechanisms, and applications. *Mol. Cancer* **2019**, *18*, 41. [CrossRef]
48. Roy, S.; Kanda, M.; Nomura, S.; Zhu, Z.; Toiyama, Y.; Taketomi, A.; Goldenring, J.; Baba, H.; Kodera, Y.; Goel, A. Diagnostic efficacy of circular RNAs as noninvasive, liquid biopsy biomarkers for early detection of gastric cancer. *Mol. Cancer* **2022**, *21*, 42. [CrossRef]
49. Qiu, S.; Li, B.; Xia, Y.; Xuan, Z.; Li, Z.; Xie, L.; Gu, C.; Lv, J.; Lu, C.; Jiang, T.; et al. CircTHBS1 drives gastric cancer progression by increasing INHBA mRNA expression and stability in a ceRNA- and RBP-dependent manner. *Cell Death Dis.* **2022**, *13*, 266. [CrossRef]
50. Liu, P.; Cai, S.; Li, N. Circular RNA-hsa-circ-0000670 promotes gastric cancer progression through the microRNA-384/SIX4 axis. *Exp. Cell Res.* **2020**, *394*, 112141. [CrossRef]
51. Togasaki, K.; Sugimoto, S.; Ohta, Y.; Nanki, K.; Matano, M.; Takahashi, S.; Fujii, M.; Kanai, T.; Sato, T. Wnt Signaling Shapes the Histologic Variation in Diffuse Gastric Cancer. *Gastroenterology* **2021**, *160*, 823–830. [CrossRef] [PubMed]
52. Nienhuser, H.; Kim, W.; Malagola, E.; Ruan, T.; Valenti, G.; Middelhoff, M.; Bass, A.; Der, C.J.; Hayakawa, Y.; Wang, T.C. Mist1+ gastric isthmus stem cells are regulated by Wnt5a and expand in response to injury and inflammation in mice. *Gut* **2021**, *70*, 654–665. [CrossRef] [PubMed]
53. Pouyafar, A.; Rezabakhsh, A.; Rahbarghazi, R.; Heydarabad, M.Z.; Shokrollahi, E.; Sokullu, E.; Khaksar, M.; Nourazarian, A.; Avci, C.B. Treatment of cancer stem cells from human colon adenocarcinoma cell line HT-29 with resveratrol and sulindac induced mesenchymal-endothelial transition rate. *Cell Tissue Res.* **2019**, *376*, 377–388. [CrossRef] [PubMed]
54. Yang, C.; Han, S. The circular RNA circ0005654 interacts with specificity protein 1 via microRNA-363 sequestration to promote gastric cancer progression. *Bioengineered* **2021**, *12*, 6305–6317. [CrossRef] [PubMed]

Disclaimer/Publisher's Note: The statements, opinions and data contained in all publications are solely those of the individual author(s) and contributor(s) and not of MDPI and/or the editor(s). MDPI and/or the editor(s) disclaim responsibility for any injury to people or property resulting from any ideas, methods, instructions or products referred to in the content.

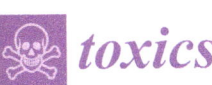

Article

A UPLC Q-Exactive Orbitrap Mass Spectrometry-Based Metabolomic Study of Serum and Tumor Tissue in Patients with Papillary Thyroid Cancer

Bo Xu [1,†], Wei Gao [2,†], Ting Xu [2], Cuiping Liu [3], Dan Wu [2,*] and Wei Tang [2,*]

1. State Key Laboratory of Reproductive Medicine, School of Public Health, Nanjing Medical University, Nanjing 211166, China
2. Department of Endocrinology, Nanjing Medical University Affiliated Geriatric Hospital, Nanjing 210024, China
3. Bank of Biological Samples, First Affiliated Hospital of Nanjing Medical University, Nanjing 210029, China
* Correspondence: danw0301@126.com (D.W.); drtangwei@njmu.edu.cn (W.T.); Tel.: +86-25-83712838 (D.W. & W.T.)
† These authors contributed equally to this work.

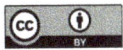

Citation: Xu, B.; Gao, W.; Xu, T.; Liu, C.; Wu, D.; Tang, W. A UPLC Q-Exactive Orbitrap Mass Spectrometry-Based Metabolomic Study of Serum and Tumor Tissue in Patients with Papillary Thyroid Cancer. *Toxics* 2023, *11*, 44. https://doi.org/10.3390/toxics11010044

Academic Editor: Panagiotis Georgiadis

Received: 2 December 2022
Revised: 24 December 2022
Accepted: 27 December 2022
Published: 31 December 2022

Copyright: © 2022 by the authors. Licensee MDPI, Basel, Switzerland. This article is an open access article distributed under the terms and conditions of the Creative Commons Attribution (CC BY) license (https://creativecommons.org/licenses/by/4.0/).

Abstract: Objective: To find the metabolomic characteristics of tumor or para-tumor tissues, and the differences in serums from papillary thyroid cancer (PTC) patients with or without lymph node metastasis. Methods: We collected serums of PTC patients with/without lymph node metastasis (SN1/SN0), tumor and adjacent tumor tissues of PTC patients with lymph node metastasis (TN1 and PN1), and without lymph node metastasis (TN0 and PN0). Metabolite detection was performed by ultra-high performance liquid chromatography combined with Q-Exactive orbitrap mass spectrometry (UPLC Q-Exactive). Results: There were 31, 15 differential metabolites in the comparisons of TN1 and PN1, TN0 and PN0, respectively. Seven uniquely increased metabolites and fourteen uniquely decreased metabolites appeared in the lymph node metastasis (TN1 and PN1) group. Meanwhile, the results indicated that four pathways were co-owned pathways in two comparisons (TN1 and PN1, TN0 and PN0), and four unique pathways presented in the lymph node metastasis (TN1 and PN1) group. Conclusions: Common or differential metabolites and metabolic pathways were detected in the lymph node metastasis and non-metastatic group, which might provide novel ways for the diagnosis and treatment of PTC.

Keywords: papillary thyroid cancer; metabolomics; lymph node metastasis; tumor tissue; serum

1. Introduction

Thyroid cancer is the most common endocrine malignancy disease. Papillary thyroid cancer (PTC), the major subtype, is derived from thyroid follicular cells [1]. The 30-year recurrence rate (29.4%) and cause-specific mortality (8.6%) of PTC still raise concern [2]. As PTC is most likely to metastasize to cervical lymph nodes in 30% to 90% of patients [3,4], lymph node metastasis is a critical risk factor for PTC recurrence and distant metastasis [5]. At present, ultrasound is the most commonly used diagnostic method for thyroid cancer [6–9]. The sensitivity and specificity of ultrasound detection in predicting central lymph node metastasis of PTC ranged from 40.4% to 92.9% and from 39.7% to 79.4%, respectively [10]. In addition, there is still no consensus on the supplementary diagnosis markers; for example, the predictive value of HBME-1 in lymph node metastasis of PTC is still conflict [11,12], and the mutations of BRAF and TERT promoter in predicting lymph node metastasis of PTC are still controversial [10,13–17]. Therefore, it is necessary to seek new markers of PTC with lymph node metastasis. Metabolic change is one of the important markers of tumors [18]. Metabolomics is an analytical study of multiple low-molecular-weight metabolites, and it is also downstream of gene expression and protein activity [19].

At the moment, metabolomics is widely used in disease prediction, mechanism exploration, and for providing new diagnostic molecular markers and therapeutic targets [20,21].

The metabolomics of PTC have been studied by gas chromatography–mass spectrometry (GC–MS) [22] and nuclear magnetic resonance (NMR) [23]. However, different analytical platforms have different metabolic coverage, which can provide various metabolomics information [24]. Liquid chromatography–mass spectrometry (LC–MS) is a commonly used technology in metabolomics analysis with high sensitivity and broad coverage [25]. There were insufficient published metabolomic studies on PTC using LC–MS. In addition, the understanding of metabolomics alterations with respect to lymph node metastasis is still deficient. Given these facts, it is necessary to adopt LC–MS-based metabolomics technology to observe the detailed metabolic changes and disordered metabolic pathways in PTC patients with lymph node metastasis.

Therefore, we performed the current study using an ultra-high performance liquid chromatography tandem Q-Exactive mass spectrometry (UPLC Q-Exactive MS) to detect the differences in serum and tumor tissue metabolism profiles between PTC patients with and without lymph node metastasis, looking for metabolic markers that could serve as diagnostic and prognostic indicators for PTC and new therapeutic targets for PTC.

2. Materials and Methods

2.1. Subjects Recruitment

This study was approved by the Ethics Committee of the First Affiliated Hospital of Nanjing Medical University. All the participants signed the informed consent forms. All the participants had undergone thyroidectomy between February 2013 and May 2017. Histological assessment was carried out according to the criteria established by the World Health Organization [26]. Pathological diagnosis was performed independently by two pathologists.

We set inclusion criteria as following: (1) patients who were 18 to 65 years old; (2) patients without distant metastasis. There were 34 patients that provided both tissue samples and serum samples. We excluded patients with other malignant tumors, hypertension, diabetes, thyroid dysfunction or other diseases which might influence metabolism, and patients who had long-term use of drugs. A total of 12 patients were excluded, including 2 patients with diabetes, 5 patients with hypertension, 2 patients with diabetes and hypertension, 2 patients with thyroid dysfunction and 1 patient with other malignant tumor.

Finally, there were 8 patients with lymph node metastasis that provided tumor tissues (TN1), para-tumor tissues (PN1) and blood serum (SN1). For patients without lymph node metastasis, there were 14 individuals that provided tumor tissues (TN0), para-tumor tissues (PN0) and blood serum (SN0). The workflow for this study is shown in Figure S1.

2.2. Metabolomic Analysis

Samples were prepared according to the previous literature [27]. The tissue preparation steps were as follows: 50 mg of frozen tissue was cut with surgical scissors, then mixed with 750 µL ultra-pure water and ultrasonicated (power: 60%). The supernatant was obtained after centrifugation (16,000× g, 15 min, 4 °C). Then, internal standards were added. The dried residues were reconstituted for metabolomic analysis. Serum sample preparation steps were as follows: 40 µL methanol and internal standards were added into 10 µL of serum. After centrifugation (16,000× g, 15 min, 4 °C), the supernatant was obtained. Then, the dried residues were reconstituted for metabolomic analysis.

The metabolomic analysis was performed as a previous report [27]. Briefly, UPLC Q-Exactive MS analysis was performed using a UPLC Ultimate 3000 system (Dionex, Germering, Germany) plus a Q-Exactive mass spectrometer (Thermo Fisher Scientific, Bremen, Germany) in both positive and negative modes with fullscan acquisition (70–1050 m/z). The instrument performed at 70,000 resolution. A multistep gradient (mobile phase A: 0.1% formic acid in ultra-pure water, mobile phase B: 0.1% formic acid in pure CAN) was operated at a flow rate of 0.4 mL/min, and the runtime was 15 min. The metabolite identification was based on the comparisons of retention time and accurate mass with metabolite standards. All samples were analyzed in a randomized manner to avoid effects induced by the injection order.

2.3. Statistical Analysis and Bioinformatics Analysis

Data collation was performed with Excel. Data analysis was performed with IBM SPSS Statistics Premium V25.0 and R. Patients' clinical information between groups was analyzed with a t test and Fisher's exact test. According to the relative quantification of metabolites, differential metabolites were screened with a t-test after log transformation. Metabolite pathway and enrichment analysis were performed using MetaboAnalyst 5.0. Statistical significance was defined using a Benjamini-Hochberg (B-H) FDR <0.05. A visualization of altered metabolites in the global metabolic network was constructed with iPath 3.0. A Venn diagram was made with jvenn.

3. Results

3.1. Population Characteristics

The tissue and serum samples (n = 22, male/female: 3/19, metastasis/no metastasis: 8/14) of PTC patients were collected. The clinical information of each group was presented in Table S1. No significant differences in gender, age and body mass index were found. The difference in maximum tumor diameter (cm) between the two groups was statistically significant, which revealed that the size of PTC tumors affects the lymph node metastasis of PTC to some extent. Our result was consistent with a previous study [28].

3.2. The Altered Metabolites

Finally, a total of 152 metabolites and 129 metabolites were annotated from the detected spectral features from UPLC Q-Exactive in tissues and serums respectively. In total, 31 metabolites were significantly altered ($p < 0.05$ and FDR < 0.05) in the comparison between TN1 and PN1. Among these altered metabolites, 23 metabolites decreased and 8 metabolites increased (Table 1). We found 15 metabolites were significantly altered ($p < 0.05$ and FDR < 0.05) in the comparison between TN0 and PN0. When compared to the PN0 group, 13 metabolites were significantly down-regulated, while 2 metabolites were significantly up-regulated in the TN0 group (Table 2). We identified two increased metabolites and two decreased metabolites in the SN1 group compared with the SN0 group ($p < 0.05$), while there was no altered metabolite found after FDR calibration (Table 3).

Table 1. List of the altered metabolites identified in the comparison between TN1 and PN1.

Metabolites	Fold Change	p	FDR
Thyroxine	0.020	4.815×10^{-3}	3.485×10^{-2}
Deoxycholic acid	0.023	2.784×10^{-3}	2.645×10^{-2}
Allantoin	0.024	6.246×10^{-3}	3.921×10^{-2}
Iodotyrosine	0.027	4.068×10^{-4}	1.030×10^{-2}
5-Hydroxymethyl-2-Deoxyuridine	0.033	1.370×10^{-5}	1.041×10^{-3}
Erucic acid	0.041	1.027×10^{-3}	1.562×10^{-2}
Cytidine monophosphate	0.062	3.140×10^{-3}	2.808×10^{-2}
Cis-Aconitic acid	0.071	1.573×10^{-3}	2.146×10^{-2}
Citric acid	0.085	2.250×10^{-5}	1.140×10^{-3}
Glycerophosphocholine	0.150	6.354×10^{-3}	3.921×10^{-2}
Uridine	0.159	4.870×10^{-5}	1.480×10^{-3}
Glycolic acid	0.183	8.537×10^{-4}	1.442×10^{-2}
Gallic acid	0.242	2.610×10^{-3}	2.645×10^{-2}
Tryptamine	0.261	9.285×10^{-3}	4.599×10^{-2}
Glyceraldehyde	0.262	3.640×10^{-5}	1.383×10^{-3}
Syringic acid	0.267	4.436×10^{-3}	3.393×10^{-2}

Table 1. Cont.

Metabolites	Fold Change	p	FDR
Glucose 6-phosphate	0.269	8.055×10^{-3}	4.535×10^{-2}
D-Glyceraldehyde 3-phosphate	0.284	6.449×10^{-3}	3.921×10^{-2}
Sorbitol	0.320	4.972×10^{-4}	1.080×10^{-2}
Gamma-Linolenic acid	0.324	9.380×10^{-3}	4.599×10^{-2}
Rhamnose	0.332	6.122×10^{-4}	1.163×10^{-2}
Inosine	0.375	8.844×10^{-3}	4.599×10^{-2}
Acetaminophen	0.585	1.912×10^{-3}	2.146×10^{-2}
L-Proline	1.539	7.248×10^{-3}	4.237×10^{-2}
L-Tryptophan	1.747	4.464×10^{-3}	3.393×10^{-2}
5-Hydroxylysine	2.817	6.362×10^{-3}	3.921×10^{-2}
3-Methylhistidine	2.839	4.259×10^{-3}	3.393×10^{-2}
N-Alpha-acetyllysine	3.222	1.877×10^{-3}	2.146×10^{-2}
Deoxycytidine	3.236	8.773×10^{-3}	4.599×10^{-2}
Uracil	8.363	1.270×10^{-5}	1.041×10^{-3}
Carnosine	32.324	1.977×10^{-3}	2.146×10^{-2}

Table 2. List of the altered metabolites identified in comparison between TN0 and PN0.

Metablolites	Fold Change	p	FDR
cis-Aconitic acid	0.051	3.330×10^{-5}	2.386×10^{-3}
Allantoin	0.096	3.694×10^{-4}	7.019×10^{-3}
Iodotyrosine	0.128	1.420×10^{-5}	2.158×10^{-3}
Isocitric acid	0.144	2.484×10^{-3}	2.696×10^{-2}
Thyroxine	0.192	1.255×10^{-3}	1.734×10^{-2}
Cytidine monophosphate	0.216	7.922×10^{-4}	1.204×10^{-2}
Trizma Acetate	0.226	1.865×10^{-4}	4.724×10^{-3}
Uridine	0.259	4.710×10^{-5}	2.386×10^{-3}
Glycolic acid	0.274	2.966×10^{-3}	3.005×10^{-2}
Citric acid	0.299	3.094×10^{-4}	6.718×10^{-3}
Gluconolactone	0.329	1.368×10^{-4}	4.724×10^{-3}
N-Acetylglutamic acid	0.360	1.447×10^{-3}	1.833×10^{-2}
Rhamnose	0.378	7.166×10^{-4}	1.204×10^{-2}
Ureidopropionic acid	2.808	2.299×10^{-3}	2.688×10^{-2}
Carnosine	4.734	1.807×10^{-4}	4.724×10^{-3}

Table 3. List of the altered metabolites identified in the comparison between SN1 and SN0.

Metabolite Name	Fold Change	p	FDR
L-Malic acid	0.187	2.310×10^{-2}	0.923
Thyroxine	0.649	2.102×10^{-2}	0.923
Carnosine	1.605	4.933×10^{-2}	0.923
Docosahexaenoic acid	1.632	4.614×10^{-2}	0.923

3.3. The Co-Owned Metabolic Changes

We found nine significantly decreased metabolites and one significantly increased metabolite in two comparisons (TN1 and PN1, TN0 and PN0).

3.4. Differential Metabolites between Two Comparisons (TN1 and PN1, TN0 and PN0)

We found that the PTC patients with lymph node metastasis (TN1 and PN1) had more differential metabolites than those without lymph node metastasis (TN0 and PN0). A visualization of the altered metabolic coverage based on iPath 3.0 is shown in Figure 1A. The detailed differential metabolites are as follows: 7 uniquely increased metabolites and 14 uniquely decreased metabolites appeared in the TN1 group when compared with the PN1 group (Figure 1B).

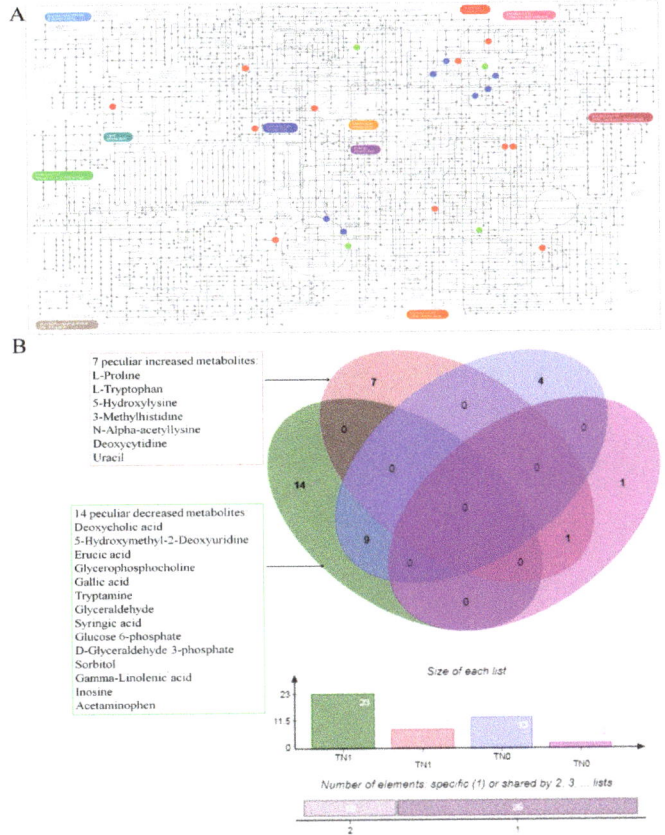

Figure 1. The altered metabolites. (**A**) Visualization of the altered metabolite coverage based on iPath 3.0. The blue points represent the co-owned metabolites in two groups (TN1 and PN1, TN0 and PN0), the red points represent the specific metabolites detected in the lymph node metastasis (TN1 and PN1) group, and the green points represent the specific metabolites detected in the group without lymph node metastasis (TN0 and PN0). The metabolites which are not indicated in the general pathway map are not shown. (**B**) This Venn diagram displays overlaps of differential metabolites between two groups (TN1 and PN1, TN0 and PN0).

3.5. The Altered Pathways

Metabolic pathway analysis and enrichment analysis of differential metabolites between TN1 and PN1 showed that there were statistical differences ($p < 0.05$ and FDR < 0.05) in pyrimidine metabolism, histidine metabolism, neomycin, kanamycin and gentamicin biosynthesis, fructose and mannose metabolism, citrate cycle (TCA cycle), beta-alanine metabolism, fructose and mannose degradation and thyroid hormone synthesis. Compared with PN0, there were six significantly altered ($p < 0.05$ and FDR < 0.05) pathways in TN0 as follows: citrate cycle (TCA cycle), glyoxylate and dicarboxylate metabolism, pyrimidine metabolism, beta-alanine metabolism, tyrosine metabolism and thyroid hormone synthesis (Figure 2, Table S2). Our results indicated that four pathways (pyrimidine metabolism, beta-alanine metabolism, thyroid hormone synthesis and citrate cycle) were co-owned pathways in the comparisons between TN1 and PN1, and between TN0 and PN0. On the other hand, we identified four unique pathways (histidine metabolism, neomycin, kanamycin and gentamicin biosynthesis, fructose and mannose metabolism, fructose and mannose degradation) presented in the TN1 group when compared with the PN1 group, and two unique pathways (glyoxylate and dicarboxylate metabolism, tyrosine metabolism) presented in the TN0 group when compared with the PN0 group (Figure 2E).

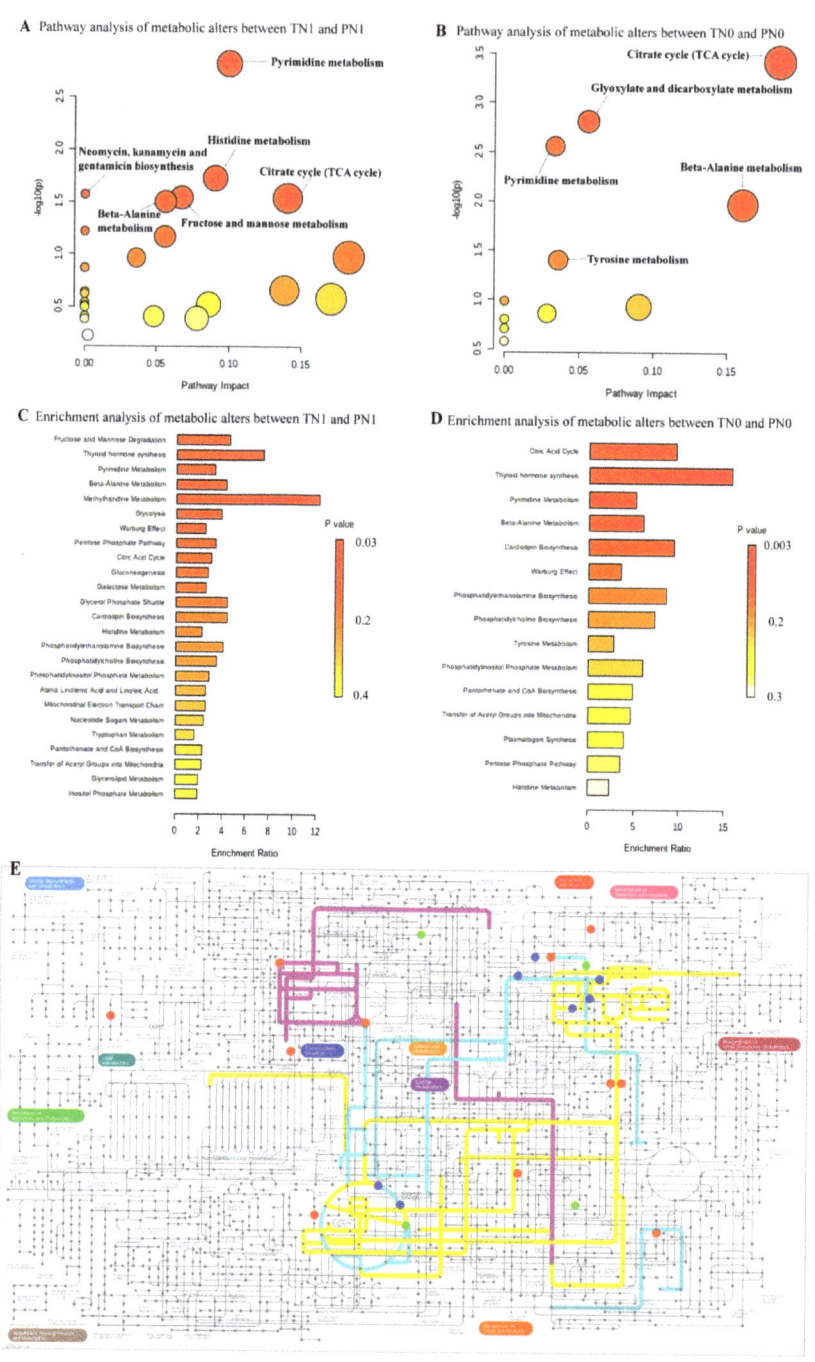

Figure 2. The altered pathways. (**A**) Pathway analysis of metabolic alterations between TN1 and

PN1. (**B**) Pathway analysis of metabolic alterations between TN0 and PN0. (**C**) Enrichment analysis of metabolic alterations between TN1 and PN1. (**D**) Enrichment analysis of metabolic alterations between TN0 and PN0. (**E**) The metabolic network of the differential metabolites and altered metabolic pathways in the KEGG general metabolic pathway map. The cyan lines represent the co-owned pathways in two groups (TN1 and PN1, TN0 and PN0), the purple lines represent the specific metabolites detected in the lymph node metastasis (TN1 and PN1) group, and the yellow lines represent the specific metabolites detected in the group without lymph node metastasis (TN0 and PN0). The metabolites which are not indicated in the general pathway map are not shown.

4. Discussion

Our UPLC-HRMS study examined both serums and tissues of PTC patients with or without lymph node metastasis, and we found co-owned and differential metabolites/metabolite pathways.

First of all, in the comparisons (TN1 and PN1, TN0 and PN0), we found nine co-owned decreased metabolites (thyroxine, allantoin, iodotyrosine, cytidine monophosphate, cis-aconitic acid, citric acid, uridine, glycolic acid, rhamnose) and one co-owned increased metabolite (carnosine). Among these metabolites, allantoin has been implicated in prostate, colon, intestinal ovarian and breast cancer protection [29], and decreased citric acid has been found in prostate cancer [30]. Thyroxine is a hormone made in the thyroid gland. A large population study showed that L-thyroxine treatment was associated with a decreased frequency of PTC, so the decreased thyroxine of PTC in our study is reasonable. Our results indicated that the ability of the thyroid to synthesize thyroxine is affected after carcinogenesis [31]. Carnosine is a low-molecular-weight hydrophilic antioxidant, and it is important for many normal body functions. It has been suggested that carnosine may not display the same function in different tissues and may even play several functions within one tissue [32]. Although some studies have shown that carnosine has a positive effect on disease treatment [33], carnosine can also exert negative effects under certain conditions [34]. Our results suggest that these metabolites might be important metabolite markers of PTC.

Furthermore, we found 7 uniquely increased metabolites (L-proline, L-tryptophan, 5-hydroxylysine, 3-methylhistidine, N-alpha-acetyllysine, deoxycytidine, uracil) and 14 uniquely decreased metabolites (deoxycholic acid, 5-hydroxymethyl-2-deoxyuridine, erucic acid, glycerophosphocholine, gallic acid, tryptamine, glyceraldehyde, syringic acid, glucose 6-phosphate, D-glyceraldehyde 3-phosphate, Sorbitol, gamma-linolenic acid, inosine, acetaminophen) in the lymph node metastasis (TN1 and PN1) group when compared with the group without lymph node metastasis (TN0 and PN0). Most of the seven uniquely increased metabolites have been verified to possibly promote the progression of other tumors; for example, L-proline addition and L-tryptophan metabolism promote tumor invasion and metastasis and accelerate cancer progression [35,36]. The concentrations of 5-hydroxylysine and 3-methylhistidine have been identified as significant prognostic factors for overall survival in oral squamous cell carcinoma [37]. We speculated that these metabolites might promote the lymph node metastasis of PTC. On the other hand, among the 14 uniquely decreased metabolites, most of them have been reported to possibly inhibit the progression of other cancers. For instance, deoxycholic acid, erucic acid and syringic acid act in an anti-tumoral way in human colorectal cancer cells, neuroblastoma/glioblastoma and gallbladder cancer separately [38–40]. A switch from high to low levels of glycerophosphocholine could induce ovarian tumor aggressiveness [41]. Gallic acid and sorbitol could induce apoptosis of human small cell lung cancer cells/human gastric adenocarcinoma cells and human colorectal cancer cells separately [42–44]. The intratumoral injection of tryptamine was certified to reduce tumor growth and tumor sizes in vivo [45]. Gamma-linolenic acid can inhibit the invasion of human colon cancer cells [46]. These metabolites might also have inhibitory effects on PTC metastasis; future studies are warranted to assess these biomarkers as candidate biomarkers.

Our results indicated that four pathways (pyrimidine metabolism, beta-alanine metabolism, thyroid hormone synthesis and citrate cycle) were co-owned pathways in the comparisons of TN1 and PN1, and TN0 and PN0. Pyrimidine metabolism is required for tumor cells to maintain high proliferation. A previous study showed that pyrimidine metabolism was significantly altered in PTC tumor tissues, which supported our results [47]. Beta-alanine metabolism, as well as pyrimidine metabolism, is a crucial process in carbohydrate metabolism. Consistent with our findings, the regulation of beta-alanine catabolism in cancer has been demonstrated in previous works [48,49]. Disturbance of thyroid hormone synthesis is the most common endocrine affliction. For thyroid hormone synthesis, an adequate supply of essential micronutrients to the thyroid gland is crucial [50]. Thyroid hormone synthesis is affected after carcinogenesis.. The consistent pathway changes also included the citric acid cycle. Our results showed that several molecules in the citric acid cycle were decreased, which indicated that citric acid cycle activity in PTC tumor tissues had decreased; therefore, the cancer cells might depend on high levels of aerobic glycolysis (the Warburg effect) as the major source for ATP to support cellular proliferation [51]. The disturbance of these pathways might be potential mechanisms of PTC.

As for the four unique pathways presented in the lymph node metastasis (TN1 and PN1) group, histidine metabolism has been shown to be an important pathway in distinguishing metastatic from extratumoral tissue in cutaneous melanoma, and can reflect carcinogenesis and cancer progression [52]. Mannose, closely related to fructose, is necessary for glycosylation [53]. Altered glycosylation is characteristic of aggressive cancers [54]. Therefore, histidine metabolism and fructose and mannose metabolism might be the possible mechanisms of the lymph node metastasis of PTC.

In short, our work may provide new clues for the underlying mechanisms regarding PTC with/without lymph node metastasis as well as potential therapeutic targets. However, the sample size of our study is small, and further studies are warranted in larger-scale populations.

5. Conclusions

This study found the distinct metabolites and metabolic pathways in PTC patients with/without lymph node metastasis. Co-owned metabolites presented in the comparisons (TN1 and PN1, TN0 and PN0) were potential markers of PTC. Unique metabolites presented in the lymph node metastasis group might be predictors and potential therapeutic targets of lymph node metastasis. The disturbance of pyrimidine metabolism, beta-alanine metabolism, thyroid hormone synthesis and citric acid cycle might be potential mechanisms of PTC. Unique pathways presented in the lymph node metastasis (TN1 and PN1) group might be the possible mechanisms of lymph node metastasis of PTC. Knowing these altered metabolites and metabolic pathways is helpful in determining therapeutic targets.

Supplementary Materials: The following supporting information can be downloaded at: https://www.mdpi.com/article/10.3390/toxics11010044/s1, Figure S1: Strategy for the metabolomic study regarding PTC; Table S1: The clinical information of patients in different groups; Table S2. Altered pathways in comparisons (TN1 and PN1,TN0 and PN0) by pathway analysis and enrichment analysis.

Author Contributions: W.T. and D.W. conceived and led the design of the study. B.X., W.G. and T.X. conducted the experiments and wrote the first draft of the article. C.L. collected samples and subject data. All authors have read and approved the final article. All authors have read and agreed to the published version of the manuscript.

Funding: This work was supported by grants from the National Natural Science Foundation of China (81770773) and the Natural Science Foundation of Jiangsu Province (BK20211375).

Institutional Review Board Statement: The study was conducted in accordance with the Declaration of Helsinki and approved by Ethics Committee of the First Affiliated Hospital of Nanjing Medical University (2010-SR-091.A1).

Informed Consent Statement: Informed consent was obtained from all subjects involved in the study. Written informed consent has been obtained from the patients to publish this paper.

Data Availability Statement: The data presented in this study are available on request from the corresponding author. The data are not publicly available due to privacy or ethical restrictions.

Conflicts of Interest: The authors declare no conflict of interest.

References

1. Cabanillas, M.E.; McFadden, D.G.; Durante, C. Thyroid cancer. *Lancet* **2016**, *388*, 2783–2795. [CrossRef] [PubMed]
2. Dong, W.; Horiuchi, K.; Tokumitsu, H.; Sakamoto, A.; Noguchi, E.; Ueda, Y.; Okamoto, T. Time-Varying Pattern of Mortality and Recurrence from Papillary Thyroid Cancer: Lessons from a Long-Term Follow-Up. *Thyroid* **2019**, *29*, 802–808. [CrossRef] [PubMed]
3. Caron, N.R.; Clark, O.H. Papillary thyroid cancer: Surgical management of lymph node metastases. *Curr. Treat. Options Oncol.* **2005**, *6*, 311–322. [CrossRef]
4. Sivanandan, R.; Soo, K.C. Pattern of cervical lymph node metastases from papillary carcinoma of the thyroid. *Br. J. Surg.* **2001**, *88*, 1241–1244. [CrossRef]
5. Ito, Y.; Kudo, T.; Kobayashi, K.; Miya, A.; Ichihara, K.; Miyauchi, A. Prognostic factors for recurrence of papillary thyroid carcinoma in the lymph. *World J. Surg.* **2012**, *36*, 1274–1278. [CrossRef] [PubMed]
6. Lew, J.I.; Solorzano, C.C. Use of ultrasound in the management of thyroid cancer. *Oncologist.* **2010**, *15*, 253–258. [CrossRef]
7. Sipos, J.A. Advances in ultrasound for the diagnosis and management of thyroid cancer. *Thyroid* **2009**, *19*, 1363–1372. [CrossRef]
8. Wong, K.T.; Ahuja, A.T. Ultrasound of thyroid cancer. *Cancer Imaging* **2005**, *5*, 157–166. [CrossRef]
9. Lew, J.I.; Rodgers, S.E.; Solorzano, C.C. Developments in the use of ultrasound for thyroid cancer. *Curr. Opin. Oncol.* **2010**, *22*, 11–16. [CrossRef]
10. Chen, J.; Li, X.L.; Zhao, C.K.; Wang, D.; Wang, Q.; Li, M.X.; Wei, Q.; Guo, J.; Xu, H.X. Conventional Ultrasound, Immunohistochemical Factors and BRAF(V600E) Mutation in Predicting Central Cervical Lymph Node Metastasis of Papillary Thyroid Carcinoma. *Ultrasound Med. Biol.* **2018**, *44*, 2296–2306. [CrossRef]
11. Chen, Y.J.; Zhao, R.M.; Zhao, Q.; Li, B.Y.; Ma, Q.Y.; Li, X.; Chen, X. Diagnostic significance of elevated expression of HBME-1 in papillary thyroid carcinoma. *Tumour Biol.* **2016**, *37*, 8715–8720. [CrossRef] [PubMed]
12. Cui, W.; Sang, W.; Zheng, S.; Ma, Y.; Liu, X.; Zhang, W. Usefulness of cytokeratin-19, galectin-3, and Hector Battifora mesothelial-1 in the diagnosis of benign and malignant thyroid nodules. *Clin. Lab.* **2012**, *58*, 673–680. [PubMed]
13. O'Neill, C.J.; Bullock, M.; Chou, A.; Sidhu, S.B.; Delbridge, L.W.; Robinson, B.G.; Gill, A.J.; Learoyd, D.L.; Clifton-Bligh, R.; Sywak, M.S. BRAF(V600E) mutation is associated with an increased risk of nodal recurrence requiring reoperative surgery in patients with papillary thyroid cancer. *Surgery* **2010**, *148*, 1139–1145, discussion 1145-6. [CrossRef] [PubMed]
14. Dutenhefner, S.E.; Marui, S.; Santos, A.B.; de Lima, E.U.; Inoue, M.; Neto, J.S.B.; Shiang, C.; Fukushima, J.T.; Cernea, C.R.; Friguglietti, C.U. BRAF: A tool in the decision to perform elective neck dissection? *Thyroid* **2013**, *23*, 1541–1546. [CrossRef]
15. Han, P.A.; Kim, H.S.; Cho, S.; Fazeli, R.; Najafian, A.; Khawaja, H.; McAlexander, M.; Dy, B.; Sorensen, M.; Aronova, A.; et al. Association of BRAF V600E Mutation and MicroRNA Expression with Central Lymph Node Metastases in Papillary Thyroid Cancer: A Prospective Study from Four Endocrine Surgery Centers. *Thyroid* **2016**, *26*, 532–542. [CrossRef]
16. Ren, H.; Shen, Y.; Hu, D.; He, W.; Zhou, J.; Cao, Y.; Mao, Y.; Dou, Y.; Xiong, W.; Xiao, Q.; et al. Co-existence of BRAF(V600E) and TERT promoter mutations in papillary thyroid. *Cancer Manag. Res.* **2018**, *10*, 1005–1013. [CrossRef]
17. Liu, R.; Li, Y.; Chen, W.; Cong, J.; Zhang, Z.; Ma, L.; Chu, L.; Xiao, H.; Zhang, Y.; Liu, Y.; et al. Mutations of the TERT promoter are associated with aggressiveness and recurrence/distant metastasis of papillary thyroid carcinoma. *Oncol. Lett.* **2020**, *20*, 50. [CrossRef]
18. Pavlova, N.N.; Thompson, C.B. The Emerging Hallmarks of Cancer Metabolism. *Cell Metab.* **2016**, *23*, 27–47. [CrossRef]
19. Gomase, V.S.; Changbhale, S.S.; Patil, S.A.; Kale, K.V. Metabolomics. *Curr. Drug Metab.* **2008**, *9*, 89–98. [CrossRef]
20. Puchades-Carrasco, L.; Pineda-Lucena, A. Metabolomics Applications in Precision Medicine: An Oncological Perspective. *Curr. Top. Med. Chem.* **2017**, *17*, 2740–2751. [CrossRef]
21. Johnson, C.H.; Ivanisevic, J.; Siuzdak, G. Metabolomics: Beyond biomarkers and towards mechanisms. *Nat. Rev. Mol. Cell Biol.* **2016**, *17*, 451–459. [CrossRef] [PubMed]
22. Chen, M.; Shen, M.; Li, Y.; Liu, C.; Zhou, K.; Hu, W.; Xu, B.; Xia, Y.; Tang, W. GC-MS-based metabolomic analysis of human papillary thyroid carcinoma tissue. *Int. J. Mol. Med.* **2015**, *36*, 1607–1614. [CrossRef] [PubMed]
23. Li, Y.; Chen, M.; Liu, C.; Xia, Y.; Xu, B.; Hu, Y.; Chen, T.; Shen, M.; Tang, W. Metabolic changes associated with papillary thyroid carcinoma: A nuclear magnetic resonance-based metabolomics study. *Int. J. Mol. Med.* **2018**, *41*, 3006–3014. [CrossRef] [PubMed]
24. Zhang, A.; Sun, H.; Wang, P.; Han, Y.; Wang, X. Modern analytical techniques in metabolomics analysis. *Analyst* **2012**, *137*, 293–300. [CrossRef] [PubMed]
25. Tautenhahn, R.; Böttcher, C.; Neumann, S. Highly sensitive feature detection for high resolution LC/MS. *BMC Bioinform.* **2008**, *9*, 504. [CrossRef]
26. DeLellis, R.A.; Heitz, L.R.; Eng, C. *Pathology and Genetics of Tumours of Endocrine Organs, Vol. 8*; World Health Organization; IARC Press: Lyon, France, 2004.

27. Zhou, K.; Ding, X.; Yang, J.; Hu, Y.; Song, Y.; Chen, M.; Sun, R.; Dong, T.; Xu, B.; Han, X.; et al. Metabolomics Reveals Metabolic Changes Caused by Low-Dose 4-Tert-Octylphenol in mice liver. *Int. J. Environ. Res. Public Health* **2018**, *15*, 2686. [CrossRef]
28. Song, M.; Huang, Z.; Wang, S.; Huang, J.; Shi, H.; Liu, Y.; Huang, Y.; Yin, Y.; Wu, Z. Predictive factors of lateral lymph node metastasis in conventional papillary thyroid carcinoma. *Gland Surg.* **2020**, *9*, 1000–1007. [CrossRef]
29. Marzook, F.; Marzook, E.; El-Sonbaty, S. Allantoin may modulate aging impairments, symptoms and cancers. *Pak. J. of Pharm. Sci.* **2021**, *34*, 1377–1384.
30. Buszewska-Forajta, M.; Monedeiro, F.; Gołębiowski, A.; Adamczyk, P.; Buszewski, B. Citric Acid as a Potential Prostate Cancer Biomarker Determined in Various Biological Samples. *Metabolites.* **2022**, *12*, 268. [CrossRef]
31. Fiore, E.; Rago, T.; Provenzale, M.A.; Scutari, M.; Ugolini, C.; Basolo, F.; Coscio, G.D.; Miccoli, P.; Grasso, L.; Pinchera, A.; et al. L-thyroxine-treated patients with nodular goiter have lower serum TSH and lower frequency of papillary thyroid cancer: Results of a cross-sectional study on 27 914 patients. *Endocr. Relat. Cancer* **2010**, *17*, 231–239. [CrossRef]
32. Boldyrev, A.A.; Aldini, G.; Derave, W. Physiology and pathophysiology of carnosine. *Physiol. Rev.* **2013**, *93*, 1803–1845. [CrossRef]
33. Budzeń, S.; Rymaszewska, J. The biological role of carnosine and its possible applications in medicine. *Adv. Clin. Exp. Med.* **2013**, *22*, 739–744. [PubMed]
34. Prokopieva, V.D.; Yarygina, E.G.; Bokhan, N.A.; Ivanova, S.A. Use of Carnosine for Oxidative Stress Reduction in Different Pathologies. *Oxid. Med. Cell. Longev.* **2016**, *2016*, 2939087. [CrossRef] [PubMed]
35. Liu, Y.; Mao, C.; Wang, M.; Liu, N.; Ouyang, L.; Liu, S.; Tang, H.; Cao, Y.; Liu, S.; Wang, X.; et al. Cancer progression is mediated by proline catabolism in non-small cell lung. *Oncogene* **2020**, *39*, 2358–2376. [CrossRef]
36. Lemos, H.; Huang, L.; Prendergast, G.C.; Mellor, A.L. Immune control by amino acid catabolism during tumorigenesis and therapy. *Nat. Rev. Cancer* **2019**, *19*, 162–175. [CrossRef] [PubMed]
37. Shikawa, S.; Sugimoto, M.; Konta, T.; Kitabatake, K.; Ueda, S.; Edamatsu, K.; Okuyama, N.; Yusa, K.; Iino, M. Salivary Metabolomics for Prognosis of Oral Squamous Cell Carcinoma. *Front. Oncol.* **2022**, *11*, 789248. [CrossRef]
38. Lin, R.; Zhan, M.; Yang, L.; Wang, H.; Shen, H.; Huang, S.; Huang, X.; Xu, S.; Zhang, Z.; Li, W.; et al. Deoxycholic acid modulates the progression of gallbladder cancer through N6-methyladenosine-dependent microRNA maturation. *Oncogene* **2020**, *39*, 4983–5000. [CrossRef]
39. Altinoz, M.A.; Elmaci, İ.; Hacimuftuoglu, A.; Ozpinar, A.; Hacker, E.; Ozpinar, A. PPARδ and its ligand erucic acid may act anti-tumoral, neuroprotective, and myelin protective in neuroblastoma, glioblastoma, and Parkinson's disease. *Mol. Asp. Med.* **2021**, *78*, 100871. [CrossRef] [PubMed]
40. Abaza, M.S.; Al-Attiyah, R.A.; Bhardwaj, R.; Abbadi, G.; Koyippally, M.; Afzal, M. Syringic acid from Tamarix aucheriana possesses antimitogenic and chemo-sensitizing activities in human colorectal cancer cells. *Pharm. Biol.* **2013**, *51*, 1110–1124. [CrossRef] [PubMed]
41. Iorio, E.; Ricci, A.; Bagnoli, M.; Pisanu, M.E.; Castellano, G.; Di Vito, M. Alterations of choline phospholipid metabolism in ovarian tumor progression. *Cancer Res.* **2005**, *65*, 9369–9376. [CrossRef]
42. Wang, R.; Ma, L.; Weng, D.; Yao, J.; Liu, X.; Jin, F. Gallic acid induces apoptosis and enhances the anticancer effects of cisplatin in human small cell lung cancer H446 cell line via the ROS-dependent mitochondrial apoptotic pathway. *Oncol. Rep.* **2016**, *35*, 3075–3083. [CrossRef] [PubMed]
43. Tsai, C.L.; Chiu, Y.M.; Ho, T.Y.; Hsieh, C.T.; Shieh, D.C.; Lee, Y.J.; Tsay, G.J.; Wu, Y.Y. Gallic Acid Induces Apoptosis in Human Gastric Adenocarcinoma Cells. *Anticancer Res.* **2018**, *38*, 2057–2067. [CrossRef] [PubMed]
44. Lu, X.; Li, C.; Wang, Y.K.; Jiang, K.; Gai, X.D. Sorbitol induces apoptosis of human colorectal cancer cells via p38 MAPK signal transduction. *Oncol. Lett.* **2014**, *7*, 1992–1996. [CrossRef] [PubMed]
45. Li, Z.; Ding, B.; Ali, M.R.; Zhao, L.; Zang, X.; Lv, Z. Dual Effect of Tryptamine on Prostate Cancer Cell Growth Regulation: A Pilot Study. *Int. J. Mol. Sci.* **2022**, *23*, 11087. [CrossRef]
46. Jiang, W.G.; Hiscox, S.; Hallett, M.B.; Scott, C.; Horrobin, D.F.; Puntis, M.C.A. Inhibition of hepatocyte growth factor-induced motility and in vitro invasion of human colon cancer cells by gamma-linolenic acid. *Br. J. Cancer* **1995**, *71*, 744–752. [CrossRef]
47. Xu, Y.; Zheng, X.; Qiu, Y.; Jia, W.; Wang, J.; Yin, S. Distinct Metabolomic Profiles of Papillary Thyroid Carcinoma and Benign Thyroid adenoma. *J. Proteome Res.* **2015**, *14*, 3315–3321. [CrossRef]
48. Xie, Z.; Li, X.; He, Y.; Wu, S.; Wang, S.; Sun, J.; He, Y.; Lun, Y.; Zhang, J. Immune Cell Confrontation in the Papillary Thyroid Carcinoma Microenvironment. *Front. Endocrinol.* **2020**, *11*, 570604. [CrossRef]
49. Budczies, J.; Brockmöller, S.F.; Müller, B.M.; Barupal, D.K.; Richter-Ehrenstein, C.; Kleine-Tebbe, A.; Griffin, J.L.; Orešič, M.; Dietel, M.; Denkert, C.; et al. Comparative metabolomics of estrogen receptor positive and estrogen receptor negative breast cancer: Alterations in glutamine and beta-alanine metabolism. *J. Proteom.* **2013**, *94*, 279–288. [CrossRef]
50. Brix, K.; Führer, D.; Biebermann, H. Molecules important for thyroid hormone synthesis and action-known facts and future perspectives. *Thyroid Res.* **2011**, *4* (Suppl. 1). [CrossRef]
51. Porporato, P.E.; Filigheddu, N.; Pedro, J.M.B.S.; Kroemer, G.; Galluzzi, L. Mitochondrial metabolism and cancer. *Cell Res.* **2018**, *28*, 265–280. [CrossRef]
52. Taylor, N.J.; Gaynanova, I.; Eschrich, S.A.; Welsh, E.A.; Garrett, T.J.; Beecher, C.; Sharma, R.; Koomen, J.M.; Smalley, K.S.M.; Messina, J.L.; et al. Metabolomics of primary cutaneous melanoma and matched adjacent extratumoral microenvironment. *PLoS ONE* **2020**, *15*, e0240849. [CrossRef] [PubMed]

53. Lieu, E.L.; Kelekar, N.; Bhalla, P.; Kim, J. Fructose and Mannose in Inborn Errors of Metabolism and Cancer. *Metabolites* **2021**, *11*, 479. [CrossRef] [PubMed]
54. Pinho, S.S.; Reis, C.A. Glycosylation in cancer: Mechanisms and clinical implications. *Nat. Rev. Cancer* **2015**, *15*, 540–555. [CrossRef] [PubMed]

Disclaimer/Publisher's Note: The statements, opinions and data contained in all publications are solely those of the individual author(s) and contributor(s) and not of MDPI and/or the editor(s). MDPI and/or the editor(s) disclaim responsibility for any injury to people or property resulting from any ideas, methods, instructions or products referred to in the content.

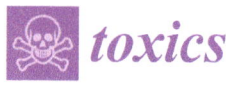

Article

Exposure to Molybdate Results in Metabolic Disorder: An Integrated Study of the Urine Elementome and Serum Metabolome in Mice

Kun Zhou [1,2,3,†], Miaomiao Tang [1,2,†], Wei Zhang [4,†], Yanling Chen [1,2,†], Yusheng Guan [1,2], Rui Huang [1,2], Jiawei Duan [1,2], Zibo Liu [1,2], Xiaoming Ji [1,2], Yingtong Jiang [1,2], Yanhui Hu [4], Xiaoling Zhang [5], Jingjing Zhou [1,2] and Minjian Chen [1,2,*]

[1] State Key Laboratory of Reproductive Medicine and Offspring Health, Center for Global Health, School of Public Health, Nanjing Medical University, Nanjing 211166, China; zk@njmu.edu.cn (K.Z.); tmm_2023@163.com (M.T.); cyanling9211@163.com (Y.C.); guanys000@163.com (Y.G.); hrye0928@163.com (R.H.); jwduan1997@163.com (J.D.); liuzibo@njmu.edu.cn (Z.L.); jxmnjmu@163.com (X.J.); ytjiang61@163.com (Y.J.); zhou_jingjing56@163.com (J.Z.)
[2] Key Laboratory of Modern Toxicology of Ministry of Education, School of Public Health, Nanjing Medical University, Nanjing 211166, China
[3] Department of Epidemiology, Center for Global Health, School of Public Health, Nanjing Medical University, Nanjing 211166, China
[4] Sir Run Run Hospital of Nanjing Medical University, Nanjing 211166, China; wzhang_nj@foxmail.com (W.Z.); njjshyh@126.com (Y.H.)
[5] Department of Hygienic Analysis and Detection, Nanjing Medical University, Nanjing 211166, China; zhangxl3@njmu.edu.cn
* Correspondence: minjianchen@njmu.edu.cn
† These authors contributed equally to this work.

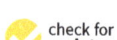

Citation: Zhou, K.; Tang, M.; Zhang, W.; Chen, Y.; Guan, Y.; Huang, R.; Duan, J.; Liu, Z.; Ji, X.; Jiang, Y.; et al. Exposure to Molybdate Results in Metabolic Disorder: An Integrated Study of the Urine Elementome and Serum Metabolome in Mice. Toxics 2024, 12, 288. https://doi.org/10.3390/toxics12040288

Academic Editors: Samuel Caito and Demetrio Raldúa

Received: 29 December 2023
Revised: 4 April 2024
Accepted: 12 April 2024
Published: 14 April 2024

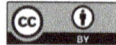

Copyright: © 2024 by the authors. Licensee MDPI, Basel, Switzerland. This article is an open access article distributed under the terms and conditions of the Creative Commons Attribution (CC BY) license (https://creativecommons.org/licenses/by/4.0/).

Abstract: The increasing use of molybdate has raised concerns about its potential toxicity in humans. However, the potential toxicity of molybdate under the current level of human exposure remains largely unknown. Endogenous metabolic alterations that are caused in humans by environmental exposure to pollutants are associated with the occurrence and progression of many diseases. This study exposed eight-week-old male C57 mice to sodium molybdate at doses relevant to humans (0.01 and 1 mg/kg/day) for eight weeks. Inductively coupled plasma mass spectrometry (ICP-MS) and ultra-performance liquid chromatography tandem mass spectrometry (UPLC-MS) were utilized to assess changes in urine element levels and serum metabolites in mice, respectively. A total of 838 subjects from the NHANES 2017–2018 population database were also included in our study to verify the associations between molybdenum and cadmium found in mice. Analysis of the metabolome in mice revealed that four metabolites in blood serum exhibited significant changes, including 5-aminolevulinic acid, glycolic acid, l-acetylcarnitine, and 2,3-dihydroxypropyl octanoate. Analysis of the elementome revealed a significant increase in urine levels of cadmium after molybdate exposure in mice. Notably, molybdenum also showed a positive correlation with cadmium in humans from the NHANES database. Further analysis identified a positive correlation between cadmium and 2,3-dihydroxypropyl octanoate in mice. In conclusion, these findings suggest that molybdate exposure disrupted amino acid and lipid metabolism, which may be partially mediated by molybdate-altered cadmium levels. The integration of elementome and metabolome data provides sensitive information on molybdate-induced metabolic disorders and associated toxicities at levels relevant to human exposure.

Keywords: molybdate; cadmium; elementome; metabolomics; toxicity

1. Introduction

Molybdenum is an essential trace element for microorganisms, plants, and animals, playing a crucial role in maintaining metabolic homeostasis [1]. In the form of molybdate, the element molybdenum finds extensive applications in food, industry, and medicine. For instance, it is utilized in the production of promising nanomaterials and layered structural materials [2,3]. Common routes of molybdenum exposure in the general population include air, soil, water, and food [4]. The absorption rate of molybdenum in the human body depends on the solubility of the various forms of molybdenum, such as molybdenum disulfide (MoS_2, insoluble in water) and sodium molybdate (water solubility: 840 g/L in water at 100 °C) [5]. Molybdenum is primarily absorbed from the gastrointestinal tract in the form of the molybdate anion, which subsequently binds with albumin and is predominantly excreted through urine [6]. For the percentage of molybdate absorbed from the gastrointestinal tract, it has been reported that molybdenum was very efficiently absorbed (88–93%), at all dietary molybdenum intakes [6]. The widespread use of molybdenum can only cause increased human exposure if there is an exposure pathway (e.g., inhalation of molybdenum containing dust) [7]. Molybdenum is an essential element, excessive exposure to molybdate has been associated with adverse health outcomes [8]. The literature reports have indicated the harmful effects of high-dose molybdate exposure (10–50 mg/kg) in animal models [9,10]. Considering the narrow safety range of essential trace elements, it is crucial to investigate the potential toxic effects of molybdate at human exposure levels. However, our current understanding of these effects remains significantly limited.

Excessive molybdate exposure can trigger changes in endogenous metabolism in the human body, which may contribute to the development of various diseases such as obesity, diabetes, cardiovascular diseases, reproductive abnormalities, and cancer [11]. For instance, lipid metabolism disorders are linked to cardiovascular diseases, while oxidative stress is associated with organ damage. Therefore, investigating the metabolic disorders caused by molybdate exposure is crucial, as it can indicate the potential toxicity of molybdate. In recent years, metabolomics has emerged as a complementary technology to genomics, transcriptomics, and proteomics, focusing on revealing gene expression outcomes [12,13]. Metabolomics, being closer to the organism's phenotype, enables the simultaneous observation of changes in numerous metabolites [14]. As metabolomics can reflect the physiological or pathological state of organisms, it plays a vital role in studying the effects and underlying mechanisms of environmental chemical toxicity [15]. Liquid chromatography coupled to tandem mass spectrometry (LC-MS) is a powerful tool for identifying and classifying metabolomes for its high sensitivity and wide range of chemical detection coverage [16]. Therefore, it is necessary to employ metabolomics technology to investigate the effects of molybdate exposure on the body's endogenous metabolism.

One of the major mechanisms underlying the toxicity of metals is their interaction with other elements in the body [17]. However, the effect of molybdate exposure on other elements is still largely unknown [18,19]. Importantly, altered exposure to elements can lead to metabolic changes in the body. For example, long-term exposure to copper can interfere with lipid metabolism [20]. Iron overload induces free radical formation, lipid peroxidation, DNA and protein damage, leading to carcinogenesis or ferroptosis [21]. Magnesium, as an essential cofactor, actively participates in carbohydrate metabolism and regulates energy metabolism and blood sugar control [22]. Therefore, the metabolic disorders resulting from molybdate exposure may be caused by disruptions in element levels in the body. Elementomics is an emerging omics technology that aims to analyze dozens of elements simultaneously, providing a comprehensive understanding of changes in their concentration in various body fluids. Hence, it is necessary to investigate the detailed effects of molybdate exposure on different elements using elementomics analysis.

Urine is a commonly used matrix for studying the body's exposure burden, while blood samples can be used to explore general metabolic changes in the body. The novel integration of elementomics and metabolomics can provide information on the disruption of the metabolome through the elementome, which has been rarely reported in previous studies.

This study utilized an animal model to investigate the effects of molybdate exposure at levels relevant to human exposure. It examined the influence of molybdate exposure on the elementome and metabolome, revealing a potential association between molybdate exposure and metabolic disorders. Meanwhile, the major findings between molybdate exposure and elementome were also verified in humans. These findings provide a novel perspective on the potential toxicity of molybdate and contribute to our understanding of this issue.

2. Materials and Methods

2.1. Experimental Materials

Sodium molybdate (purity $\geq$ 99%) was purchased from Rhawn Reagent [Shanghai, China, https://www.rhawn.cn (accessed on 21 December 2023)]. Methanol (purity $\geq$ 99%) (Merck, Darmstadt, Germany) and acetonitrile (purity $\geq$ 99%) (Merck, Darmstadt, Germany) were utilized in this study. The standard compounds were purchased from Sigma-Aldrich (St. Louis, MO, USA), Adamas Reagent Co., Ltd. (Shanghai, China), and Aladdin Reagent Company (Shanghai, China). Deionized water (resistivity $\geq$ 18.2 MΩ cm) was obtained using a Milli-Q system (Millipore, Milford, MA, USA). Nitric acid (65–70%, w/w, $\geq$99.9999%, trace metals basis) was purchased from Alfa Aesar Ltd. (Tianjin, China). The Multielementary solutions including IV-ICPMS-71A (10 ppm 43 Element (Al, As, Ba, Be, Cd, Ca, Ce, Cr, Co, Cu, Dy, Er, Eu, Gd, Ga, Ho, Fe, La, Pb, Lu, Mg, Mn, Nd, Ni, P, K, Pr, Rb, Sm, Se, Ag, Na, Sr, S, Tl, Th, Tm, U, V, Yb, Zn, Cs, and B), 3% v/v Nitric Acid), IV-ICPMS-71B (10 ppm Refractory Element (Sb, Ge, Hf, Mo, Nb, Si, Ta, Te, Sn, Ti, W, and Zr), 3% v/v Nitric Acid/trace Hydrofluoric Acid), IV-ICPMS-71C (10 ppm Precious Metal (Au, Os, Pt, Rh, Ir, Pd, Re, and Ru), 30% v/v Hydrochloric Acid), CCS-4 (100 ppm Aklali, Alkaline Earth, Non-Transition Elements (Al, As, Ba, Be, Bi, Ca, Cs, Ga, In, Li, Mg, K, Rb, Se, Na, and Sr), 7% v/v Nitric Acid), AAHG1 (1000 µg/mL mercury, 5% v/v Nitric Acid), MSAU (100 µg/mL gold HCl, 10% v/v Hydrochloric Acid), MSLI (100 µg/mL lithium, 0.1% v/v Nitric Acid), and an internal standard IV-ICPMS-71D (10 ppm 6 Element (Bi, In, Sc, Tb, Y, and ^{6}Li), 3% v/v Nitric Acid) were purchased from Inorganic Ventures (Christiansburg, VA, USA). The elements in the solutions can be found on the website [https://www.inorganicventures.com (accessed on 21 December 2023)].

2.2. Animal Experiment

Eight-week-old male C57 mice, bred under specific pathogen-free (SPF) conditions, were obtained from the Laboratory Animal Center of Nanjing Medical University in Nanjing, China. To avoid the impact of estrous cycle on metabolism in female mice, only male mice were selected. After one week of adaptive feeding, the mice were randomly divided into control and treatment groups. The administration was conducted via gavage. The control, low-exposure, and high-exposure groups were given sodium molybdate at doses of 0, 0.01, and 1 mg/kg/day, respectively, corresponding to human exposure levels. The selection of the low dose of 0.01 mg/kg/day was based on its ability to generate a toxicity burden similar to tolerable upper intake level (UL) and minimal risk level (MRL) in humans. The European Commission's Scientific Committee on Food has set the UL of molybdenum at 0.6 mg/day for adults, which is equivalent to 0.01 mg/kg/day considering an average weight of 60 kg [23]. This dose is also close to the previously reported MRL of 0.008 mg/kg/day [24]. The dose of 1 mg/kg/day was selected based on the range of human occupational exposure [25]. The exposure period lasted for 8 weeks. To improve statistical power, the ratio of the number of mice in the treatment group to the control group was set at 1:1.5. Based on animal welfare considerations and sample size estimation using 3Rs-Reduction.co.uk, 5 mice were used in the control group, and 3 mice were used in each of the treatment groups. This sample size was determined based on a signal-to-noise ratio of the toxic effects including metabolite and the element changes ranging from 2.0 to 2.8 observed in our pilot study. All mice had ad libitum access to food and water and were housed in a controlled and standardized laboratory environment with a temperature ranging from 20 to 26 °C, relative humidity ranging from 40 to 70%, and a 12 h light/dark cycle. The body weights of the mice were recorded weekly. Fasting urine and blood samples were collected, and the mice were then sacrificed. The organs, including the heart, lung, liver, spleen, kidney, and intestine, were weighed. This study strictly adhered to international standards on animal welfare and the guidelines of the Institute for Laboratory Animal Research of Nanjing Medical University. All procedures conducted in this study were approved by the Animal Ethical and Welfare Committee of Nanjing Medical University (IACUC-2008055).

2.3. Histological Examination

Heart, liver, spleen, lung, kidney, and intestine samples were collected, fixed in 4% paraformaldehyde and then embedded in paraffin [26]. Afterwards, the tissues were cut into sections (5 μm), which were deparaffinized, rehydrated, and stained with hematoxylin (0.1%) for 10 min, and eosin (0.1%) for 5 min. Hematoxylin and eosin (HE) stained sections were digitalized with the whole-slide Pannoramic MIDI scanner (3DHISTECH Ltd., Budapest, Hungary) at 20× magnification and analyzed with Pannoramic Viewer software (3DHISTECH, Budapest, Hungary).

2.4. Analysis of Elementome in Urine

The detection of the elementome in urine using the standard curve method for quantification was conducted following our previous reports [27]. Prior to the experiment, all glassware was soaked in 10% nitric acid for 24 h, rinsed with deionized water 8 to 10 times, and dried in a vacuum drying cabinet at 37 °C for later use. For each sample, 10 μL of urine was added to 485 μL of 1% dilute nitric acid, and 5 μL of internal standard IV-ICPMS-71D (10 ppm 6 Element (Bi, In, Sc, Tb, Y, and ^{6}Li), 3% v/v Nitric Acid) (Inorganic Ventures, Christiansburg, VA, USA) at the concentration of 1 mg/L was added. The mixture was thoroughly mixed. The samples were then quantified using an iCAP Qc inductively coupled plasma mass spectrometry (ICP-MS) instrument (Thermo Fisher Scientific, Bremen, Germany). The Multielementary solutions (Inorganic Ventures, Christiansburg, VA, USA) were used in elementome analysis. The employed ICP-MS was equipped with a collision cell, and helium (99.999% grade) at 5.0 mL/min was used for the collision cell to remove polyatomic interferences. Quality control samples and blank samples were analyzed in parallel with the study samples. The limit of detection (LOD) was calculated as 3 times the standard deviation for 10 consecutive blank samples [28]. The concentration of undetectable urinary elements was imputed with LOD/2 according to the previous report [29]. The recoveries of the detected elements were between 86.8% and 107%.

2.5. Analysis of Metabolome in Serum

The blood serum metabolomics detection was conducted following our previously reported method [30]. Blood was collected by retro-orbital bleed into 1.5 mL Eppendorf tubes directly and allowed to clot for 30 min, followed by centrifugation at 3000× g for 10 minutes at 4 °C to collect serum (200–300 μL). Then, protein precipitation of blood serum (20 μL) was performed using methanol at a volume ratio of 1:3. After centrifugation at 20,000× g for 15 min at 4 °C, the supernatant was transferred. The target analytes were dried in a vacuum concentrator (Labconco, MO, USA) at room temperature and reconstituted with 20 μL deionized water for further analysis. Ultra-high performance liquid chromatography (UPLC) (Dionex, Germering, Germany) equipped with a Hypersil GOLD C18 column (100 mm × 2.1 mm, 1.9 μm, column temperature at 40 °C) and tandem Q Exactive Orbitrap and triple quadrupole mass spectrometry (Thermo Fisher Scientific, Bremen, Germany) were used in the analysis. The full scan mode was employed, ranging from 70 m/z to 1050 m/z, at a resolution of 70,000 with the heated electrospray ionization (HESI) source. For UPLC analysis, a multistep gradient was used with mobile phase A consisting of 0.1% formic acid in water and mobile phase B consisting of 0.1% formic acid in acetonitrile. The flow rate was set at 0.4 mL/min over a run time of 17 min. Gradient program was conducted as follows: 0–3 min, 1% mobile phase B and 99% mobile phase A; 3–10 min, 1–99% mobile phase B and 99–1% mobile phase A; 10–15 min, 99% mobile phase B and 1% mobile phase A; 15–17 min, 1% mobile phase B and 99% mobile phase A. The autosampler temperature was maintained at 4 °C, and the injection volume was 10 µL. The mass spectrometer parameters were set as follows: for the positive mode, a spray voltage of 3.5 kV; for the negative mode, a spray voltage of 2.5 kV; for both modes, a capillary temperature of 300 °C; a sheath gas flow of 50 arbitrary units (AU); an auxiliary gas flow of 13 AU; a sweep gas flow of 0 AU; and an S-Lens RF level of 60. Metabolite identification was based on the comparison of accurate mass and retention time with authentic metabolite standards. The analysis was conducted in a randomized fashion to avoid complications related to the injection order. An equivalent volume from each serum sample was mixed to create quality control (QC) samples. The same procedural steps applied to the test samples were followed for the QC samples, which were injected after every fifth sample injection during the analysis.

2.6. Human NHANES Population Study

We conducted an analysis using NHANES data from 2017 to 2018, which included years with available urine metal exposure data. The participant selection process is illustrated in Figure 1A. Specifically, to avoid the impact of menstrual cycles on metabolism, we included only adult male subjects who had complete data for total molybdenum and cadmium in urine. Ultimately, a total of 838 subjects were included in our study. All data can be downloaded from the official website [https://www.cdc.gov/nchs/nhanes (accessed on 21 December 2023)]. The Centers for Disease Control and Prevention (CDC) Research Ethics Review Board approved the project, and all participants gave informed consent.

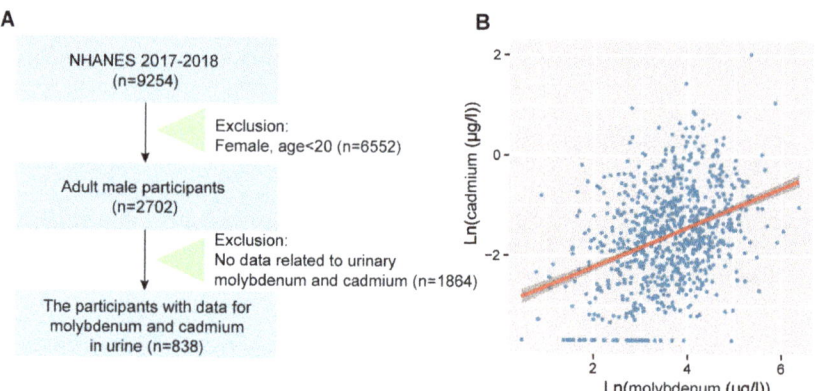

Figure 1. Correlation analysis of urinary molybdenum and cadmium in the NHANES population. (**A**) Participant screening process for NHANES 2017–2018. (**B**) Scatter plot illustrating the linear regression between molybdenum and cadmium. Data of molybdenum and cadmium were ln-transformed before analysis.

2.7. Assessment of Molybdenum and Cadmium Exposure in NHANES

Spot urine samples were analyzed for molybdenum and cadmium using inductively coupled plasma-dynamic reaction mass spectrometry (ICP-DRC-MS) at the National Center for Environmental Health, CDC. For values below the LOD, imputation was performed using the LOD value divided by the square root of two for each metal. The laboratory analyses followed the protocols described in the previous study [31].

2.8. Statistical Analysis

For the animal study, a *t*-test was used to analyze the differences between the two groups. When the comparison involved three groups, one-way analysis of variance (ANOVA) followed by Dunnett's test was employed. The normality and homogeneity of variance for all data were assessed using the Kolmogorov–Smirnov test. To improve the robustness of the differential metabolites based on the dose–effect relationship, Spearman's correlation analysis was conducted to investigate associations between molybdate and elementome, and molybdate and metabolome in the animal study. Pearson's correlation test was used to explore the associations between differential elements and differential metabolites. In the population study using NHANES data, Spearman's correlation analysis, and univariate and multivariate linear regression models were applied to study the association between molybdenum and cadmium. To account for potential confounding variables, age, race, education, smoking status, and BMI were included for adjustments in multivariate linear regression. Age was included as a continuous variable, and race, education, smoking status, and BMI were included as categorical variables. Model 1 was unadjusted; model 2 was controlled for age and race; model 3 was controlled for age, race, education, smoking status and BMI. The statistical analysis was performed using R (Version 4.0.5). Partial Least Squares Discrimination Analysis (PLS-DA) was utilized for dimensionality reduction analysis of elementome and metabolome data by SIMCA version 14.1 (Umetrics, Umea, Sweden). The statistical significance threshold was set at $p < 0.05$. The visualization of the metabolite network was established using iPath [https://pathways.embl.de (accessed on 21 December 2023)]. The study design can be found in Figure 2.

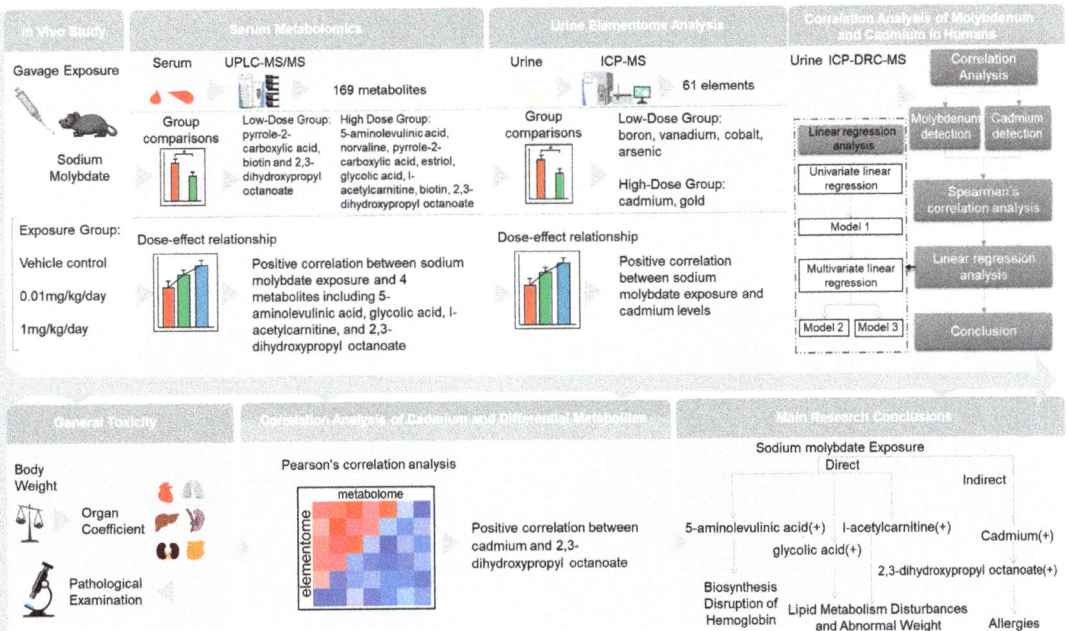

Figure 2. Overview of the study design and proposed effects of molybdate exposure on metabolic disorders associated toxicities, either directly or indirectly, through disruption of element. "+" indicates a positive correlation; * $p < 0.05$. The control group is represented by red column, the 0.01 mg/kg/day group by green column, and the 1 mg/kg/day group by blue column in the dose-effect relationship analysis.

3. Results

3.1. The Effect of Molybdate Exposure on Body Weight, Organ Coefficients, and Histopathological Examination in Mice

In this study, we investigated the effect of molybdate exposure on various parameters in mice, including body weight, organ coefficients (weight of the organ (g)/total body weight (g) × 100), and histopathological examinations. During the exposure period, no significant differences in body weight were observed among mice in different groups at each time point (Figure S1A). Molybdate exposure did not lead to significant differences in the organ coefficients of the heart, liver, spleen, lung, kidney, and intestine in mice (Figure S1B). In the pathological analysis of the heart, liver, spleen, lung, kidney, and intestine, no evident histopathological changes were observed (Figure S1C). Overall, these results suggest that molybdate exposure does not significantly affect body weight, organ coefficients, or induce histopathological changes in the examined organs of mice.

3.2. The Effect of Molybdate Exposure on the Serum Metabolome in Mice

In this study, our hypothesis was that molybdate exposure could potentially influence metabolite profiles in mice. To explore this hypothesis, we conducted metabolomics analysis on serum samples. A total of 169 metabolites were quantified in mouse serum. The score plots of the PLS-DA model (Figure 3A) clearly demonstrated a distinct separation between the control and exposed groups ($R^2X = 0.649$, $R^2Y = 0.993$, $Q^2 = 0.430$), indicating a significant impact of molybdate exposure on the metabolome profile in mice. To gain an overview of the detected metabolites, iPath was used to construct metabolic pathways (Figure S2). The metabolites were mainly enriched in amino acid metabolism, metabolism of cofactor and vitamin, and lipid metabolism (Figure 3B). Further analysis focused on the differential metabolites between the control and molybdate exposure groups. A total of eight different metabolites were identified (Figure 3B, C, Table 1). Pyrrole-2-carboxylic acid was decreased ($p < 0.001$) in the molybdate-0.01 mg/kg/day group compared to the control group, while biotin and 2,3-dihydroxypropyl octanoate were increased ($p < 0.05$). In the molybdate-1 mg/kg/day group, norvaline was slightly decreased ($p < 0.05$) and pyrrole-2-carboxylic acid was decreased ($p < 0.05$), while 5-aminolevulinic acid, estriol, glycolic acid, l-acetylcarnitine, biotin, and 2,3-dihydroxypropyl octanoate were increased ($p < 0.05$). Spearman's correlation analysis between molybdate doses and metabolite levels revealed positive dose–effect correlations between molybdate and 5-aminolevulinic acid, glycolic acid, l-acetylcarnitine, and 2,3-dihydroxypropyl octanoate, respectively ($r = 0.691$, $p < 0.05$; $r = 0.882$, $p < 0.05$; $r = 0.682$, $p < 0.05$; $r = 0.636$, $p < 0.05$) (Table 1). These results significantly contribute to our understanding of the metabolic perturbations induced by molybdate exposure in mice, and identified 5-aminolevulinic acid, glycolic acid, l-acetylcarnitine, and 2,3-dihydroxypropyl octanoate as robust metabolic changes.

Table 1. Different metabolites in serum of mice caused by molybdate exposure.

Metabolite	0.01 mg/kg/day		1 mg/kg/day		0, 0.01, 1 mg/kg/day [a]	
	Fold Change	p	Fold Change	p	r	p
5-aminolevulinic acid	1.145	0.100	1.100	0.041 *	0.691	0.019 *
norvaline	0.828	0.195	0.763	0.026 *	−0.573	0.066
pyrrole-2-carboxylic acid	0.397	0.000 *	0.504	0.011 *	−0.473	0.142
estriol	13.253	0.066	8.636	0.042 *	0.309	0.355
glycolic acid	2.458	0.056	2.422	0.008 *	0.882	0.000 *
l-acetylcarnitine	1.446	0.145	1.600	0.045 *	0.682	0.021 *
biotin	1.790	0.033 *	1.783	0.043 *	0.473	0.142
2,3-dihydroxypropyl octanoate	1.406	0.041 *	1.732	0.035 *	0.636	0.035 *

* $p < 0.05$. [a] Spearman correlation test using data from the 0, 0.01, 1 mg/kg/day groups.

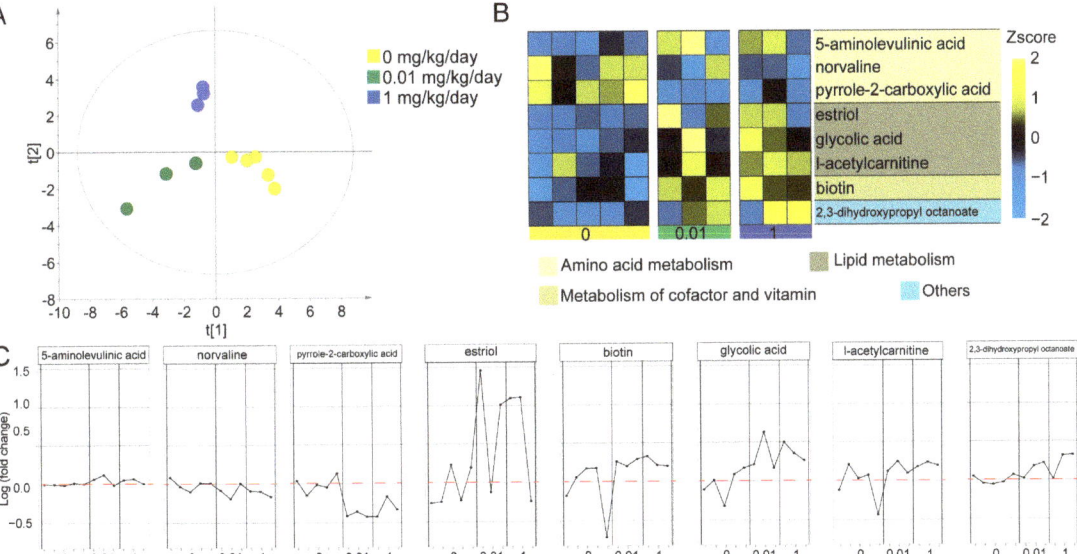

Figure 3. Overview of the effect of molybdate exposure on the serum metabolome. (**A**) PLS-DA score plots of metabolites, with each point representing a serum sample and colored according to the treatment groups. The control group is represented by yellow, the 0.01 mg/kg/day group by green, and the 1 mg/kg/day group by blue. The t [1] score on the X-axis represents the scores of the samples on the first latent variable (LV1) obtained from the PLS-DA model. The t [2] score on the Y-axis represents the scores of the samples on the second latent variable (LV2) obtained from the PLS-DA model. (**B**) Heatmap of differential metabolites. Yellow and blue colors represent increased and decreased levels of metabolites, respectively. (**C**) Changes in different metabolites in each sample of the different groups. A Z-score is a statistical measure that quantifies how many standard deviations a particular metabolite's concentration is from the mean concentration of that metabolite across a set of samples. The Z-score is calculated using the formula: $Z = (X - M)/SD$. Z is the Z-score; X is the level of the metabolite; M is the mean level of the metabolite; and SD is the standard deviation of the level of the metabolite.

3.3. Molybdate Exposure Increased the Urinary Molybdenum Content and Affected the Urine Elementome in Mice

In this study, we investigated the internal exposure level following exposure of mice to molybdate and its impact on the urinary elementome profile in mice using ICP-MS analysis. After exposure to molybdate, a significant increase in total molybdenum levels was observed in mice in the 0.01 mg/kg/day group ($p < 0.05$) and the 1 mg/kg/day group ($p < 0.01$), as depicted in Figure 4A. PLS-DA was performed on the elementome data obtained from the urine samples. The score plots of the PLS-DA model (Figure 4B) clearly demonstrated a distinct separation between the control and exposed mice ($R^2X = 0.429$, $R^2Y = 0.718$, $Q^2 = 0.436$), indicating a significant influence of molybdate exposure on the elementome profile in mice. Elementome analysis conducted on the urine samples detected a total of 61 elements (Figure 4C). As shown in Table 2, the results revealed a significant increase in the levels of boron, vanadium, cobalt, and arsenic after exposure to 0.01 mg/kg/day of molybdate ($p < 0.05$). Additionally, cadmium levels were found to be increased, while the levels of gold were decreased in the group treated with 1 mg/kg/day of molybdate ($p < 0.05$). Spearman's correlation analysis between molybdate doses and element levels showed a positive correlation between molybdate and cadmium ($r = 0.786$, $p < 0.05$) (Table 2). These findings significantly contribute to our understanding of the elementome response to molybdate exposure in mice, especially the effect of molybdate on the body's handling of cadmium.

Table 2. Different elements in urine of mice caused by molybdate exposure.

Element	0.01 mg/kg/day		1 mg/kg/day		0, 0.01, 1 mg/kg/day [c]		LOD [b] (µg/L)
	Fold Change	p	Fold Change	p	r	p	
Boron	2.106	0.028 *	1.566	0.089	0.409	0.212	2.12
Vanadium	1.969	0.008 *	1.472	0.120	0.145	0.670	0.03
Cobalt	1.798	0.036 *	1.244	0.230	0.027	0.937	0.01
Arsenic	1.931	0.032 *	1.376	0.197	0.382	0.247	0.04
Cadmium	1.000	NA [a]	25.578	0.000 *	0.786	0.004 *	0.08
Gold	0.533	0.296	0.192	0.037 *	−0.477	0.138	0.01

[a] Cadmium was not detectable in the molybdate-0.01 mg/kg/day group. [b] The limit of detection. [c] Spearman correlation test using data from the 0, 0.01, 1 mg/kg/day groups. * $p < 0.05$.

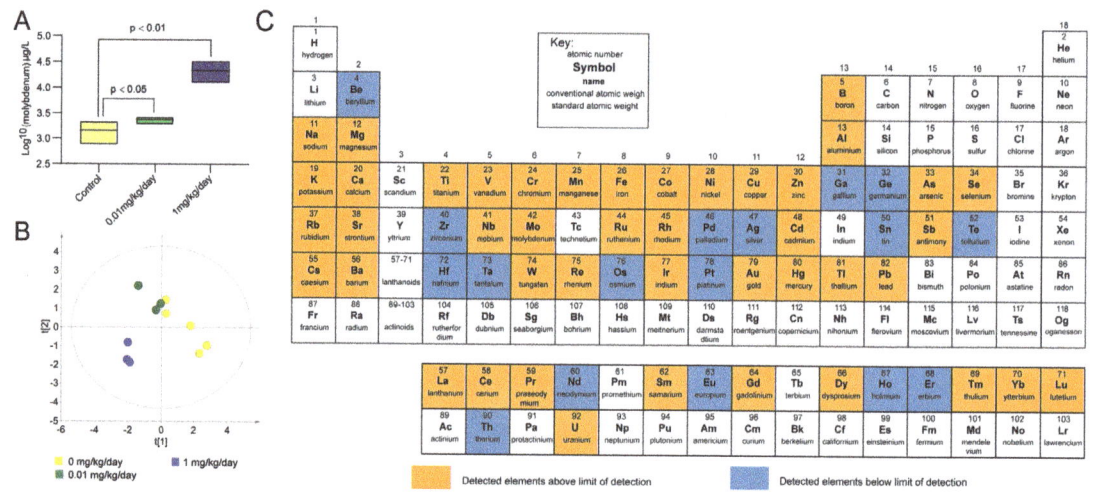

Figure 4. Overview of the effect of molybdate exposure on the urine elementome. (A) Box plots illustrating the total urinary molybdenum concentration in mice following molybdate treatment. (B) PLS-DA score plots of elements, with each point representing a urine sample and colored according to the treatment groups. The control group is represented by yellow, the 0.01 mg/kg/day group by green, and the 1 mg/kg/day group by blue. The x-axis and y-axis represent the scores obtained from the PLS-DA model. These scores are derived from the latent variables that capture the maximum covariance between the predictor variables (element levels) and the response variable (groups). The t [1] score on the X-axis represents the scores of the samples on the first latent variable (LV1) obtained from the PLS-DA model. The t [2] score on the Y-axis represents the scores of the samples on the second latent variable (LV2) obtained from the PLS-DA model. (C) Summary of the elements texted in urine.

3.4. Validation of the Positive Correlation between Urinary Molybdenum and Cadmium in Humans

To validate the correlation between molybdenum and cadmium observed in mice, we conducted a population study using NHANES data from 2017 to 2018 to analyze the relationship between urinary molybdenum levels and cadmium content. The study included 838 eligible participants, and their basic characteristics are presented in Table S1. The average age of the participants was 52.14 (±17.81) years. Among male adults, non-Hispanic whites (34.4%) constituted the largest ethnic group. In terms of education level, 22.1% had completed high school or below, while 26.1% were high school graduates or held a GED equivalent. Approximately 28.0% had some college education or an associate's degree, and 23.6% were college graduates or held higher degrees. Among adult males, 47.3% had never smoked, 32.2% reported past smoking but were not currently smoking, and 20.5% reported current smoking. A large proportion of individuals (38.2%) were classified as obese based on their BMI. The means (standard deviations (SDs)) of cadmium and molybdenum were 0.34 (0.46) and 53.40 (51.70) µg/L, respectively.

Spearman's correlation analysis revealed a positive correlation between urinary molybdenum and cadmium ($r = 0.32$, $p < 0.01$). In the present study, univariate and multivariate linear regression analyses were performed, and the results of model 1, model 2, and model 3 are presented in Table 3. In model 1, a significant positive correlation between molybdenum and cadmium was observed ($\beta = 0.39$, 95% CI 0.32–0.46). To account for potential confounding variables, additional linear regression models were constructed. Model 2 was partially adjusted for age and race, while model 3 was fully adjusted for age, race, education, smoking status, and BMI. The results demonstrated a significant positive correlation between cadmium and molybdenum in both model 2 ($\beta = 0.44$, 95% CI 0.38–0.50) and model 3 ($\beta = 0.47$, 95% CI 0.41–0.52, Figure 1B). These findings further support the validated positive correlation between urinary molybdenum and cadmium in the population. Consequently, we conducted further investigations to explore the impact of molybdate exposure on key metabolisms through the perturbations in cadmium.

Table 3. Multivariable associations of urinary molybdenum with cadmium.

Element	No.	Model 1 β (95%CI)	p	No.	Model 2 β (95%CI)	p	No.	Model 3 β (95%CI)	p
Cadmium	838	0.39 (0.32, 0.46)	$p < 0.01$	838	0.44 (0.38, 0.50)	$p < 0.01$	822	0.47 (0.41, 0.52)	$p < 0.01$

Model 1: unadjusted model. Model 2: adjusted for age and race. Model 3: adjusted for age, race, education, smoking status, and BMI.

3.5. Correlation between Urinary Cadmium and Differential Serum Metabolites in Mice

It has been reported [32] that exposure to inorganic mercury can influence the elementome, leading to subsequent changes in the metabolome of organisms. Based on this, we proposed a hypothesis that molybdate exposure could potentially modify the metabolome of mice by altering their elemental composition in urine. Then, based on the elementome and metabolome results, we observed a dose-dependent change ($p < 0.05$) in cadmium, 5-aminolevulinic acid, glycolic acid, l-acetylcarnitine, and 2,3-dihydroxypropyl octanoate after molybdate exposure. Consequently, we specifically examined the correlation between cadmium and the above four differential metabolites by Pearson's correlation analysis. As shown in Table 4, 2,3-dihydroxypropyl octanoate showed a positive correlation with cadmium ($r = 0.782$, $p < 0.01$), suggesting that the increase in 2,3-dihydroxypropyl octanoate induced by molybdate exposure might be mediated by cadmium (Figure 2).

Table 4. Correlation between urinary cadmium and differential serum metabolites.

Metabolite	Cadmium	
	r	p
5-aminolevulinic acid	0.025	0.942
glycolic acid	0.176	0.606
l-acetylcarnitine	0.413	0.207
2,3-dihydroxypropyl octanoate	0.782	0.004 *

* $p < 0.05$.

4. Discussion

In this study, we did not observe any significant effects of molybdate exposure on body weight, organ coefficients, and histopathological examinations in mice. However, the analysis of the association between molybdate and the metabolome revealed four dose-related metabolite changes after exposure. These findings highlighted the sensitivity of omics technologies in detecting the effects of molybdate exposure and its potential toxicity, even at levels relevant to human exposure. Moreover, the integrated multi-omics analysis identified potential metabolic disturbances resulting from the altered levels of elements caused by molybdate exposure.

4.1. The Direct Effects of Molybdate Exposure on Serum Metabolome

Correlation analysis between molybdate exposure and the metabolome revealed that molybdate exposure mainly affects the levels of several metabolites involved in amino acid metabolism and lipid metabolism. Since these metabolic pathways are associated with various biochemical processes, it indicates that molybdate-induced metabolic disorders can lead to certain metabolic toxic effects. Molybdate can directly influence the levels of various metabolites, partially due to its role as a cofactor of flavoenzymes involved in diverse metabolic pathways. Exposure to molybdate can have significant effects on organisms by disrupting metabolism. In our study, we observed significant changes in four metabolites including 5-aminolevulinic acid, glycolic acid, l-acetylcarnitine, and 2,3-dihydroxypropyl octanoate following molybdate exposure in a dose-related manner.

5-aminolevulinic acid is an amino acid that plays a crucial role in the biosynthesis of heme, an essential component of hemoglobin [33]. Interestingly, when humans were exposed to molybdate at normal levels, there was a significant increase in the serum levels of 5-aminolevulinic acid, a key metabolite involved in the biosynthesis of hemoglobin [34]. Another study demonstrated that 5-aminolevulinic acid has the ability to affect the synthesis of porphyrin and hemoglobin, suggesting that 5-aminolevulinic acid may have a potential role in affecting erythropoiesis and changing hemoglobin production in certain conditions related to impaired red blood cell formation [35]. These findings provided evidence supporting previous reports that molybdenum, as a trace element, plays a crucial role in affecting the synthesis and function of hemoglobin [18].

Molybdate has the ability to form a complex with glycolic acid [36], which inhibits the normal excretion of glycolic acid, thereby explaining the increased levels of glycolic acid caused by molybdate. Glycolic acid, the smallest α-hydroxy acid, has effects on changes in human skin condition [37]. Simultaneously, glycolic acid can contribute to obesity by inhibiting the activity of lipase [38]. Glycolic acid has been used to distinguish between metabolically unhealthy obese participants and metabolically healthy obese subjects in a previous study [39]. L-acetylcarnitine (also known as acetyl-l-carnitine or ALCAR) is a compound derived from l-carnitine [40]. It has been studied for its potential effects on lipid metabolism and obesity [41]. Several studies have suggested that l-acetylcarnitine may play a potential role in weight changes through regulating fat oxidation and energy expenditure [42].

4.2. The Effects of Molybdate Exposure on Urine Elementome

Previous studies have demonstrated the potential of molybdate to influence the concentration of other elements within an organism [43]. Molybdenum functions as an active cofactor for molybdenum enzymes, playing a crucial role in various metabolic processes [44]. Furthermore, molybdate can influence the absorption and excretion of other elements, thereby leading to fluctuations in tissue element levels [45]. Notably, a positive correlation was found between molybdenum and cadmium in urine of mice and humans in this study. Cadmium is a non-essential element known for its toxicity. Once cadmium enters the body, it is challenging to eliminate completely, due to the absence of an efficient excretion mechanism, leading to potential accumulation [46]. It has been demonstrated that ducks fed with basal diet with different concentrations of molybdenum or/and cadmium influenced the concentration of trace elements in the digestive organs, in which a strongly positive correlation between molybdenum and cadmium was observed [47]. There are also other studies indicating a positive correlation between molybdenum and cadmium in humans [48]. Cadmium is a food-chain contaminant that has high rates of soil-to-plant transference, which makes dietary Cd intake unavoidable in both humans and animals. In this study, we randomly selected mice into different groups, used a high purity sodium molybdate standard (purity $\geq$ 99%), and no differences in food and water consumption among different mice groups were detected, confirming that the change of urinary cadmium was caused by molybdate exposure. In line with these findings, we also observed a positive correlation between molybdate and cadmium in mice, and this positive correlation was validated in the human population, suggesting that molybdate may impact the toxic element cadmium and exert toxic effects.

4.3. The Indirect Effects of Molybdate on Serum Metabolome through Urine Elementome

2,3-dihydroxypropyl octanoate, also known as caprylic acid triglyceride or octanoic acid triglyceride [49], is a triglyceride composed of three caprylic acid molecules esterified to a glycerol backbone [50]. It is a common lipid molecule in biological samples [51]. It has been reported that certain individuals may experience allergies with increased 2,3-dihydroxypropyl octanoate [52]. Interestingly, it is reported that alloys containing molybdenum may induce allergies such as eczema and impaired wound [53], suggesting that the up-regulation of 2,3-dihydroxypropyl octanoate caused by molybdate exposure in this study might promote allergies in mice. Notably, a study shed light on the potential role of cadmium in modulating allergic reactions and suggested a possible correlation between cadmium intake and allergies including ear swelling and edema in rats [54], suggesting that molybdate may affect 2,3-dihydroxypropyl octanoate through its association with cadmium and ultimately induce allergies.

5. Conclusions

In this study, a mouse model was used to investigate the effects of molybdate exposure, which is relevant to human exposure levels. By employing a novel approach that integrates elementome and metabolome data, a comprehensive understanding of the impact of molybdate exposure on body elements and metabolic profiles was obtained. While no significant change was observed at the given doses of molybdate in body weight, organ coefficients, and histopathological examinations, sensitive changes in the toxicity related metabolome were detected. Specifically, molybdate exposure disrupted amino acid and lipid metabolism in serum, which may be partially mediated by molybdate-altered cadmium levels. This study provides valuable insights into the potential toxicity and mechanisms of molybdate at levels relevant to human exposure. It also highlights the significance of integrating elementome and metabolome analyses in future toxicological research, particularly for studying metabolic disturbances and the underlying mechanisms related to elements.

Supplementary Materials: The following supporting information can be downloaded at: https://www.mdpi.com/article/10.3390/toxics12040288/s1, Figure S1: General toxicity of molybdenum exposure in vivo; Figure S2: Detected metabolites in the general metabolic pathway based on iPath 3.0 [https://pathways.embl.de (accessed on 21 December 2023)]; Table S1: Participant characteristics.

Author Contributions: Conceptualization, M.C.; methodology, K.Z. and M.C.; software, Y.C. and M.C.; validation, M.T. and W.Z. and Z.L.; formal analysis, Y.C., Y.G. and J.D.; investigation, Y.G., R.H., J.D. and J.Z.; resources, W.Z., X.J., Y.H., X.Z. and M.C.; data curation, K.Z.; writing—original draft preparation, K.Z., M.T., Y.G. and Y.J.; writing—review and editing, M.C.; visualization, Y.C., Y.G., R.H. and J.D.; supervision, M.C.; project administration, M.C.; funding acquisition, M.C. All authors have read and agreed to the published version of the manuscript.

Funding: This research was funded by China National Key Research & Development (R&D) Plan (grant number: 2021YFC2700600), Natural Science Foundation of China (grant numbers: 82273668, 81872650), Excellent Young Backbone Teachers of "Qinglan Project" of Colleges and Universities in Jiangsu Province, the Wuxi City Health Committee top-notch talent (grant number: BJ2020077), Practice and Innovation Training Programs for Jiangsu Province College Students (grant numbers: 202310312011Z, 202110312072Y), and the Priority Academic Program Development of Jiangsu Higher Education Institutions (PAPD).

Institutional Review Board Statement: This study strictly adhered to international standards on animal welfare and the guidelines of the Institute for Laboratory Animal Research of Nanjing Medical University. All procedures conducted in this study were approved by the Animal Ethical and Welfare Committee of Nanjing Medical University (IACUC-2008055).

Informed Consent Statement: Not applicable.

Data Availability Statement: Data are contained within the article.

Conflicts of Interest: The authors declare no conflicts of interest.

References

1. Himoto, T.; Masaki, T. Current Trends of Essential Trace Elements in Patients with Chronic Liver Diseases. *Nutrients* **2020**, *12*, 2084. [CrossRef]
2. Sobańska, Z.; Zapór, L.; Szparaga, M.; Stępnik, M. Biological effects of molybdenum compounds in nanosized forms under in vitro and in vivo conditions. *Int. J. Occup. Med. Environ. Health* **2020**, *33*, 1–19. [CrossRef] [PubMed]
3. Imani Yengejeh, S.; Liu, J.; Kazemi, S.A.; Wen, W.; Wang, Y. Effect of Structural Phases on Mechanical Properties of Molybdenum disulfide. *ACS Omega* **2020**, *5*, 5994–6002. [CrossRef] [PubMed]
4. Lozano, M.; Murcia, M.; Soler-Blasco, R.; Casas, M.; Zubero, B.; Riutort-Mayol, G.; Gil, F.; Olmedo, P.; Grimalt, J.O.; Amorós, R.; et al. Exposure to metals and metalloids among pregnant women from Spain: Levels and associated factors. *Chemosphere* **2022**, *286*, 131809. [CrossRef] [PubMed]
5. Stafford, J.M.; Lambert, C.E.; Zyskowski, J.A.; Engfehr, C.L.; Fletcher, O.J.; Clark, S.L.; Tiwary, A.; Gulde, C.M.; Sample, B.E. Dietary toxicity of soluble and insoluble molybdenum to northern bobwhite quail (*Colinus virginianus*). *Ecotoxicology* **2016**, *25*, 291–301. [CrossRef]
6. Turnlund, J.R.; Keyes, W.R.; Peiffer, G.L. Molybdenum absorption, excretion, and retention studied with stable isotopes in young men at five intakes of dietary molybdenum. *Am. J. Clin. Nutr.* **1995**, *62*, 790–796. [CrossRef]
7. Mohamed, H.R.H.; El-Atawy, R.H.; Ghoneim, A.M.; El-Ghor, A.A. Induction of fetal abnormalities and genotoxicity by molybdenum nanoparticles in pregnant female mice and fetuses. *Environ. Sci. Pollut. Res. Int.* **2020**, *27*, 23950–23962. [CrossRef]
8. Toxicological Profile for Molybdenum; Agency for Toxic Substances and Disease Registry (ATSDR) Toxicological Profiles: Atlanta, GA, USA, 2020. Available online: https://wwwn.cdc.gov/TSP/ToxProfiles/ToxProfiles.aspx?id=1482&tid=289 (accessed on 21 December 2023).
9. Zhang, C.; Wang, X.; Pi, S.; Wei, Z.; Wang, C.; Yang, F.; Li, G.; Nie, G.; Hu, G. Cadmium and molybdenum co-exposure triggers autophagy via CYP450s/ROS pathway in duck renal tubular epithelial cells. *Sci. Total Environ.* **2021**, *759*, 143570. [CrossRef]
10. Pandey, R.; Singh, S.P. Effects of molybdenum on fertility of male rats. *Biometals* **2002**, *15*, 65–72. [CrossRef]
11. Schwarz, G.; Belaidi, A.A. Molybdenum in human health and disease. *Met. Ions Life Sci.* **2013**, *13*, 415–450. [CrossRef]
12. McKenzie, A. Reading e-journal article pdf files—Turn your laptop into an electronic book. *Anaesth Intensive Care* **2006**, *34*, 519. [PubMed]
13. Dumas, M.E. Metabolome 2.0: Quantitative genetics and network biology of metabolic phenotypes. *Mol. Biosyst.* **2012**, *8*, 2494–2502. [CrossRef] [PubMed]
14. Bouhifd, M.; Beger, R.; Flynn, T.; Guo, L.; Harris, G.; Hogberg, H.; Kaddurah-Daouk, R.; Kamp, H.; Kleensang, A.; Maertens, A.; et al. Quality assurance of metabolomics. *ALTEX* **2015**, *32*, 319–326. [CrossRef] [PubMed]
15. Li, Q.; Wang, Y.; Wu, S.; Zhou, Z.; Ding, X.; Shi, R.; Thorne, R.F.; Zhang, X.D.; Hu, W.; Wu, M. CircACC1 Regulates Assembly and Activation of AMPK Complex under Metabolic Stress. *Cell Metab.* **2019**, *30*, 157–173.e157. [CrossRef] [PubMed]
16. Harvey, F.C.; Collao, V.; Bhattacharya, S.K. High-Resolution Liquid Chromatography-Mass Spectrometry for Lipidomics. *Methods Mol. Biol.* **2023**, *2625*, 57–63. [CrossRef] [PubMed]
17. López Alonso, M.; Prieto Montaña, F.; Miranda, M.; Castillo, C.; Hernández, J.; Luis Benedito, J. Interactions between toxic (As, Cd, Hg and Pb) and nutritional essential (Ca, Co, Cr, Cu, Fe, Mn, Mo, Ni, Se, Zn) elements in the tissues of cattle from NW Spain. *Biometals* **2004**, *17*, 389–397. [CrossRef] [PubMed]
18. Feng, J.; Chen, J.; Xing, C.; Huang, A.; Zhuang, Y.; Yang, F.; Zhang, C.; Hu, G.; Mao, Y.; Cao, H. Molybdenum Induces Mitochondrial Oxidative Damage in Kidney of Goats. *Biol. Trace Elem Res.* **2020**, *197*, 167–174. [CrossRef] [PubMed]
19. Mendel, R.R.; Kruse, T. Cell biology of molybdenum in plants and humans. *Biochim. Biophys. Acta* **2012**, *1823*, 1568–1579. [CrossRef] [PubMed]
20. Meng, X.L.; Li, S.; Qin, C.B.; Zhu, Z.X.; Hu, W.P.; Yang, L.P.; Lu, R.H.; Li, W.J.; Nie, G.X. Intestinal microbiota and lipid metabolism responses in the common carp (*Cyprinus carpio* L.) following copper exposure. *Ecotoxicol. Environ. Saf.* **2018**, *160*, 257–264. [CrossRef]
21. Wang, Y.; Yu, L.; Ding, J.; Chen, Y. Iron Metabolism in Cancer. *Int. J. Mol. Sci.* **2018**, *20*, 95. [CrossRef]
22. Mooren, F.C. Magnesium and disturbances in carbohydrate metabolism. *Diabetes Obes. Metab.* **2015**, *17*, 813–823. [CrossRef] [PubMed]
23. European Commission Scientific Committee on Food. *Opinion of the Scientific Committee on Food on the Tolerable Upper Intake Level of Molybdenum*; European Commission: Brussels, Belgium, 2000.

24. Todd, G.D.; Keith, S.; Faroon, O.; Buser, M.; Ingerman, L.; Hard, C.; Citra, M.J.; Nguyen, A.; Klotzbach, J.M.; Diamond, G.L. Toxicological profile for molybdenum: Draft for public comment. 2017. Available online: https://stacks.cdc.gov/view/cdc/46170 (accessed on 21 December 2023).
25. Bernasconi, L.; Brolli, B.; Negro, A.; Zoino, J.L.; Schicchi, A.; Petrolini, V.M.; Lonati, D.; Ronchi, A.; Locatelli, C.A. Accidental ingestion of sodium molybdate at the workplace followed by short-term biomonitoring. *Med. Lav.* **2022**, *113*, e2022015. [CrossRef]
26. Slaoui, M.; Fiette, L. Histopathology procedures: From tissue sampling to histopathological evaluation. *Methods Mol. Biol.* **2011**, *691*, 69–82. [CrossRef] [PubMed]
27. Wang, X.; Sun, X.; Zhang, Y.; Chen, M.; Dehli Villanger, G.; Aase, H.; Xia, Y. Identifying a critical window of maternal metal exposure for maternal and neonatal thyroid function in China: A cohort study. *Environ. Int.* **2020**, *139*, 105696. [CrossRef]
28. Silver, M.K.; Arain, A.L.; Shao, J.; Chen, M.; Xia, Y.; Lozoff, B.; Meeker, J.D. Distribution and predictors of 20 toxic and essential metals in the umbilical cord blood of Chinese newborns. *Chemosphere* **2018**, *210*, 1167–1175. [CrossRef]
29. Chen, M.; Tang, R.; Fu, G.; Xu, B.; Zhu, P.; Qiao, S.; Chen, X.; Xu, B.; Qin, Y.; Lu, C.; et al. Association of exposure to phenols and idiopathic male infertility. *J. Hazard Mater.* **2013**, *250–251*, 115–121. [CrossRef] [PubMed]
30. Zhang, H.; Lu, T.; Feng, Y.; Sun, X.; Yang, X.; Zhou, K.; Sun, R.; Wang, Y.; Wang, X.; Chen, M. A metabolomic study on the gender-dependent effects of maternal exposure to fenvalerate on neurodevelopment in offspring mice. *Sci. Total Environ.* **2020**, *707*, 136130. [CrossRef]
31. Guo, X.; Li, N.; Wang, H.; Su, W.; Song, Q.; Liang, Q.; Liang, M.; Sun, C.; Li, Y.; Lowe, S.; et al. Combined exposure to multiple metals on cardiovascular disease in NHANES under five statistical models. *Environ. Res.* **2022**, *215*, 114435. [CrossRef]
32. García-Sevillano, M.A.; García-Barrera, T.; Navarro, F.; Gailer, J.; Gómez-Ariza, J.L. Use of elemental and molecular-mass spectrometry to assess the toxicological effects of inorganic mercury in the mouse *Mus musculus*. *Anal. Bioanal. Chem.* **2014**, *406*, 5853–5865. [CrossRef]
33. Hendawy, A.O.; Khattab, M.S.; Sugimura, S.; Sato, K. Effects of 5-Aminolevulinic Acid as a Supplement on Animal Performance, Iron Status, and Immune Response in Farm Animals: A Review. *Animals* **2020**, *10*, 1352. [CrossRef]
34. Hara, T.; Koda, A.; Nozawa, N.; Ota, U.; Kondo, H.; Nakagawa, H.; Kamiya, A.; Miyashita, K.; Itoh, H.; Nakajima, M.; et al. Combination of 5-aminolevulinic acid and ferrous ion reduces plasma glucose and hemoglobin A1c levels in Zucker diabetic fatty rats. *FEBS Open Bio.* **2016**, *6*, 515–528. [CrossRef]
35. Malik, Z.; Djaldetti, M. 5-Aminolevulinic acid stimulation of porphyrin and hemoglobin synthesis by uninduced Friend erythroleukemic cells. *Cell Differ.* **1979**, *8*, 223–233. [CrossRef] [PubMed]
36. Modec, B.; Dolenc, D.; Kasunic, M. Complexation of molybdenum(V) with glycolic acid: An unusual orientation of glycolato ligand in $\{Mo_2O_4\}^{2+}$ complexes. *Inorg. Chem.* **2008**, *47*, 3625–3633. [CrossRef]
37. Valle-González, E.R.; Jackman, J.A.; Yoon, B.K.; Mokrzecka, N.; Cho, N.J. pH-Dependent Antibacterial Activity of Glycolic Acid: Implications for Anti-Acne Formulations. *Sci. Rep.* **2020**, *10*, 7491. [CrossRef] [PubMed]
38. Liu, T.T.; Su, W.C.; Chen, Q.X.; Shen, D.Y.; Zhuang, J.X. The inhibitory kinetics and mechanism of glycolic acid on lipase. *J. Biomol. Struct. Dyn.* **2020**, *38*, 2021–2028. [CrossRef] [PubMed]
39. Chen, H.H.; Tseng, Y.J.; Wang, S.Y.; Tsai, Y.S.; Chang, C.S.; Kuo, T.C.; Yao, W.J.; Shieh, C.C.; Wu, C.H.; Kuo, P.H. The metabolome profiling and pathway analysis in metabolic healthy and abnormal obesity. *Int. J. Obes.* **2015**, *39*, 1241–1248. [CrossRef] [PubMed]
40. Khaw, S.C.; Wong, Z.Z.; Anderson, R.; Martins da Silva, S. l-carnitine and l-acetylcarnitine supplementation for idiopathic male infertility. *Reprod. Fertil.* **2020**, *1*, 67–81. [CrossRef]
41. Asbaghi, O.; Kashkooli, S.; Amini, M.R.; Shahinfar, H.; Djafarian, K.; Clark, C.C.T.; Shab-Bidar, S. The effects of L-carnitine supplementation on lipid concentrations inpatients with type 2 diabetes: A systematic review and meta-analysis of randomized clinical trials. *J. Cardiovasc. Thorac. Res.* **2020**, *12*, 246–255. [CrossRef] [PubMed]
42. Gómez, L.A.; Heath, S.H.; Hagen, T.M. Acetyl-L-carnitine supplementation reverses the age-related decline in carnitine palmitoyltransferase 1 (CPT1) activity in interfibrillar mitochondria without changing the L-carnitine content in the rat heart. *Mech. Ageing Dev.* **2012**, *133*, 99–106. [CrossRef]
43. Zhou, S.; Zhang, C.; Xiao, Q.; Zhuang, Y.; Gu, X.; Yang, F.; Xing, C.; Hu, G.; Cao, H. Effects of Different Levels of Molybdenum on Rumen Microbiota and Trace Elements Changes in Tissues from Goats. *Biol. Trace Elem. Res.* **2016**, *174*, 85–92. [CrossRef]
44. Schwarz, G.; Mendel, R.R. Molybdenum cofactor biosynthesis and molybdenum enzymes. *Annu. Rev. Plant Biol.* **2006**, *57*, 623–647. [CrossRef] [PubMed]
45. Wang, C.; Nie, G.; Yang, F.; Chen, J.; Zhuang, Y.; Dai, X.; Liao, Z.; Yang, Z.; Cao, H.; Xing, C.; et al. Molybdenum and cadmium co-induce oxidative stress and apoptosis through mitochondria-mediated pathway in duck renal tubular epithelial cells. *J. Hazard Mater.* **2020**, *383*, 121157. [CrossRef] [PubMed]
46. Bhardwaj, J.K.; Panchal, H.; Saraf, P. Cadmium as a testicular toxicant: A Review. *J. Appl. Toxicol.* **2021**, *41*, 105–117. [CrossRef] [PubMed]
47. Liao, Z.; Cao, H.; Dai, X.; Xing, C.; Xu, X.; Nie, G.; Zhang, C. Molybdenum and Cadmium exposure influences the concentration of trace elements in the digestive organs of Shaoxing duck (*Anas platyrhyncha*). *Ecotoxicol. Environ. Saf.* **2018**, *164*, 75–83. [CrossRef] [PubMed]
48. Meeker, J.D.; Rossano, M.G.; Protas, B.; Diamond, M.P.; Puscheck, E.; Daly, D.; Paneth, N.; Wirth, J.J. Cadmium, lead, and other metals in relation to semen quality: Human evidence for molybdenum as a male reproductive toxicant. *Environ. Health Perspect.* **2008**, *116*, 1473–1479. [CrossRef]

49. Umerska, A.; Cassisa, V.; Matougui, N.; Joly-Guillou, M.L.; Eveillard, M.; Saulnier, P. Antibacterial action of lipid nanocapsules containing fatty acids or monoglycerides as co-surfactants. *Eur. J. Pharm. Biopharm.* **2016**, *108*, 100–110. [CrossRef] [PubMed]
50. Spink, C.H. Differential scanning calorimetry. *Methods Cell Biol.* **2008**, *84*, 115–141. [CrossRef] [PubMed]
51. Barupal, D.K.; Fiehn, O. Generating the Blood Exposome Database Using a Comprehensive Text Mining and Database Fusion Approach. *Environ. Health Perspect.* **2019**, *127*, 97008. [CrossRef] [PubMed]
52. Polat Yemiş, G.; Delaquis, P. Natural Compounds With Antibacterial Activity Against Cronobacter spp. in Powdered Infant Formula: A Review. *Front. Nutr.* **2020**, *7*, 595964. [CrossRef]
53. Thomas, P.; Weik, T.; Roider, G.; Summer, B.; Thomsen, M. Influence of Surface Coating on Metal Ion Release: Evaluation in Patients With Metal Allergy. *Orthopedics* **2016**, *39*, S24–S30. [CrossRef]
54. Tucovic, D.; Kulas, J.; Mirkov, I.; Popovic, D.; Zolotarevski, L.; Despotovic, M.; Kataranovski, M.; Aleksandra, P.A. Oral Cadmium Intake Enhances Contact Allergen-induced Skin Reaction in Rats. *Biomed. Environ. Sci.* **2022**, *35*, 1038–1050. [CrossRef] [PubMed]

Disclaimer/Publisher's Note: The statements, opinions and data contained in all publications are solely those of the individual author(s) and contributor(s) and not of MDPI and/or the editor(s). MDPI and/or the editor(s) disclaim responsibility for any injury to people or property resulting from any ideas, methods, instructions or products referred to in the content.

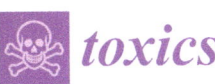

Article

Multi-Omics Analyses Reveal the Mechanisms of Early Stage Kidney Toxicity by Diquat

Huazhong Zhang [1,2], Jinsong Zhang [1,2], Jinquan Li [1,2], Zhengsheng Mao [2], Jian Qian [3], Cheng Zong [4], Hao Sun [1,2,*] and Beilei Yuan [4,*]

1. Department of Emergency, The First Affiliated Hospital of Nanjing Medical University, Nanjing 210029, China
2. Institute of Poisoning, Nanjing Medical University, Nanjing 211100, China
3. Department of Urology, The First Affiliated Hospital of Nanjing Medical University, Nanjing 210029, China
4. College of Safety Science and Engineering, Nanjing Tech University, Nanjing 211816, China
* Correspondence: haosun@njmu.edu.cn (H.S.); yuanbeilei@163.com (B.Y.)

Abstract: Diquat (DQ), a widely used bipyridyl herbicide, is associated with significantly higher rates of kidney injuries compared to other pesticides. However, the underlying molecular mechanisms are largely unknown. In this study, we identified the molecular changes in the early stage of DQ-induced kidney damage in a mouse model through transcriptomic, proteomic and metabolomic analyses. We identified 869 genes, 351 proteins and 96 metabolites that were differentially expressed in the DQ-treated mice relative to the control mice ($p < 0.05$), and showed significant enrichment in the PPAR signaling pathway and fatty acid metabolism. Hmgcs2, Cyp4a10, Cyp4a14 and Lpl were identified as the major proteins/genes associated with DQ-induced kidney damage. In addition, eicosapentaenoic acid, linoleic acid, palmitic acid and (R)-3-hydroxybutyric acid were the major metabolites related to DQ-induced kidney injury. Overall, the multi-omics analysis showed that DQ-induced kidney damage is associated with dysregulation of the PPAR signaling pathway, and an aberrant increase in Hmgcs2 expression and 3-hydroxybutyric acid levels. Our findings provide new insights into the molecular basis of DQ-induced early kidney damage.

Keywords: diquat; kidney injury; multi-omics; fatty acid metabolism; PPAR signaling pathway

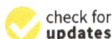

Citation: Zhang, H.; Zhang, J.; Li, J.; Mao, Z.; Qian, J.; Zong, C.; Sun, H.; Yuan, B. Multi-Omics Analyses Reveal the Mechanisms of Early Stage Kidney Toxicity by Diquat. Toxics 2023, 11, 184. https://doi.org/10.3390/toxics11020184

Academic Editor: Panagiotis Georgiadis

Received: 23 December 2022
Revised: 11 February 2023
Accepted: 14 February 2023
Published: 16 February 2023

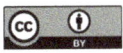

Copyright: © 2023 by the authors. Licensee MDPI, Basel, Switzerland. This article is an open access article distributed under the terms and conditions of the Creative Commons Attribution (CC BY) license (https://creativecommons.org/licenses/by/4.0/).

1. Introduction

Pesticides are the leading cause of poisoning-related accidental deaths in China. Following the discontinuation of paraquat, diquat (DQ) has become the preferred bipyridyl herbicide. However, cases of DQ poisoning have continued to increase in recent years, and the predominant route of exposure is the gastrointestinal tract [1]. The kidney is the main excretory organ as well as the primary target of DQ, and the toxic effects of the latter mainly involve the renal tubules, eventually leading to acute kidney injury (AKI) [2]. The incidence of AKI in patients with DQ poisoning is 73.3%, which is significantly higher compared to that caused by paraquat or other pesticides.

Previous studies have shown that DQ is selectively toxic to the kidneys, and has a similar chemical structure to that of the highly nephrotoxic orellanine [2]. Renal tubular dysfunction is the initial manifestation of DQ toxicity [3], and obvious renal tubular epithelial cell damage has been observed during autopsy [4]. The offspring of DQ-intoxicated rats exhibit renal duct damage. Furthermore, the prognosis of patients with DQ poisoning is closely related to AKI, which is usually reversible in the early stage. However, given the narrow time window for treatment, the incidence of endpoint events (death or uremia) exceeds 30%. Therefore, early detection and prevention of AKI are crucial in cases of DQ poisoning [5–7].

The clinical diagnosis of AKI is currently based on elevated blood creatinine (Scr) and blood urea nitrogen (BUN), along with low urine output [7]. However, the rise in Scr and BUN is increased when renal function has already declined by nearly 50%, while the urine output is susceptible to multiple factors such as diuretics and blood volume. Moreover, Scr and BUN are easily cleared by continuous renal replacement therapy (CRRT) and the urine volume varies with the ultrafiltration volume of CRRT. Thus, none of these indicators can accurately reflect the changes in renal function during CRRT [8]. Therefore, it is unclear whether using high Scr and oliguria as the clinical criteria for the initiation of CRRT delays the clearance of nephrotoxic substances such as DQ, and whether hemoperfusion (HP) combined with early CRRT improves prognosis [2,8]. Therefore, it is crucial to identify novel biomarkers and effector molecules for early detection and progression of kidney injury, and to guide hemodialysis treatment.

In this study, we used integrated metabolomics, transcriptomics and proteomics to explore the molecular mechanisms underlying DQ-induced nephrotoxicity at the very early stage. Based on multi-omics analyses, we found that DQ induced aberrant gene expression at the mRNA, protein, and metabolite levels. Our findings provide novel insights into DQ-induced kidney injury and identify novel biomarkers.

2. Materials and Methods

2.1. Animals and Chemical Reagents Treatments

Male C57BL/6 J mice aged 28 weeks and weighing 25–30 g were bought from Nanjing Medical University (NYD-L-2020082601). The mice were kept in a specialized pathogen-free environment (22–26 °C, 40%–60% humidity, and 12 h light/dark cycles) with food and water provided ad libitum. The feed used in this experiment meets the national standard. The feed mainly contains energy, protein, fat, amino acid, minerals, etc. All mice were given the same food. The mice were randomly divided into the control, low-dose DQ (200 mg/kg) and high-dose DQ (350 mg/kg) groups after one week of acclimatization ($N = 30$ per group). DQ and saline (control) were administered via the intragastric route. The mice were euthanized on days 1, 3 and 7 after induction, and kidney tissue samples were collected from 10 mice of each group. Ten kidney samples were used for metabolomics analysis, three were used for proteomics analysis, and three for transcriptomic analysis. Diquat (DQ) was purchased from Aladdin (D101258-100 mg).

2.2. Histopathologic Examination

The kidney tissues were fixed in 4% paraformaldehyde for 24 h, dehydrated in an ethanol gradient and embedded in paraffin. The paraffin blocks were cut into 5 μm-thick slices, which were stained using hematoxylin and eosin (H&E). Instrument information: Tissue-tekvip6 automatic tissue processor (Sakura, Japan), HistoStar tissue burying machine (Thermo, US), Thermo Finesse E+ paraffin microtome (Thermo, US), Gemini AS automatic dyeing machine (Thermo, US), Olympus BX53 optical microscope (Olympus, Japan), and DP72 image analysis system (Olympus, Japan).

2.3. Transcriptome Analysis

RNA sequencing (RNA-seq) was performed on three biological replicates of the DQ-treated and control group kidney tissues by Biotree Biotech Co., Ltd. (Shanghai, China). Briefly, total RNA was extracted and reverse transcribed, and the double-stranded cDNA was used to construct libraries. After quality control, the libraries are pooled and sequenced on the Illumina Novaseq 6000 platform (Thermo, US). The clean reads were filtered from the raw sequencing data after checking for the sequencing error rate and the distribution of GC content. The gene expression levels were calculated as the number of fragments per kilobase of transcript per million reads (FPKM). The expression matrix of all samples was generated, and differentially expressed genes (DEGs) between the control and DQ-treated samples were screened using the edgeR program with $Padj < 0.05$ as the criterion. The DEGs were then functionally annotated by gene ontology (GO) analysis in terms of molecular functions (MF), biological processes (BP) and cellular components (CC), as well as Kyoto Encyclopedia of Genes and Genomes (KEGG) pathway enrichment analyses using the clusterProfiler (http://www.bioconductor.org/packages/release/bioc/html/

clusterProfiler.html) program, (accessed on 31 December 2021). The GO terms related to molecular function, biological process and cellular component were analyzed.

2.4. Proteomics Analysis

Total protein was extracted from the kidney tissues of three biological replicates from the control and DQ-treated groups, quantified and stored at −80 °C. Proteomic sequencing and analysis were conducted by Biotree Biotech Co., Ltd. (Shanghai, China). Briefly, the extracted proteins were first quantified by the BCA assay, precipitated using acetone, and then subjected to reduction, alkylation, digestion, TMT labeling, SDC cleanup, peptide desalting and high-pH pre-fractionation. For nanoLC–MS/MS analysis, 2 μg total peptides from each sample was separated and analyzed using a nano-UPLC (EASY-nLC1200) coupled to Orbitrap Exploris 480 (Thermo Fisher Scientific) with a nano-electrospray ion source. Data-dependent acquisition (DDA) was performed in profile and the positive mode with Orbitrap analyzer for 90 min. The Tandem Mass Tag (TMT) was used to identify the proteins and screen for unique peptides with p-Value < 0.05 (Student's t test) and fold change > 1.5 as the criteria. The proteins were subjected to principal component analysis (PCA), volcano plot analysis, hierarchical clustering analysis, GO and KEGG analyses, and protein–protein interaction (PPI) network analysis.

2.5. Untargeted LC–MS Metabolomics Analysis

The kidney tissue samples from the control and DQ-treated groups (10 biological replicates per group) were prepared as previously described [9]. Metabolomic sequencing and analysis were performed by Biotree Biotech Co. Ltd. (Shanghai, China). The metabolic profiles were acquired using Quadrupole-Electrostatic Field Orbitrap Mass Spectrometer (Thermo Fisher Scientific). The single peak corresponding to each metabolite was filtered, and the missing values in the original data were reproduced. The internal standard was utilized for normalization, and the outliers were filtered based on the relative standard deviation. Partial least squares discriminant analysis (PLS-DA) and unsupervised principal component analysis (PCA) were used to identify the differential metabolites between two groups, with VIP > 1 and $p < 0.05$ as the criteria. The differential metabolites were subjected to correlation analysis, KEGG pathway analysis, and hierarchical clustering.

2.6. Statistical Analysis

Data visualization was performed using GraphPad Prism 5. The data were expressed as the mean ± standard deviation of the mean (SD). Data were processed by GraphPad Prism 5. The mean values were statistically analyzed by unpaired t-tests and the significant differences among different groups were assessed by a non-parametric test. Differences were considered statistically significant at $p < 0.05$.

3. Results

3.1. Establishment and Validation of DQ-Treated Mouse Model

We established a mouse model of DQ-induced kidney injury to study the early stages of AKI (Figure 1a). While DQ did not affect serum Scr levels on day 1, serum BUN levels were not affected by 200 mg/kg or 350 mg/kg DQ. The serum UREA levels were significantly higher in mice treated with 350 mg/kg DQ compared to the control group. In contrast, 200 mg/kg DQ had no significant effect on the urea level. Subsequently, both Scr and BUN continued to rise, and significant differences were observed on the 3rd and 7th days (Figure 1b,c). Furthermore, while no substantial lesions were observed in the kidney tissues of the DQ-treated mice in the first day of exposure, the renal tubules exhibited vacuolation and necrosis 3 days later (Figure S1). Based on these results, we selected the dose of 200 mg/kg to simulate the early stage DQ-induced kidney damage.

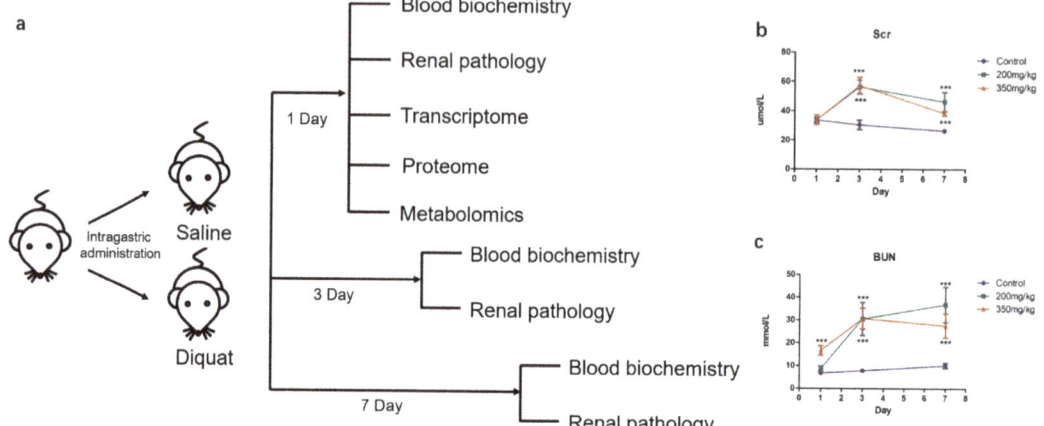

Figure 1. Establishment and validation of DQ-treated mice. (**a**) Outline of animal experiments. (**b**) The concentration of Scr (*** $p < 0.001$). (**c**) The concentration of BUN (*** $p < 0.001$).

3.2. Transcriptomic Analysis of DQ-Treated Mice

As shown in the UpSet graph in Figure 2a, 16,927 genes were expressed in all samples. Furthermore, 869 genes were differentially expressed in the DQ-treated samples relative to the control, of which 473 genes were downregulated and 396 genes were upregulated (Figure 2b and Table S1). The DEGs were enriched in GO terms related to fatty acid metabolism, extracellular structure organization, sulfur compound metabolism (Figure 2c), extracellular matrix, collagen-containing extracellular matrix (Figure 2d), extracellular matrix structural constituent, and sulfur compound binding (Figure 2e). Furthermore, KEGG analysis revealed that these DEGs were significantly associated with pathways of drug metabolism, drug metabolism-cytochrome P450, glutathione metabolism and retinol metabolism (Figure 2f). These results indicate that DQ might dysregulate numerous pathways in the kidneys.

3.3. Proteomic Analysis of DQ-Treated Mice

We used TMT-based quantitative proteomics analysis to identify the differentially expressed proteins (DEPs) that might be linked to DQ-induced kidney damage. PCA revealed notable differences in protein abundance between the DQ and control groups (Figure 3a). There were 351 DEPs between the two groups, of which 133 proteins were upregulated and 218 proteins were downregulated in the DQ-treated mice (Figure 3b and Table S2). The DEPs were mainly enriched in pathways associated with Parkinson's disease, Salmonella infection, chemical carcinogenesis, PPAR signaling, phagosome, tuberculosis, ribosome, bile secretion and retinol metabolism (Figure 3c). According to the GO enrichment analysis, DEPs were primarily associated with terms such as intracellular, intracellular part, organelle, intracellular organelle, cytoplasm, membrane-bounded organelle, intracellular membrane-bounded organelle, cytoplasm part, organelle part and intracellular organelle part (Figure 3d).

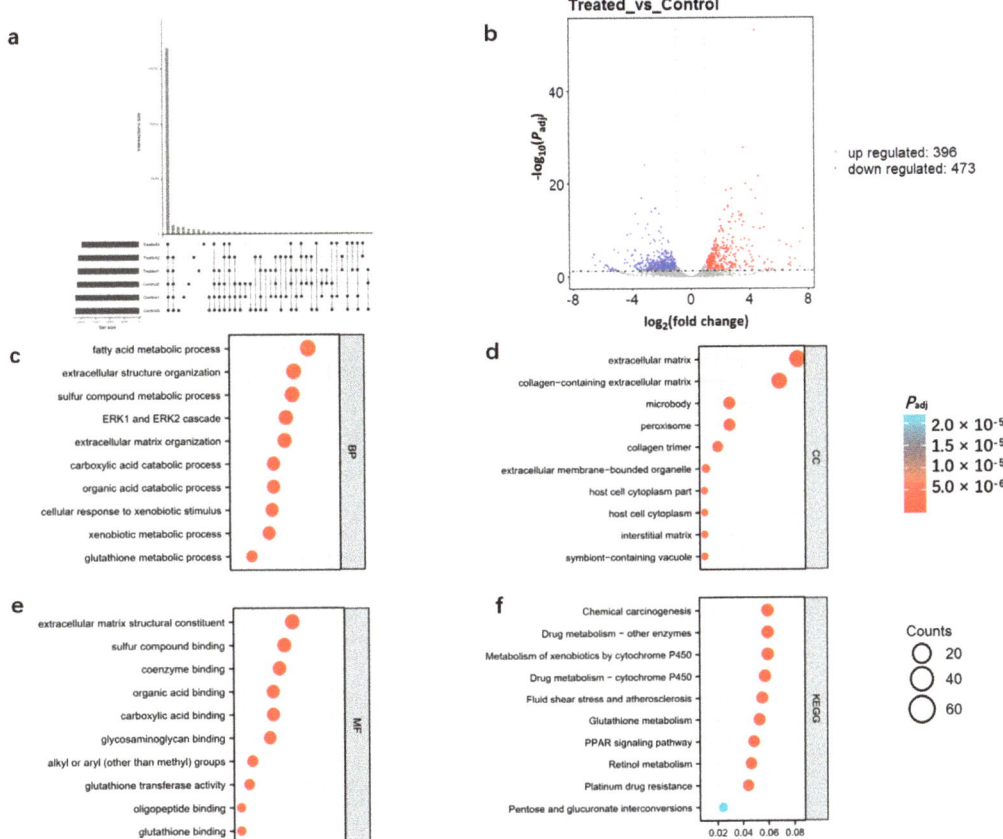

Figure 2. Transcriptome profiles of control and DQ-treated kidney tissues. (**a**) Summary of transcriptome datasets: 16,927 genes were expressed in all samples, N = 3. (**b**) The volcano plot of differentially expressed genes (DEGs) between the control and DQ-treated groups. (**c**) The enriched biological processes of DEGs. (**d**) The enriched cellular components of DEGs. (**e**) The enriched molecular function of DEGs. (**f**) The top 10 enriched Kyoto Encyclopedia of Genes pathways of DEGs and their contraction.

Furthermore, a protein–protein interaction (PPI) network was constructed using the STRING database. As shown in the network in Figure 3e, DQ exposure altered ribonucleoprotein complex biogenesis (Bop1, Tarbp2, Imp4, Pqbp1, Pop4, Snrpf, Las1l, Mrpl1, Utp18, Ddx49, Prpf39), ncRNA processing (Bop1, Mettl1, Tarbp2, Imp4, Pop4, Las1l, Mrpl1, Utp18, Ddx49), ncRNA metabolic process (Bop1, Mettl1, Tarbp2, Imp4, Pop4, Las1l, Mrpl1, Utp18, Ddx49), response to wounding (Aqp1, Fcer1g, Pdpn, Grn, Jak2, Scnn1b, Tarbp2, Map2k1, Arhgap35), mitochondrial protein complex (Cox4i1, Grpel2, Mrps25, Chchd1, Dnajc15, Sdhd, Ndufa11, Mrpl1, Mrpl30), ribosome (Rpl37a, Uba52, Rps26, Mrps25, Chchd1, Rpl37, Mrpl1, Mrpl30, Rpl17), enzyme activator activity (Apoa2, Bcl10, Thy1, Map2k1, Dnajc15, Tab1, Cwf19l1, Arhgap35, Depdc5), organic hydroxy compound transport (Apoa2, Aqp1, Aqp3, Fcer1g, Slc10a2, Apom, Sdhd, Slc51a), fatty acid metabolic process (Adh7, Apoa2, Cyp2a4, Cyp4a10, Pdpn, Lpl, Gstm7, Acsl3), and positive regulation of cell activation (Bcl10, Fcer1g, Pdpn, Jak2, Thy1, Lgals8, Dnaja3, Hamp). In summary, DQ-induced kidney injury is likely mediated by dysregulated proteins involved in metabolism.

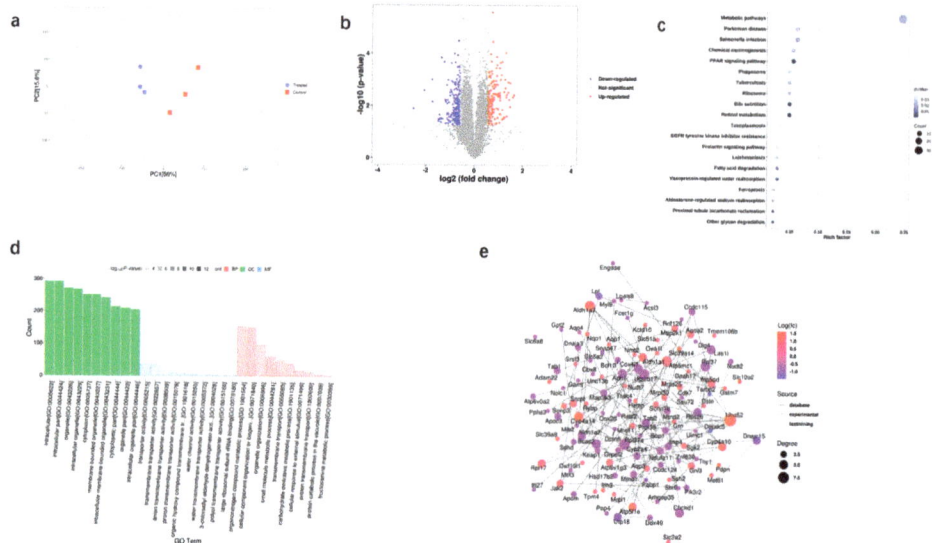

Figure 3. Proteomic profiles of control and DQ-treated kidney tissues. (**a**) PCA of the proteomes of DQ-treated and control kidney samples indicated two distinct clusters ($N = 3$). (**b**) Volcano plot of differentially expressed proteins (DEPs) between the control and DQ-treated groups. (**c**) Kyoto Encyclopedia of Genes and (**d**) Genomes pathways of DEPs and their contraction. (**e**) PPI network of the DEPs. The red circles represent significantly upregulated proteins, and the purple circles represent significantly downregulated proteins. The size of the circle is positively correlated with the degree of connection.

3.4. Integrated Transcriptome and Proteome Datasets

Integration of the transcriptome and proteome datasets revealed that 34 genes were substantially altered by DQ exposure (Table S3). KEGG pathway analysis showed that these genes are significantly associated with the PPAR signaling pathway, retinol metabolism, asthma, cholesterol metabolism, fatty acid degradation, valine/leucine and isoleucine degradation, fatty acid metabolism, and kidney injury caused by DQ (Figure 4a). Furthermore, GSEA consistently demonstrated that these DEGs and DEPs were substantially enriched for metabolism-related pathways, including the drug metabolism cytochrome P450, the PPAR signaling pathway, retinol metabolism, metabolism of lipids, amino acid metabolism, glutathione metabolism and fatty acid metabolism (Figure 4b). Taken together, the aforementioned pathways are likely targeted by DQ during kidney injury.

3.5. Metabolomic Analysis of DQ-Treated Mice

The metabolic by-products that may contribute to DQ-induced kidney injury were identified by untargeted LC–MS. The results of PCA and OPLS-DA clearly showed distinct metabolic patterns of the control and DQ-treated mice (Figure 5a,b). Overall, 96 metabolites were differentially expressed between the control and DQ-treated groups (adjusted $p < 0.05$), of which 40 were elevated and 56 were decreased in the latter (Figure 5c, Table S4). Furthermore, five of these differentially regulated metabolites are involved in purine metabolism, three in biosynthesis of unsaturated fatty acids, two in primary bile acid biosynthesis, one in fatty acid biosynthesis, and one in fatty acid metabolism (Figure 5d). To ascertain which metabolic pathways were most affected by DQ exposure, we performed KEGG pathway enrichment analysis. As shown in Figure 5d, the top 10 pathways were those related to purine metabolism, biosynthesis of unsaturated fatty acids, primary bile acid biosynthesis, nicotinate and nicotinamide metabolism, taurine and hypotaurine metabolism, fatty acid metabolism, amino sugar and nucleotide sugar metabolism, glycine, serine and threonine metabolism, porphyrin and chlorophyll metabolism, fatty acid elongation in mitochondria.

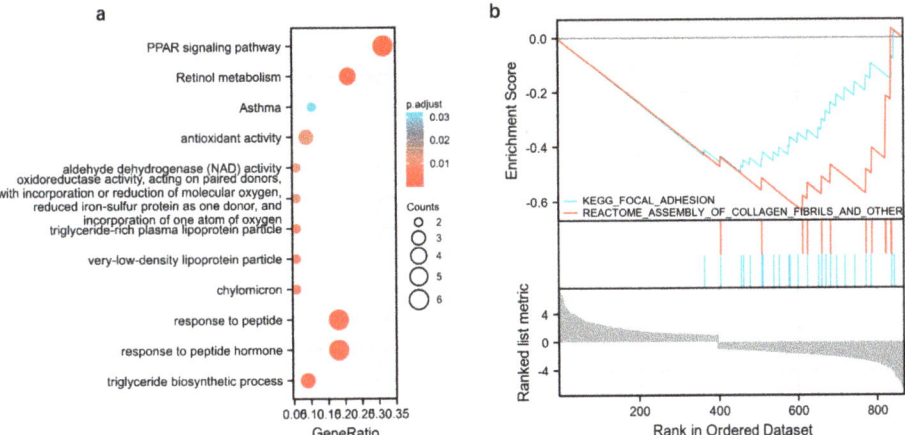

Figure 4. Gene set enrichment analysis (GSEA)-based analysis. (**a**) Pathways enriched in the 34 overlapping genes. (**b**) Results of GSEA.

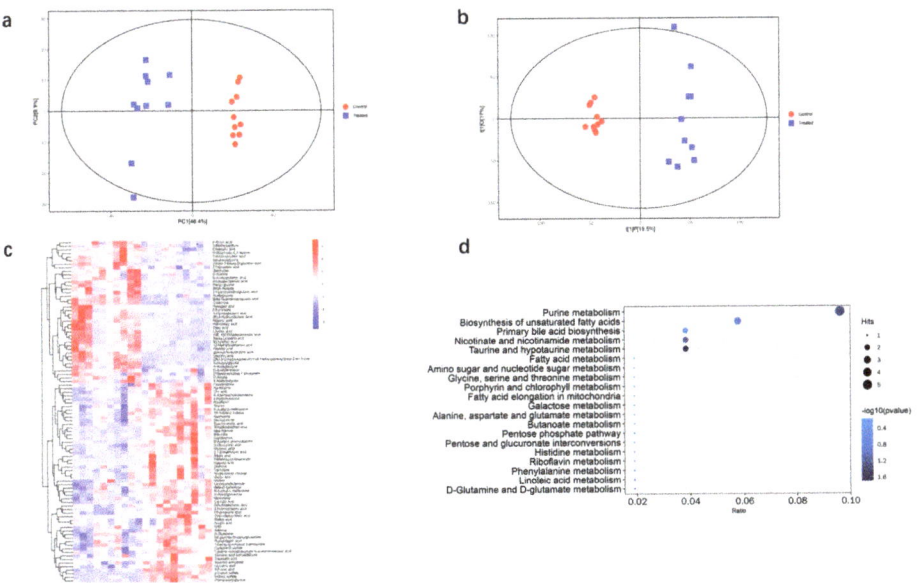

Figure 5. Metabolomic analysis of DQ-treated mice. (**a**) PCA of the metabolic profiles ($N = 10$). (**b**) Score plots of the OPLS-DA model classifying the DQ-treated and control groups. (**c**) Heatmap analysis of the differently expressed metabolites between the DQ-treated and control groups. The columns show the significantly upregulated (red) or downregulated metabolites (blue) in the different groups. (**d**) KEGG pathway analysis based on the differently expressed metabolites identified in the DQ-treated and control groups.

3.6. Integrated Transcriptomic, Proteomic and Metabolomics

We constructed a correlation network diagram of the metabolites, DEPs and DEGs to gain further insights into the molecular mechanisms underlying DQ-induced nephrotoxicity. As shown in Figure 6, the top 20 co-related genes were Gm3776, Ccl21a, Vgf, Gsta1, Fgf21, Krt20, Ugt1a9, Lrrc55, Areg, 9130409I23Rik, Ccdc180, Edil3, Prss35, Cbr3, Ccr7, Nppb, Cyp2b10, F2rl3, Gm4841, Zfp683. The top 20 co-related proteins were Q3UFS4, Q9D486, Q62314, O70324, O89050, Q62011, Q8K209, Q9CYH5, P61460, Q99JH8, Q80TE3, O70571, Q8BQM4, Q75N73, P97473, P15409, P33174, P70172, P18469 and Q8VDM1. The top 20 metabolites were hippuric acid, 5-methoxyindoleacetate, chenodeoxycholic acid, tetradecanedioic acid, indoxyl sulfate, (R)-3-hydroxybutyric acid, traumatic acid, gamma-aminobutyric acid, alpha-linolenic acid, adipic acid, phenylacetylglycine, hypotaurine, 3-hydroxybutyric acid, palmitoleic acid, caprylic acid, eicosapentaenoic acid, linoleic acid, 2-furoic acid, beta-alanine and N-acetyl-L-phenylaninex. These genes, proteins and their metabolites are mostly connected to the PPAR signaling pathway and fatty acid metabolism.

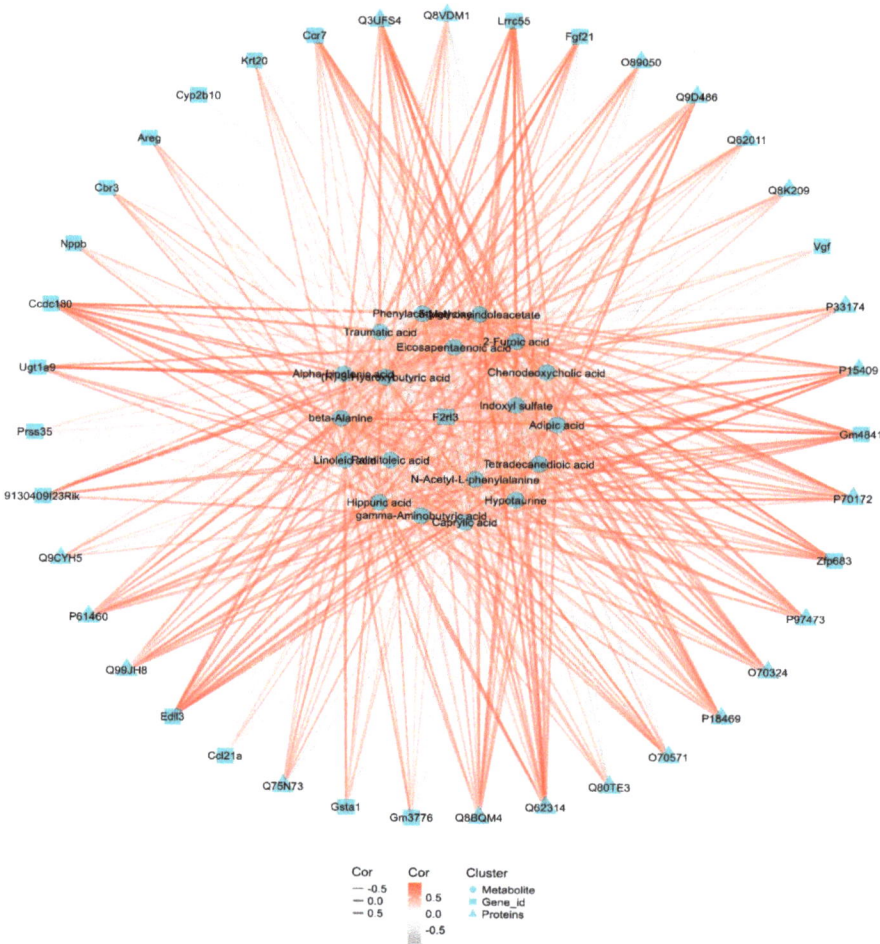

Figure 6. Integrative network of transcriptome, proteome and metabolome datasets.

4. Discussion

DQ is a highly nephrotoxic bipyridine herbicide that primarily targets the renal tubules and induces AKI. The molecular basis of DQ-induced kidney injury is cell death due to excessive production of reactive oxygen species (ROS) formed during lipid peroxidation [2,10]. The prognosis of DQ poisoning is highly correlated with AKI. Although AKI is reversible in its early stages, the therapeutic window is narrow. Therefore, it is crucial to identify the biomarkers and effectors of the incipient stages of AKI for early diagnosis of kidney damage.

We identified the time window of DQ-induced kidney damage by analyzing different time points and dosages. There was no evident renal parenchymal damage, or any changes in serum Scr or BUN levels after 24 h exposure to 200 mg/kg DQ, which corresponded to the early stage of the DQ-induced kidney damage. To identify the molecular mechanisms of DQ-induced renal damage at this stage, we used an integrated multi-omics approach, which revealed that exposure to DQ significantly affects the PPAR signaling pathway and fatty acid metabolism.

According to the integrated multi-omics data, the PPAR signaling pathway and fatty acid metabolism were associated with upregulation of Hmgcs2, Cyp4a10 and Cyp4a14, and the downregulation of Lpl mRNA and proteins in the DQ-treated kidneys. PPAR, a lipid-activated nuclear receptor, is abundantly expressed in tissues with high fatty acid metabolism, such as the kidney [11]. PPAR-deficient mice accumulate more lipids in their kidneys, which increases production of inflammatory mediators, eventually leading to kidney injury [12,13]. In addition, PPAR is also a transcription factor that controls genes involved in lipid metabolism and the mitochondrial fatty acid oxidation pathway [14], which fulfills a significant portion of the body's energy needs [15,16]. Integrated proteomic and transcriptomic analysis revealed that the fatty acid oxidation pathway, and subsequently fatty acid metabolism, were downregulated in the DQ-treated group.

The primary rate-limiting enzyme for ketogenesis is Hmgcs2 (3-hydroxy-3-methylglutaryl-CoA synthase 2). Hmgcs2 is a key rate-regulating enzyme for ketone body formation, which is related to fatty acid metabolism and mainly exists in cell mitochondria. The HMG-CoA generated by it is converted into acetoacetic acid under the action of HMG-CoA lyase, and acetoacetic acid can be converted into hydroxybutyric acid and acetone, which are called ketone bodies. Ketogenesis of cells is an important part of fatty acid metabolism, and acetyl CoA, the product of fatty acid oxidation, is the raw material for the formation of ketosomes. Therefore, Hmgcs2 may regulate the changes in fatty acid metabolism by regulating the ketogenesis process. Upregulation of Hmgcs2 in the glomeruli of high fructose-fed rats and high fructose-treated differentiated podocytes enhanced ketone bodies level, particularly that of hydroxybutyrate (3-OHB), to block histone deacetylase (HDAC) activity [17]. Hmgcs2 is likely upregulated through the PPAR-α pathway [18]. The findings imply that enhanced renal ketogenesis due to Hmgcs2 overexpression may be significant in the pathogenesis of diabetic neuropathy DN in patients with type 2 diabetes, indicating that Hmgcs2 is a potential therapeutic target for the management of diabetic renal complications [19]. We found that Hmgcs2 gene and protein expression levels increased in the kidney tissues after DQ exposure, indicating its role in DQ-induced renal damage as well.

CYP4A (cytochrome P450, family 4, subfamily a) catalyzes the hydroxylation of medium- and long-chain fatty acids [20]. One of the pathway for fatty acid degradation is through oxidation, in which dicarboxylic acids are formed and subsequently undergo β-oxidation from the omega end. This pathway is catalyzed by CYP450 enzymes and the peroxisomal β-oxidation pathway which are regulated by PPARα [21] The mouse genome contains four Cyp4a genes: Cyp4a10, Cyp4a12a, Cyp4a12b, and Cyp4a14—all of which are localized in chromosome 4 [22]. Murine Cyp4a10 and Cyp4a14 (homologous to human CYP4A22 and CYP4A11, respectively) are highly expressed in the liver and kidneys, and are known to convert the arachidonic acid to its metabolite 20-hydroxyeicosatetraenoic acid (20-HETE), which regulates the inflammatory response through the generation of

ROS [15,22]. As a result, the aberrant expression of Cyp4a10 and Cyp4a14 observed in our study may lead to fatty acid breakdown.

LPL (lipoprotein lipase) catalyzes the hydrolysis of triglyceride (TAG), which is the rate-limiting step in the lipolysis of chylomicrons and VLDL. In addition to other cell types, myocytes and adipocytes also synthesize LPL, which is then stored in the Golgi apparatus for either intracellular breakdown or secretion onto the cell surface. Patients with nephrotic syndrome often have hyperlipidemia due to the lack of LPL activators. Furthermore, the high levels of free fatty acids in the bloodstream of these patients upregulates ANGPTL4, which may inactivate LPL by either converting the active LPL dimers into inactive monomers or as a reversible non-competitive inhibitor of LPL [23]. In this study, LPL expression was downregulated in the DQ-treated kidney tissues, indicating its role in DQ-induced nephrotoxicity.

We identified eicosapentaenoic acid, linoleic acid, palmitic acid and (R)-3-hydroxybutyric acid as significant metabolites involved in DQ-related kidney injury. Eicosapentaenoic acid, linoleic acid and palmitic acid are polyunsaturated fatty acids (PUFAs), which have been linked to a number of renal disorders. One study showed that retinoic acid signaling mediates production of toxic PUFAs [24]. Increased PUFA peroxidation by ROS initiates ferroptosis, an iron-dependent form of programmed cell death. Fatty acid oxidation in the liver produced high levels of 3-hydroxybutyrate acid, which is then transferred to extrahepatic tissues including the heart, brain and muscle to be used as a fuel. As one of the ketone bodies, 3-hydroxybutyric acid can directly promotes 3-hydroxybutyrylation of some proteins and functions as an endogenous inhibitor of histone deacetylases as well as an agonist of Gpr109a [25]. β-OHB is one of the intermediate metabolites of fatty acid oxidation. In addition to being a functional vector that transfers energy from liver to peripheral tissues under starvation stress, β-OHB is also an important signaling molecule and epigenetic regulatory molecule in vivo, regulating all aspects of life function. This study showed that glomerular podocytes damage and albuminuria production caused by fructose intake showed an increase in β-OHB beginning at week 8 of modeling and continuing until week 16 of the study deadline [17]. Therefore, β-OHB is a key metabolic substance in the occurrence and development of kidney injury. Taken together, dysregulated fatty acid metabolism may induce by the nephrotoxic effects of DQ.

Overall, Hmgcs2 upregulated and subsequently may promote 3-hydroxybutyric acid levels, dysregulating the PPAR signaling pathway. Our findings offer a new insight into the mechanisms underlying DQ-induced nephrotoxicity.

5. Conclusions

Our study is the first to investigate the mechanism of the early stage of DQ-induced kidney injury using a multi-omics approach. Our findings lay the foundation for diagnosing and treating renal damage following DQ exposure, and offer new insights into the molecular basis of DQ-induced kidney damage.

Supplementary Materials: The following supporting information can be downloaded at: https://www.mdpi.com/article/10.3390/toxics11020184/s1, Figure S1: Representative results of pathologic staining. Scale bars represent 100 μm in 20 × images. Black arrowheads indicate renal tubules exhibited vacuolation and necrosis.; Table S1. Differential genes in control and DQ treated groups; Table S2. Differentially proteins in control and DQ treated groups; Table S3. Differential genes/proteins both in transcriptome and proteome; Table S4. Differential metabolites in control and DQ treated groups.

Author Contributions: H.Z. designed the experiment and carried out the molecular biologic studies. J.L. and Z.M. collected the data. C.Z. and J.Q. drafted the manuscript. H.S. participated in study design. J.Z. reviewed the manuscript. B.Y. edited the manuscript. All authors have read and agreed to the published version of the manuscript.

Funding: This research was funded by the National Natural Science Foundation of China, grant number [No.82072158, 81803274]; Key Clinical Specialty Project, grant number [Su Finance (2020) No. 155]. The APC was funded by Young Scholars Fostering Fund of the First Affiliated Hospital of Nanjing Medical University.

Institutional Review Board Statement: The animal study protocol was approved by the Institutional Animal Care and Use Committee of Nanjing Medical University (protocol code 12371 and the date of approval is 2019-05-17).

Informed Consent Statement: Informed consent was obtained from all subjects involved in the study.

Data Availability Statement: The data presented in this study are available on request from the corresponding author. The data are not publicly available due to some data are still being analyzed.

Acknowledgments: The authors would like to thank all collaborators and colleagues involved in this project for useful discussions.

Conflicts of Interest: The authors declare that they have no known competing financial interests or personal relationships that could have appeared to influence the work reported in this paper.

References

1. Yu, G.; Jian, T.; Cui, S.; Shi, L.; Kan, B.; Jian, X. Acute diquat poisoning resulting in toxic encephalopathy: A report of three cases. *Clin. Toxicol. (Phila.)* **2022**, *60*, 647–650. [CrossRef]
2. Magalhaes, N.; Carvalho, F.; Dinis-Oliveira, R.J. Human and experimental toxicology of diquat poisoning: Toxicokinetics, mechanisms of toxicity, clinical features, and treatment. *Hum. Exp. Toxicol.* **2018**, *37*, 1131–1160. [PubMed]
3. Guck, D.; Hernandez, R.; Moore, S.; Van de Louw, A.; Haouzi, P. Rapid Glomerulotubular Nephritis as an Initial Presentation of a Lethal Diquat Ingestion. *Case Rep. Nephrol.* **2021**, *2021*, 4723092. [PubMed]
4. Hantson, P.; Wallemacq, P.; Mahieu, P. A case of fatal diquat poisoning: Toxicokinetic data and autopsy findings. *J. Toxicol. Clin. Toxicol.* **2000**, *38*, 149–152. [CrossRef]
5. Petejova, N.; Martinek, A.; Zadrazil, J.; Teplan, V. Acute toxic kidney injury. *Ren. Fail.* **2019**, *41*, 576–594. [CrossRef] [PubMed]
6. Ronco, C.; Bellomo, R.; Kellum, J.A. Acute kidney injury. *Lancet* **2019**, *394*, 1949–1964.
7. Kellum, J.A.; Romagnani, P.; Ashuntantang, G.; Ronco, C.; Zarbock, A.; Anders, H.J. Acute kidney injury. *Nat. Rev. Dis. Primers.* **2021**, *7*, 52.
8. Pan, H.C.; Chen, Y.Y.; Tsai, I.J.; Shiao, C.C.; Huang, T.M.; Chan, C.K.; Liao, H.W.; Lai, T.S.; Chueh, Y.; Wu, V.C.; et al. Accelerated versus standard initiation of renal replacement therapy for critically ill patients with acute kidney injury: A systematic review and meta-analysis of RCT studies. *Crit. Care* **2021**, *25*, 5.
9. Yuan, B.; Wu, W.; Chen, M.; Gu, H.; Tang, Q.; Guo, D.; Chen, T.; Chen, Y.; Lu, C.; Song, L.; et al. From the Cover: Metabolomics Reveals a Role of Betaine in Prenatal DBP Exposure-Induced Epigenetic Transgenerational Failure of Spermatogenesis in Rats. *Toxicol. Sci.* **2017**, *158*, 356–366. [CrossRef]
10. Yu, G.; Cui, S.; Jian, T.; Kan, B.; Jian, X. Diquat poisoning in a pregnant woman resulting in a miscarriage and maternal death. *Clin. Toxicol. (Phila.)* **2021**, *59*, 1275–1277. [CrossRef]
11. Tahri-Joutey, M.; Andreoletti, P.; Surapureddi, S.; Nasser, B.; Cherkaoui-Malki, M.; Latruffe, N. Mechanisms Mediating the Regulation of Peroxisomal Fatty Acid Beta-Oxidation by PPARalpha. *Int. J. Mol. Sci.* **2021**, *22*, 8969. [CrossRef]
12. Iwaki, T.; Bennion, B.G.; Stenson, E.K.; Lynn, J.C.; Otinga, C.; Djukovic, D.; Raftery, D.; Fei, L.; Wong, H.R.; Liles, W.C.; et al. PPARalpha contributes to protection against metabolic and inflammatory derangements associated with acute kidney injury in experimental sepsis. *Physiol. Rep.* **2019**, *7*, e14078.
13. Luan, Z.L.; Zhang, C.; Ming, W.H.; Huang, Y.Z.; Guan, Y.F.; Zhang, X.Y. Nuclear receptors in renal health and disease. *EBioMedicine* **2022**, *76*, 103855. [PubMed]
14. Yin, X.; Zeng, W.; Wu, B.; Wang, L.; Wang, Z.; Tian, H.; Wang, L.; Jiang, Y.; Clay, R.; Wei, X.; et al. PPARalpha Inhibition Overcomes Tumor-Derived Exosomal Lipid-Induced Dendritic Cell Dysfunction. *Cell Rep.* **2020**, *33*, 108278. [CrossRef]
15. Marechal, L.; Sicotte, B.; Caron, V.; Brochu, M.; Tremblay, A. Fetal Cardiac Lipid Sensing Triggers an Early and Sex-related Metabolic Energy Switch in Intrauterine Growth Restriction. *J. Clin. Endocrinol. Metab.* **2021**, *106*, 3295–3311. [PubMed]
16. Zhang, H.; Yan, Q.; Wang, X.; Chen, X.; Chen, Y.; Du, J.; Chen, L. The Role of Mitochondria in Liver Ischemia-Reperfusion Injury: From Aspects of Mitochondrial Oxidative Stress, Mitochondrial Fission, Mitochondrial Membrane Permeable Transport Pore Formation, Mitophagy, and Mitochondria-Related Protective Measures. *Oxid Med. Cell Longev.* **2021**, *2021*, 6670579.
17. Fang, L.; Li, T.S.; Zhang, J.Z.; Liu, Z.H.; Yang, J.; Wang, B.H.; Wang, Y.M.; Zhou, J.; Kong, L.D. Fructose drives mitochondrial metabolic reprogramming in podocytes via Hmgcs2-stimulated fatty acid degradation. *Signal Transduct. Target Ther.* **2021**, *6*, 253.
18. Yi, W.; Xie, X.; Du, M.; Bu, Y.; Wu, N.; Yang, H.; Tian, C.; Xu, F.; Xiang, S.; Zhang, P.; et al. Green Tea Polyphenols Ameliorate the Early Renal Damage Induced by a High-Fat Diet via Ketogenesis/SIRT3 Pathway. *Oxid Med. Cell Longev.* **2017**, *2017*, 9032792.
19. Zhang, D.; Yang, H.; Kong, X.; Wang, K.; Mao, X.; Yan, X.; Wang, Y.; Liu, S.; Zhang, X.; Li, J.; et al. Proteomics analysis reveals diabetic kidney as a ketogenic organ in type 2 diabetes. *Am. J. Physiol. Endocrinol. Metab.* **2011**, *300*, E287–E295. [CrossRef]

20. Capdevila, J.H.; Falck, J.R. The arachidonic acid monooxygenase: From biochemical curiosity to physiological/pathophysiological significance. *J. Lipid Res.* **2018**, *59*, 2047–2062. [CrossRef] [PubMed]
21. Khalil, Y.; Carrino, S.; Lin, F.; Ferlin, A.; Lad, H.V.; Mazzacuva, F.; Falcone, S.; Rivers, N.; Banks, G.; Concas, D.; et al. Tissue Proteome of 2-Hydroxyacyl-CoA Lyase Deficient Mice Reveals Peroxisome Proliferation and Activation of omega-Oxidation. *Int. J. Mol. Sci.* **2022**, *23*, 987. [PubMed]
22. Yang, Z.; Smalling, R.V.; Huang, Y.; Jiang, Y.; Kusumanchi, P.; Bogaert, W.; Wang, L.; Delker, D.A.; Skill, N.J.; Han, S.; et al. The role of SHP/REV-ERBalpha/CYP4A axis in the pathogenesis of alcohol-associated liver disease. *JCI Insight.* **2021**, *6*, e140687. [CrossRef]
23. Agrawal, S.; Zaritsky, J.J.; Fornoni, A.; Smoyer, W.E. Dyslipidaemia in nephrotic syndrome: Mechanisms and treatment. *Nat. Rev. Nephrol.* **2018**, *14*, 57–70. [PubMed]
24. Sidhom, E.H.; Kim, C.; Kost-Alimova, M.; Ting, M.T.; Keller, K.; Avila-Pacheco, J.; Watts, A.J.; Vernon, K.A.; Marshall, J.L.; Reyes-Bricio, E.; et al. Targeting a Braf/Mapk pathway rescues podocyte lipid peroxidation in CoQ-deficiency kidney disease. *J. Clin. Investig.* **2021**, *131*. [CrossRef]
25. Zhang, S.J.; Li, Z.H.; Zhang, Y.D.; Chen, J.; Li, Y.; Wu, F.Q.; Wang, W.; Cui, Z.J.; Chen, G.Q. Ketone Body 3-Hydroxybutyrate Ameliorates Atherosclerosis via Receptor Gpr109a-Mediated Calcium Influx. *Adv. Sci. (Weinh.)* **2021**, *8*, 2003410. [PubMed]

Disclaimer/Publisher's Note: The statements, opinions and data contained in all publications are solely those of the individual author(s) and contributor(s) and not of MDPI and/or the editor(s). MDPI and/or the editor(s) disclaim responsibility for any injury to people or property resulting from any ideas, methods, instructions or products referred to in the content.

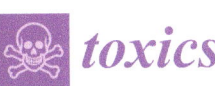

Article

Stage-Related Neurotoxicity of BPA in the Development of Zebrafish Embryos

Jianjun Liu [†], Wenyu Kong [†], Yuchen Liu [†], Qiyao Ma, Qi Shao, Liwen Zeng, Yu Chao, Xiaoyao Song * and Jie Zhang *

Department of Toxicology, School of Public Health, Medical College of Soochow University, Suzhou 215031, China
* Correspondence: xysong@suda.edu.cn (X.S.); zhangjie_78@suda.edu.cn (J.Z.)
† These authors contributed equally to this work.

Abstract: Bisphenol A (BPA) is one of the most widely produced chemicals in the world used in the production of epoxy resins and polycarbonate plastics. BPA is easily migrated from the outer packaging to the contents. Due to the lipophilic property, BPA is easily accumulated in organisms. Perinatal low-dose BPA exposure alters brain neural development in later generations. In this study, after BPA treatment, the spontaneous movement of zebrafish larvae from the cleavage period to the segmentation period (1–24 hpf) was significantly decreased, with speed decreasing by 18.97% and distance decreasing between 18.4 and 29.7% compared to controls. Transcriptomics analysis showed that 131 genes were significantly differentially expressed in the exposed group during the 1–24 hpf period, among which 39 genes were significantly upregulated and 92 genes were significantly downregulated. The GO enrichment analysis, gene function analysis and real-time quantitative PCR of differentially expressed genes showed that the mRNA level of guanine deaminase (cypin) decreased significantly in the 1–24 hpf period. Moreover, during the 1–24 hpf period, BPA exposure reduced guanine deaminase activity. Therefore, we confirmed that cypin is a key sensitive gene for BPA during this period. Finally, the cypin mRNA microinjection verified that the cypin level of zebrafish larvae was restored, leading to the restoration of the locomotor activity. Taken together, the current results show that the sensitive period of BPA to zebrafish embryos is from the cleavage period to the segmentation period (1–24 hpf), and cypin is a potential target for BPA-induced neurodevelopmental toxicity. This study provides a potential sensitive period and a potential target for the deep understanding of neurodevelopmental toxicity mechanisms caused by BPA.

Keywords: bisphenol A; zebrafish; sensitive period; guanine deaminase; locomotor behavior

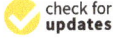

Citation: Liu, J.; Kong, W.; Liu, Y.; Ma, Q.; Shao, Q.; Zeng, L.; Chao, Y.; Song, X.; Zhang, J. Stage-Related Neurotoxicity of BPA in the Development of Zebrafish Embryos. *Toxics* **2023**, *11*, 177. https://doi.org/10.3390/toxics11020177

Academic Editor: Robyn L. Tanguay

Received: 30 December 2022
Revised: 9 February 2023
Accepted: 10 February 2023
Published: 14 February 2023

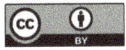

Copyright: © 2023 by the authors. Licensee MDPI, Basel, Switzerland. This article is an open access article distributed under the terms and conditions of the Creative Commons Attribution (CC BY) license (https://creativecommons.org/licenses/by/4.0/).

1. Introduction

Bisphenol A (BPA) is one of the most widely produced chemicals in the world, as an analogue of bisphenol (BP). BPA is mainly used in industry to synthesize materials such as polycarbonate and epoxy resin. It has been used in the manufacture of plastic cups, baby bottles, food and beverage cans since the 1960s [1–4]. Studies have shown that BPA is easily migrated from containers or packaging materials to food and beverages. Due to the lipophilic property ($LogK_{ow}$ = 3.3), BPA is easily accumulated in organisms. BPA has been detected in wild animals, especially fish (0.2–13,000 ng/g) [5], and can be detected in human blood and urine. A study reported that BPA was found in 46% of all blood samples analyzed, with a geometric mean (GM) concentration of 0.19 ng/mL. BPA was found in 84% of urine samples from adults, with a GM concentration of 1.01 ng/mL [0.48 μg/g creatinine (Cr)] [6–8]. According to reports, a significant positive correlation was found between serum and urine BPA levels in pregnant women and neonates [9,10]. Exposure to BPA during pregnancy induced anxiety, reduced exploratory behavior and increased depressive behavior in adult mice [11]. Similarly, perinatal low-dose BPA exposure has altered brain neural development in offspring rats [12,13]. Therefore, exposure to BPA in the early stages of life is of great concern, in which the embryo and infancy stage play a very important role in the natural development of the nervous system.

Zebrafish (Danio rerio) is a model organism widely used in toxicological evaluation [14–16]. Recent reports have shown that brain structures are homologous between zebrafish and humans such as the amygdala, hippocampus and hypothalamus [17]. Furthermore, zebrafish show a wide range of complex behavior in cognition, aggression, anxiety and social interaction [18]. Thus, zebrafish is a useful tool for elucidating the function of novel genes for neurogenesis [19] and have been used to validate the function of human candidate genes involved in autism, etc. [19–21]. After fertilization, zebrafish embryos go through seven stages to complete embryonic development [22]: the zygotic stage (0–0.75 hpf), cleavage period (0.75–2.20 hpf), blastula period (2.20–5.25 hpf), gastrula period (5.25–10 hpf), segmentation period (10–24 hpf), pharyngeal period (24–48 hpf) and hatching period (48–72 hpf). The nervous system starts to develop and form the neural plate at 6 hpf, and the neural tube and different brain regions form beginning in the 10–16 hpf period. By 24 hpf, brain morphogenesis is advanced, and the brain is divided into the forebrain, including the diencephalon and telencephalon, midbrain, hindbrain and spinal cord, while the earliest clusters of neurons are interconnected by axons [23]. There is a correspondence between the embryonic and the behavior development of zebrafish. The spontaneous contractions of trunk muscles of zebrafish can be observed at 17 hpf, tail movement appears at 21 hpf, the locomotor ability of zebrafish shows the avoidance reflex phenomenon to external stimuli at 48 hpf and the rate of swimming in response to touch becomes maximal at 36 hpf close to that of adult zebrafish [24,25]. Therefore, damage to the nervous system often results in changes in behavior [26]. Normally developed zebrafish embryos have the ability to move freely at 96–120 hpf, and their locomotor ability can be used as a sensitive endpoint for exogenous chemicals to damage the nervous development of the body [27].

In this study, we integrated transcriptomics and neurodevelopmental toxicity analysis to comprehensively study the potential biological mechanisms of BPA exposure in zebrafish during the embryonic development period. We investigated the BPA-induced neurotoxicity in different stages of the development of zebrafish embryos to reveal the possible sensitive period of the development upon exposure to BPA and to explore the potential biomarker of BPA neurodevelopmental toxicity.

2. Materials and Methods

2.1. Chemicals and Reagents Preparation

BPA powder (99%) was purchased from Sigma-Aldrich (St Louis, MO, USA). A stock solution of BPA was dissolved and diluted in dimethyl sulfoxide (DMSO) (Sigma-Aldrich, St Louis, MO, USA) to achieve BPA treatment concentrations. DEPC water (Beyotime, Nanjing, China) was used when cleaning zebrafish embryos and diluting cDNA.

2.2. BPA Exposure of Zebrafish Embryos

The workflow of the present research is in Figure 1. Zebrafish (Danio rerio) were obtained from the Zebrafish Experiment Center of Soochow University (Suzhou, China). They were raised in standard laboratory conditions at 28.5 °C with a 14:10 light/dark (LD) cycle. Zebrafish were fed three times per day. Male and female adult fish (male/female = 1/1 or 1/2) were separated by isolation boards in spawning tanks in the evening. The isolation boards were removed when the light turned on automatically the next morning; then, the embryos were collected within 2 h and rinsed with fish culture water for subsequent experiments. Healthy embryos were selected by stereomicroscopy. In total, 30 embryos per group were placed in an empty well of a 6-well plate, and then 3 mL of systemic culture water was added to each well. According to the characteristics of zebrafish embryo development, each stage of early embryo development was completed in 96 hpf, so the time point of 96 hpf was selected in the follow-up experiment. According to 96 hpf median lethal concentration, we determined that the LC_{50} was 11.4 mg/L. As design, we chose half of the LC_{50} (5.7 mg/L) as the exposure concentration. Zebrafish embryos were treated with

5.7 mg/L BPA (Figure 2) from the cleavage period to the segmentation period (1–24 hpf), pharyngula period (24–48 hpf) and hatching period (48–72 hpf); washed with fish culture water 3 times and cultured until 96 hpf (changing water every day). The DMSO solvent control (SC) group and blank control (BC) group were set up (the final concentration of DMSO was 0.1%). Each dose group had three replicates. The embryos were chorionated. The dead embryos were picked out during the culture process. All animal protocols were performed in accordance with the Guidelines on the Care and Use of Animals and with the approval of the Soochow University Animal Welfare Committee.

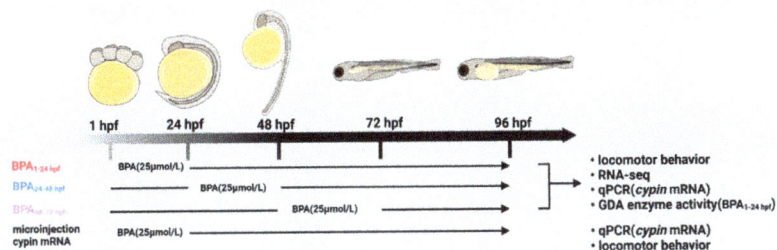

Figure 1. A workflow of the present study design.

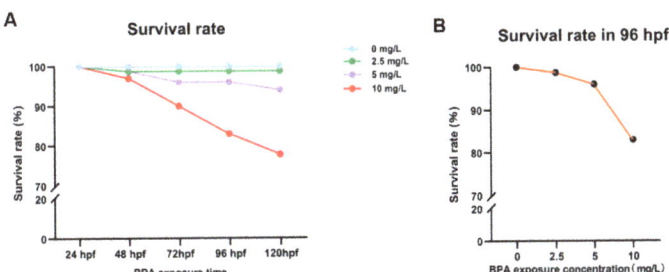

Figure 2. Survival rate of zebrafish exposed to BPA. (**A**) Survival rate of zebrafish exposed to different concentrations of BPA. (**B**) Survival rate of zebrafish exposed to different concentrations of BPA at 96hpf. The modified Kohl method was used to calculate the $LC_{50,\ 72\ hpf}$ = 12.639 mg/L, 95% confidence interval of 11.857–13.473; $LC_{50,\ 96\ hpf}$ = 10.193 mg/L, 95% confidence interval of 9.040–11.494; $LC_{50,\ 120\ hpf}$ = 9.045 mg/L, 95% confidence interval of 7.608–10.753. Data are the mean ± SD (n = 90 in each concentration).

2.3. Locomotor Behavioral Analysis

To investigate the effect of early-life exposure to BPA on the nervous system, we studied the locomotor behavioral change underlying two scenarios such as spontaneous motion and light-dark cycle stimulation. Three experimental replicated with 30 embryos were exposed. Excluding embryos that died or that had overt toxicity, we selected 8 zebrafish for each treatment group. Statistics were calculated for at least 8 zebrafish per treatment group; then, the differences in 3 replicate experiments were calculated. At 96 hpf, the normally developed zebrafish larvae were placed in a 96-well plate, one for each well, and 250 µL of systematic fish culture water was added to make sure the zebrafish larvae could swim freely. The 96-well plate was placed in a Zebralab high-throughput behavior analyzer (View PointLife Sciences, Lyon, France) to detect the changes in locomotor behavior.

For spontaneous motion detection, after the light adapting to 30 min in the system, the spontaneous movement of zebrafish larvae within 10 min was collected, and the swimming speed of zebrafish larvae was calculated automatically.

For the light-dark cycle stimulus assay, after the light adapting to 30 min in the system, the light–dark cycle was set to 90 s (90 s light/90 s dark alternating) and repeated 3 times to detect the response of zebrafish to the dark-light transition stimulus.

2.4. Transcriptomics Analysis

In order to explore the toxic mechanism of BPA in the sensitive stage of neurotoxicity, we used RNA-seq to analyze the transcriptome of zebrafish larvae in SC group and exposed group. The total genomic RNA of zebrafish exposed to BPA from the cleavage period to the segmentation period (1–24 hpf) was extracted. The cracking reagent was blown, mixed and centrifuged (13,000 rpm, 4 °C) to obtain short mRNA. The short mRNA was used as the template to synthesize cDNA1 chain, and then the cDNA2 chain was further synthesized and purified. Then, the poly A tail was added to the end of the cDNA2 chain, and the joint sequence was connected. The DNA fragment was enriched after purification and analyzed by a biological analyzer. The RIN (RNA Integrity Number) value was 8 after analyzing on the bioanalyzer. The library was constructed, and the quality inspection was carried out. The screening of differential genes was performed to calculate the read number of genes in each sample according to htseq-count software. After obtaining the raw reads in FastQ format, the 3' end adapter sequence was pruned, and the low-quality value (<20) region in the sequencing files was removed. Gene expression level was expressed by fragments per kilobase of transcript per million mapped reads (FPKM). The raw read counts were used to analyze differentially expressed genes (DEGs) using the "DESeq" package. Then, the data were standardized, the differential genes were selected according to the p value ($p < 0.05$) and fold change values larger than 1.5 of the differences, unsupervised hierarchical clustering of differential genes was performed. GO enrichment analysis of the differentially expressed genes was carried out to show the function of the differentially expressed genes.

2.5. Real-Time Quantitative PCR Analysis

Total RNA was isolated from larvae using TRIzol reagent (Beyotime). The yields of RNA samples were measured with a Nanodrop spectrophotometer (ThermoFisher Scientific, Waltham, MA, USA). All samples had an OD A_{260}/A_{280} ratio (range 1.8–2.0). A total of 1000 ng of RNA was used for the cDNA synthesis reaction using a RevertAid First Strand cDNA Synthesis Kit (ThermoFisher Scientific). Quantitative real-time PCR analysis was carried out with QuantStudio 6 (ThermoFisher Scientific) using the maxima SYBR Green qPCR Master Mix (Roche), and subjected to the following two-step RT-PCR method: 120 s at 95 °C, followed by 45 cycles of 95 °C for 20 s and 60 °C for 40 s. The transcription of β-actin was used as a housekeeping gene. Gene expression levels were measured in triplicate for each treatment. The sequences of the primers used in this study are presented in Table S1. The fold change of genes tested was calculated using the $2^{-\Delta\Delta CT}$ method.

2.6. Microinjection

Based on changes in mRNA activity in the results of the above transcriptomics analysis and real-time quantitative PCR analysis, we focused on Cypin. In order to verify the role of cypin in BPA exposure, we used rescue experiments. At the position of about 300 bp after polyA, the primer sequence of the target gene cypin was designed with the vector (pCDNA3.1-HA), restriction site (NotI, NheI) and target gene (cypin). The total RNA of the brain tissue of zebrafish was used as template and reverse transcribed into cDNA as template for PCR amplification. Zebrafish cypin fragments were amplified by designed primer sequences and analyzed by agarose gel electrophoresis. After gel recovery and homologous recombination, the recombinant plasmid was digested with NotI and NheI, and the sequencing results showed that cypin was cut by agarose gel electrophoresis. After sequencing, it was found that the sequenced recombinant plasmid was the target gene cypin plasmid, indicating that the plasmid was constructed successfully. After cypin sequencing, the promoter was amplified with T7 promoter and pCDNA3.1-HA as upstream and downstream primers. The PCR product was purified, and the mRNA of cypin was synthesized by T7 transcriptase. Agarose gel electrophoresis analysis showed that the transcription was successful. All zebrafish eggs were divided into six groups: blank control group (BC group); microinjection of DEPC water group (DEPC group); microinjection of cypin mRNA group (cypin group); BPA treatment group; BPA treatment after microinjection of DPEC water group (BPA + DEPC group); and BPA treatment after microinjection of cypin mRNA group (BPA + cypin group). The BPA treatment group, BPA + DEPC group and BPA + cypin group were exposed to BPA for 24 hpf from the cleavage period to the segmentation period (1–24 hpf). The purified mRNA was diluted to a 0.3 M injection sample with Rnase-free water. The injection pressure was adjusted so that the volume of each injection was 1–1.5 nL, and cypin was injected in the single-cell stage of zebrafish embryos. After washing with fish culture water 3 times, they were cultured to 96 hpf (changing water every day). Triplicates were set up at all concentrations, and dead fish embryos were selected in time during culture. Zebrafish behavior and qPCR analysis experiments were carried out after 96 hpf.

2.7. Guanine Deaminase Activity Assay

The guanine deaminase activity of zebrafish exposed to BPA (5.7 mg/L) from the cleavage period to the segmentation period (1–24 hpf) and of the blank control group were detected using a guanine deaminase kit (Kanglang Biotechnology, Shanghai, China). The absorbance (OD) was determined by a microplate reader (BIO-TEX, Southlake, TX, USA) at 450 nm, and the content of guanine deaminase (GDA) in zebrafish samples was calculated by a standard curve. Taking the concentration of the standards as the abscissa and the OD value as the ordinate, and the corresponding concentration was determined from the standard curve according to the OD value of the sample and then multiplied by the dilution multiple, that is, the actual concentration of the sample.

2.8. Statistical Analysis

A formal acute toxicity test was designed using the modified Kohl method (Kaber) [28]. The movement speed and distance of zebrafish were counted by EthoVisionXT10.0 analysis software (Noldus Information Technologies, Wageningen, The Netherlands), and the data were collected once a second. The experimental data were statistically analyzed by SPSS 17.0 software (IBM, Armonk, NY, USA), and the statistical results were expressed as the mean ± SD. In the rescue experiment, one-way analysis of variance (one-way ANOVA) corrected by Bonferroni was used for multiple comparisons. Guanine deaminase activity was tested by a t-test. In addition, p-values less than 0.05 was considered as statistical difference.

3. Results
3.1. Survival Rate of Zebrafish Exposed to BPA

Based on previous studies, embryos were exposed to BPA concentrations of 0, 2.5, 5 and 10 mg/L from 0 to 96 hpf, which is when embryos have crossed the hatching stage and completed early embryo development. In total, 30 zebrafish embryos were in each dose group, with 3 replicates. After that, the embryo survival rate was recorded from 24 hpf up to 120 hpf after BPA exposure (Figure 2A). According to the characteristics of zebrafish embryo development, 96 hpf zebrafish embryos have crossed the hatching stage and completed early embryo development; therefore, during the follow-up experiment, we determined 96 hpf as the end of the time of exposure. According to the $LC_{50, 96 hpf}$, the subsequent experimental concentration was determined to be about half of the median lethal concentration, that is, 5.7 mg/L.

3.2. Effects of BPA on Zebrafish Locomotor Behavior

As shown in Figure 3, the spontaneous movement speed of zebrafish in the blank control group was approximately 0.13 mm/s, while that in the exposed group from the cleavage period to the segmentation period ($BPA_{1-24hpf}$ group) decreased significantly

($p < 0.05$), at approximately 18.97% lower than control. Compared with the BC group, there were no statistical differences of spontaneous movement speed in other BPA-exposed-period groups ($p > 0.05$). Generally, larvae increase their movement when subjected to dark conditions. This increase in movement was consistent across multiple dark-light cycles (Figure 4A). However, further analysis found that from the cleavage period to the segmentation period (1–24 hpf), the moving distance in the light-dark cycle of the BPA exposure group of zebrafish larvae were significantly decreased, dropping 29.7% in the light period ($p < 0.05$, Figure 4B) and 18.4% in the dark period ($p < 0.05$, Figure 4C). There were no statistical differences in the light-dark cycle in the other groups compared with the BC group. Therefore, we confirmed that the sensitive period of BPA on the locomotor behavior of zebrafish larvae was from the cleavage to the segmentation period (1–24 hpf) in this study.

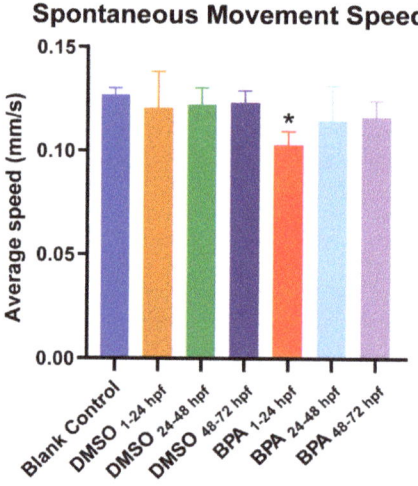

Figure 3. Effects of exposure to BPA on spontaneous movement speed of zebrafish embryos at different developmental periods. Data are the mean ± SD (n = 24 in each concentration). *, significant from blank control, $p < 0.05$.

3.3. Transcriptome Analysis of Zebrafish Larvae at Different Developmental Periods after BPA Exposure

Figure 5A shows the hierarchical cluster heatmaps of differential genes expression based on log10 of FPKM values through cluster analysis. As shown in Figure 5A, compared with the BC group, there were statistical differences in 131 differential genes in the BPA-exposed group during 1–24 hpf, of which 39 were significantly upregulated and 92 were significantly downregulated (Figure 5A). As shown in Figure 5B, we screened the differential genes of the cleavage period to the segmentation period (1–24 hpf) in the exposed group using the gene ontology (GO) analysis. Then, we listed the enrichment scores of the top 20 terms that corresponded to the differential genes. Among them, there were six entries with the highest enrichment scores corresponding to three GO terms: long-chain fatty acid decomposition in the process of biology (acadl); cypin in the guanine catabolic processes; molecular functions, including NAD transporter activity and FMN transporter activity (slc25a17), long-chain acyl coenzyme A dehydrogenase activity (acadl) and guanine catabolism (cypin). Because of the enrichment score of cypin and its enrichment in both terms, and because it was closely related to neural development, we included it as a biomarker for further investigation. As shown in Figure 5C, the results of real-time qPCR showed that the expression of cypin was significantly decreased after exposure to BPA from the cleavage period to the segmentation period (1–24 hpf) compared with the BC group ($p < 0.05$). Our transcriptome sequencing results also showed that cypin mRNA levels of

1–24 hpf zebrafish larvae were significantly downregulated in the exposed group. These results suggest that cypin might play an important role in the neural development from cleavage period to the segmentation period (1–24 hpf) of zebrafish.

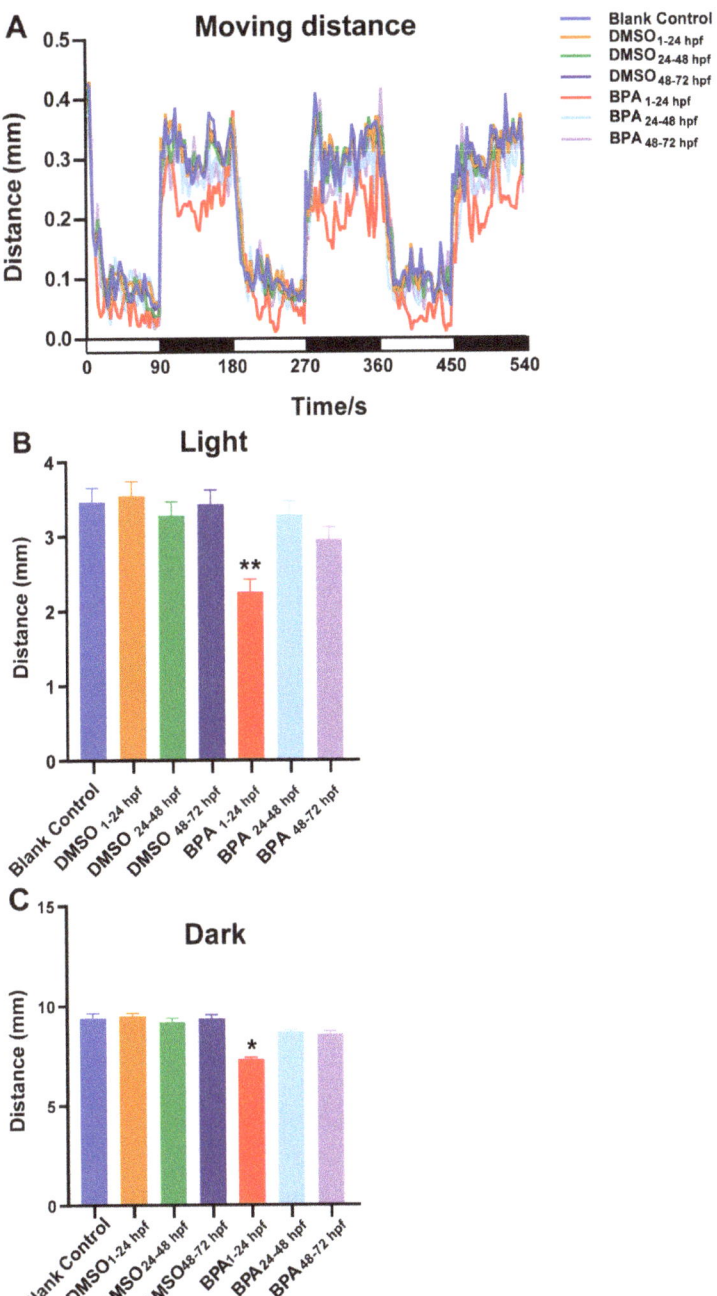

Figure 4. Effects of exposure to BPA on locomotor behavior under the light-dark cycle stimulation of zebrafish embryos at different developmental periods. (**A**) The trend of distance. (**B**,**C**) The analysis

results of the trend of the distance. Abscissa white for light, black for darkness. Data are the mean ± SD (n = 24 in each concentration). *, significant from blank control, $p < 0.05$, **, significant from blank control, $p < 0.01$.

3.4. Changes in Cypin during Zebrafish Embryonic Development

Figure 6 shows the expression of cypin in zebrafish embryos (wild-type unexposed embryos) during development (1 hpf, 24 hpf, 48 hpf, 72 hpf, 96 hpf). The results showed that, compared with 1 hpf zebrafish embryos, the expression of cypin was significantly increased at 24 hpf ($p < 0.05$) and then returned to the 1 hpf level at other points in development time. This suggests that cypin played an important role in early neural development.

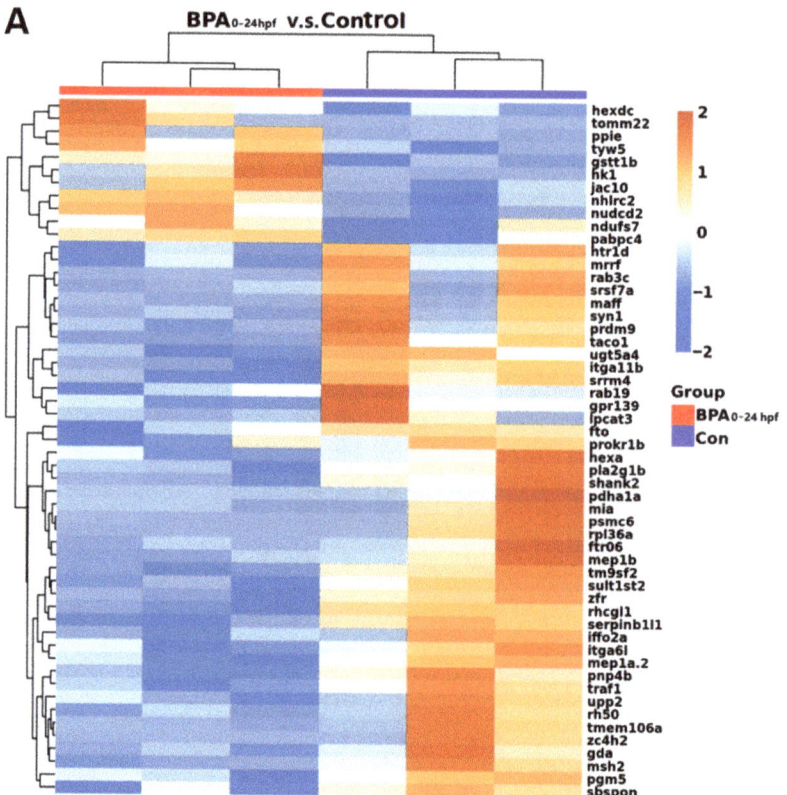

Figure 5. Cont.

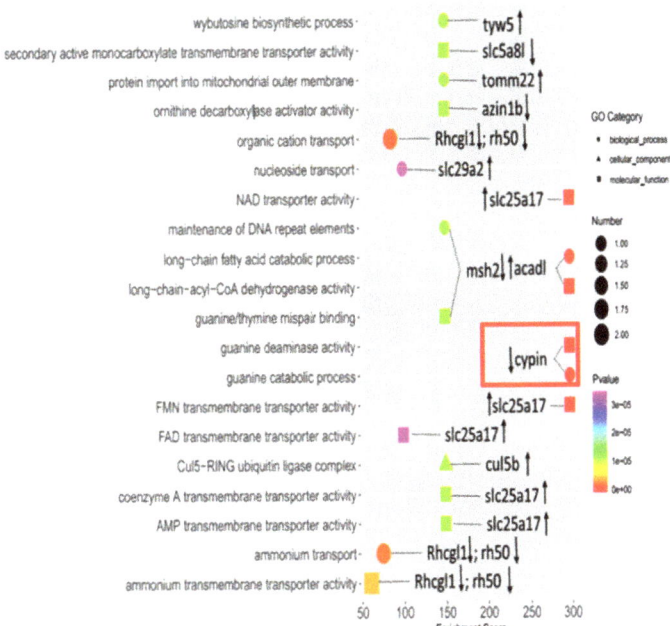

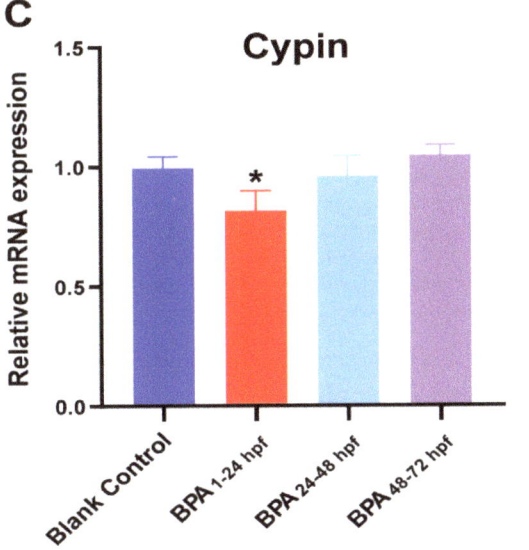

Figure 5. Transcriptome analysis of zebrafish from the cleavage period to the segmentation period (1–24 hpf), pharyngula period (24–48 hpf) and hatching period (48–72 hpf) induced by BPA. (**A**) Cluster analysis heatmap. Red indicates increased gene expression, and blue indicates decreased gene expression. (**B**) GO function enrichment analysis bubble diagram for differentially expressed genes. (**C**) The expression of cypin. Data are the mean ± SD (30 embryos per sample, and repeat three times), *, significant from blank control, $p < 0.05$.

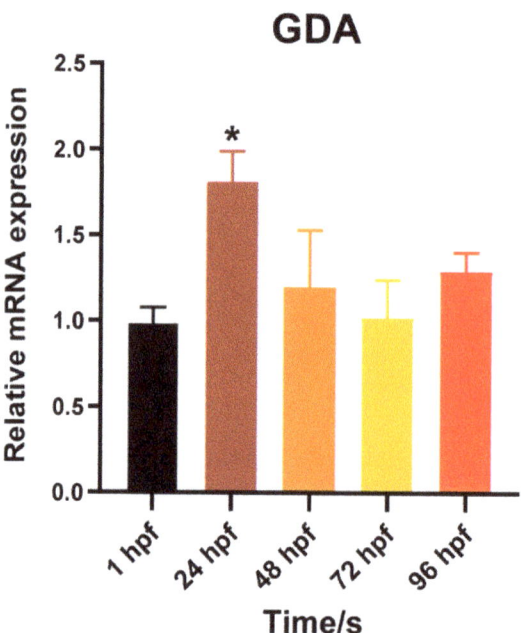

Figure 6. The expression of cypin at different developmental periods. Data are the mean ± SD, *, significant from 1 hpf, $p < 0.05$.

3.5. Effect of BPA on the Activity of Guanine Deaminase in Zebrafish Embryos during 1–24 hpf

Cypin, also known as guanine deaminase (GDA), the primary guanine deaminase in the brain, plays key roles in shaping neuronal circuits and regulating neuronal survival. Based on the above results, we found that the mRNA of cypin only decreased significantly in the stage from the cleavage period to the segmentation period (1–24 hpf). However, in the aforementioned BPA-unexposed zebrafish (Figure 6), the mRNA levels of cypin were significantly elevated at 1–24 hpf compared to those in other stages. The magnitude of cypin change was significant. Therefore, we focused on the changes of GDA activity in BPA exposure stage from the cleavage period to the segmentation period (1–24 hpf). As shown in Figure 7, since zebrafish exposed to BPA at 1-24 hpf had reduced cypin expression, we then tested whether the fish also had reduced GDA and found that the fish exposed to BPA had significantly lower GDA.

3.6. Changes in Cypin Expression after Microinjection of Cypin mRNA

Through the above experiments, we found that BPA exposure reduced the mRNA level and activity of cypin. Therefore, we wanted to confirm whether cypin was the key sensitive gene of BPA during this period by the microinjection of cypin mRNA. After the microinjection of cypin mRNA, we determined the post-injection results of mRNA using qPCR. According to Figure 8, the expression of cypin in the cypin group was significantly higher than that in the BC group. The expression of cypin in BPA treatment group and BPA+DEPC group decreased significantly compared with the BC (blank control) group, but there was no significant difference between the BC group and BPA+ cypin group, suggesting that BPA can induce the downregulation of cypin gene expression and the microinjection of cypin mRNA can reverse the downregulation of cypin gene expression induced by BPA.

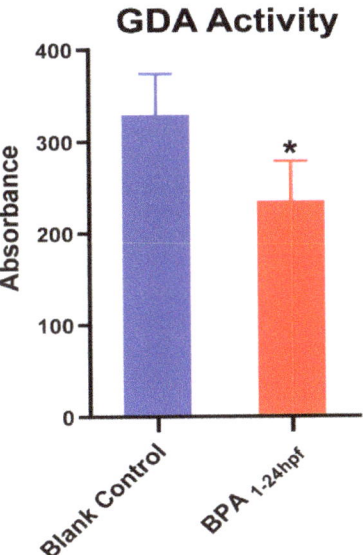

Figure 7. Effects of exposure to BPA on GDA enzyme activity in zebrafish embryos from the cleavage period to the segmentation period (1–24 hpf). Data are the mean ± SD, *, significant from blank control, $p < 0.05$.

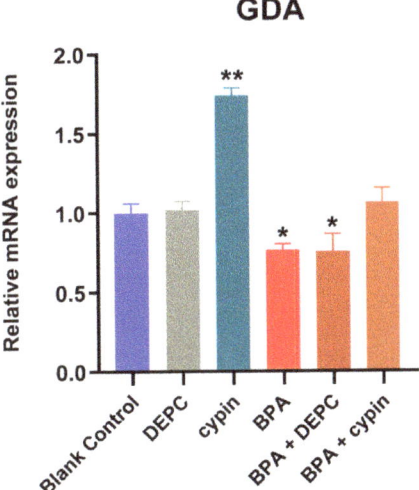

Figure 8. Expression of cypin gene after microinjection of cypin mRNA in zebrafish embryos. Data are the mean ± SD, *, significant from blank control, $p < 0.05$. **, significant from blank control, $p < 0.01$. DEPC group: microinjection of DEPC water; cypin group; microinjection of cypin mRNA; BPA treatment group: BPA treatment; BPA + DEPC group: BPA treatment after microinjection of DPEC; BPA + cypin group: BPA treatment after microinjection of cypin mRNA.

3.7. The Locomotor Behavior Change of Zebrafish Larvae after Microinjection of Cypin mRNA

After the microinjection of cypin mRNA, the spontaneous movement of zebrafish larvae was observed (Figure 9). Compared with the BC group, there was no statistical difference of spontaneous movement speed in the DEPC group, but it was significantly increased in the cypin group ($p < 0.05$), indicating that cypin could accelerate the swimming speed of zebrafish larvae. The spontaneous movement speed in the BPA treatment group and BPA + DEPC group both decreased significantly ($p < 0.05$), and that in the BPA + cypin group had no statistical difference compared to the BC group ($p > 0.05$), showing that BPA could suppress zebrafish movement speed and that cypin microinjection could reverse the BPA-induced movement speed inhibition of zebrafish larvae to normal levels.

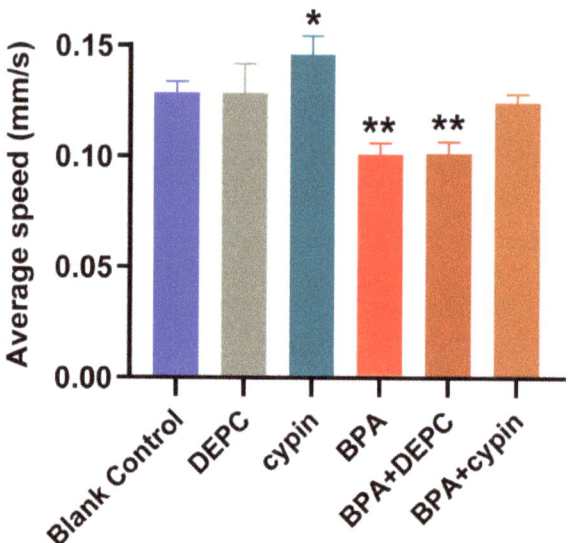

Figure 9. Effect of BPA on the spontaneous movement of zebrafish embryos after microinjection of cypin mRNA. Data are the mean ± SD (n = 24 in each concentration). *, significant from blank control, $p < 0.05$. **, significant from blank control, $p < 0.01$.

The behavioral results of light and dark stimuli were consistent with the results of spontaneous movement speed (Figure 10A–C). After microinjection, the locomotor behavior of zebrafish larvae returned to normal level. All of the abovementioned results suggested that BPA mediates neurotoxicity and affects the locomotor behavior of zebrafish larvae by inhibiting the expression of cypin mRNA from the cleavage period to the segmentation period (1–24 hpf).

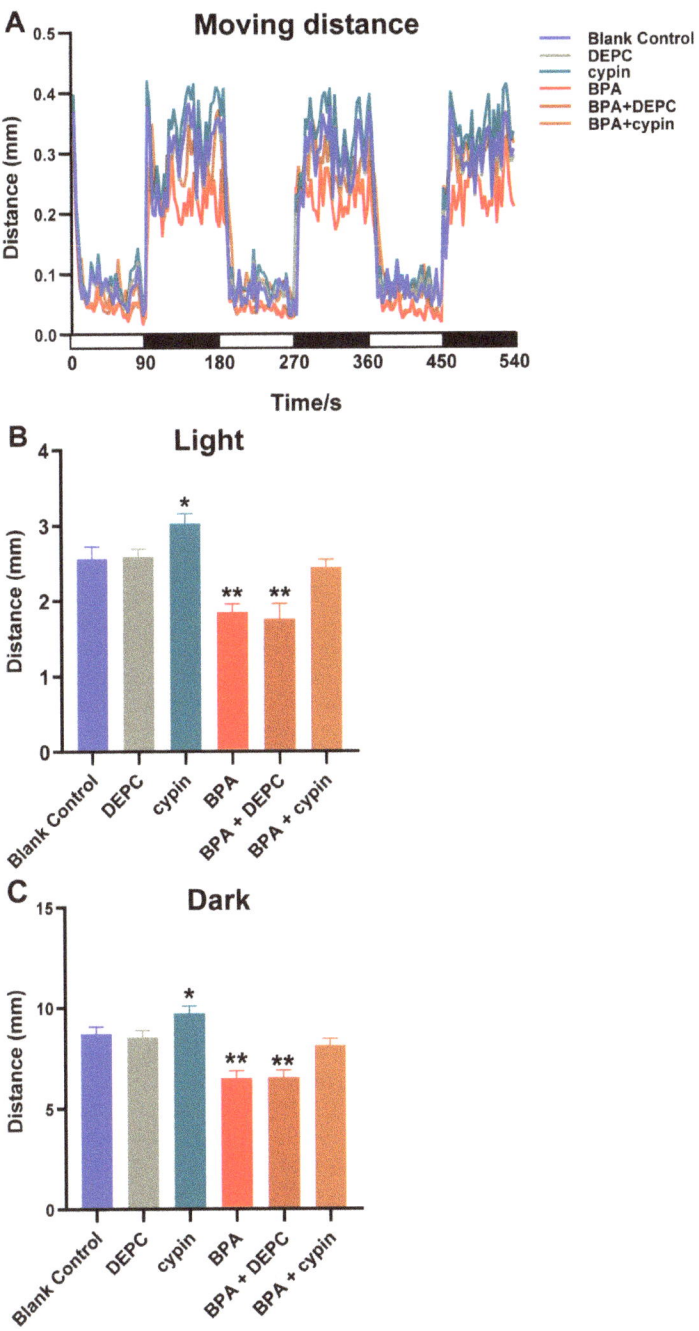

Figure 10. Effects of exposure to BPA on locomotor behavior under light-dark cycle stimulation of zebrafish embryos after microinjection of cypin mRNA. (**A**) The trend of distance. (**B**,**C**) The analysis results of the trend of the distance. Abscissa white for light, black for darkness. Data are the mean ± SD (n = 24 in each concentration). *, significant from blank control, $p < 0.01$; **, significant from blank control, $p < 0.001$.

4. Discussion

Bisphenol A is an environmental endocrine disruptor. Scientists have reached the consensus that bisphenol A could be enriched in organisms through the food chain [29]. It is structurally similar to estrogen and competes for binding to estrogen receptors α/β, thus interfering with hormone signaling in the nervous system [30–32], which is essential for brain development. Prenatal exposure to BPA can impair the neurodevelopment of children, mainly manifested as anxiety, depression and hyperactivity [33,34].

In this study, the zebrafish larvae were exposed to BPA from the cleavage period to the segmentation period (1–24 hpf). Neurodevelopment in zebrafish begins during gastrula formation (approximately 6 hpf), when nerve cells arrive in place and form neural plates [35]. The neural plate becomes tubular at the end of gastrula formation (9–10 hpf), and different brain regions are segmented in the following 6–8 h [36]. At 24 hpf, zebrafish brain partitioning is basically complete, and the initial neurons are connected by axons [23,37]. Therefore, we deduce that the cleavage period to segmentation period (1–24 hpf) of zebrafish is a very important period of nervous system development. Our result did find that BPA exposure from the cleavage period to the segmentation period significantly decreased the spontaneous movement of zebrafish larvae. There was no difference in other periods. Locomotor behavior is a relatively sensitive indicator of internal physiological changes as well as of nerve injury. Thus, we believed that BPA induced neurotoxicity mainly in segmentation period. First, cypin, a key gene targeted by BPA, was upregulated during 1–24 hpf of development (Figure 6). Second, toxicokinetic prediction modeling showed that the concentration of BPA in zebrafish embryos (chorionated) gradually increased over time, reached the highest level at 40 hpf and then began to decrease. We found that the concentration of BPA in the prediction model increased continuously at 1–24 hpf, and our results showed that the expression of cypin only increased significantly at the 1–24 hpf period during the normal development of zebrafish embryos and decreased only at this period after BPA exposure. Therefore, even if the highest concentration is not reached in the 1–24 hpf period, it still produces the most serious effect. Therefore, we speculate that the toxicokinetics of BPA itself may play a role [38]. This modeling in our study correlates with our findings and suggests that the most susceptible period for BPA to exert its neurodevelopmental toxic effects is early in life, both in terms of its own toxicokinetics and the metabolic kinetics of zebrafish.

Cypin, known as cytosolic postsynaptic density protein 95 interactor, is also called the primary guanine deaminase (GDA; Guaninase) in the brain and plays key role in shaping neuronal circuits and regulating neuronal survival [39,40]. Microchemical analysis of the brain revealed that that cypin is mainly located in the dendritic axis and synaptic neck [39]. The overexpression of cypin in hippocampal neurons increases the number of dendrites, while knockdown could reduce the dendrite number [41] that is associated with GDA activity [41] and zinc ion-binding [42]. The decrease in the number of dendrites may lead to the failure of neurons to receive information normally, leading to neural abnormalities. Neuronal dendrites play an important role in the normal reception of information by the neural signal network. To understand the role of cypin in the neuron development of zebrafish, we tested cypin gene expression in different periods of embryonic development. The qPCR results showed cypin expression fluctuated with increasing exposure time compared to 1 hpf, increasing significantly at 24 hpf and falling back to the same level as 1 hpf at 48 hpf, 72 hpf and 96 hpf. The abovementioned results were consistent with the results of the Patel MV determination of the level of cypin in the mice brain, and the expression of cypin was increased at the beginning and then decreased to normal level [43]. Another study found that reduced locomotor behavior in children with autism spectrum disorder (ASD) may be due to cypin deficiency during pregnancy [44]. All of these findings indicate that cypin plays an important role in early neural development and are consistent with our findings.

To verify the role of cypin under BPA exposure, we detected the activity of guanine deaminase (GDA) and found that BPA could decrease the activity of GDA. GDA plays a critical role in neurodevelopment, and its enzyme activity is essential for normal purine recovery and brain development and function [41]. A specific reduction in guanine to adenine nucleotide levels was also found in Lesch-Nyhan disease, where a patient had dyspraxia and intellectual disabilities [45]. Our results did find that enzymes involved in purine metabolism, such as guanine deaminase, may play an important role in regulating appropriate neuronal activity, which suggests that the decrease of BPA-induced guanine deaminase activity may lead to impaired neurodevelopment in zebrafish. In summary, we speculate that BPA affects the neural development of zebrafish by interfering with the expression of cypin during the 1–24 hpf period. To confirm this hypothesis, we used a microinjection experiment of cypin mRNA. Then, microinjected embryos were exposed to BPA up to 24 hpf. The results of PCR showed that the level of cypin mRNA returned to normal, and the spontaneous locomotor behavior of zebrafish returned to the normal level. Therefore, we speculate that that cypin plays an important role in the neural development process from the cleavage period to the segmentation period (1–24 hpf) of zebrafish. Notably, based on the critical period identified in this study (1–24 hpf), there was a motor measurement endpoint directly related to the synapse, spontaneous caudal coiling, only at 24 hpf [46]. This would be a BPA neurodevelopmental endpoint that requires further attention in this study early in life.

The limitations and prospects of this study also need to be mentioned. It has been found that PSD-95 is involved in learning and memory impairment induced by BPA in rats [47], and the binding of cypin to PSD-95 correlates with the formation of stable dendrite branches [48]. Therefore, cypin may play a role in BPA-induced neurotoxicity by binding PSD-95 to affect the neural network. In addition, the study also found that RhoA, a member of the Rho family, has been shown to regulate dendritic crystal formation, global dendritic structure and dynamic dendritic behavior [49], and activated RhoA acts as a negative regulator of dendritic branching by reducing cypin expression in a translocation-dependent manner [50]. Does BPA affect the expression of RhoA, thereby regulating the expression of cypin and thus affecting the locomotor behavior of zebrafish? Further discussion and confirmation of the mechanism are still needed in the future.

5. Conclusions

In this study, we concluded that the sensitive period of BPA to neurotoxicity in zebrafish embryos is from the cleavage period to the segmentation period (1–24 hpf), which is manifested as the inhibition of locomotor behavior in zebrafish. Moreover, BPA can mediate neurotoxicity by downregulating the expression of cypin mRNA from the cleavage period to the segmentation period (1–24 hpf) and influence the locomotor behavior of zebrafish. Therefore, we speculate that cypin gene may be a potential biomarker of neural development.

Supplementary Materials: The following supporting information can be downloaded at: https://www.mdpi.com/article/10.3390/toxics11020177/s1, Table S1: Primer sequences for target genes.

Author Contributions: Conceptualization, J.Z. and X.S.; methodology, J.L., W.K. and Y.L.; investigation, J.L.; resources, Q.M., Q.S., L.Z. and Y.C.; data curation, J.L.; writing—original draft preparation, J.L.; writing—review and editing, J.L., W.K. and Y.L.; supervision, J.Z. and X.S.; funding acquisition, J.Z. All authors have read and agreed to the published version of the manuscript.

Funding: This work was supported by the National Nature Sciences Foundation of China (Grant number: 81673203).

Institutional Review Board Statement: Soochow University Animal Welfare Committee.

Informed Consent Statement: Not applicable.

Data Availability Statement: All data generated or analyzed during this study are included in this published article (and its Supplementary Information Files).

Conflicts of Interest: The authors declare no conflict of interest.

References

1. Vandenberg, L.N.; Hauser, R.; Marcus, M.; Olea, N.; Welshons, W.V. Human exposure to bisphenol A (BPA). *Reprod. Toxicol.* **2007**, *24*, 139–177. [CrossRef]
2. Rubin, B.S. Bisphenol A: An endocrine disruptor with widespread exposure and multiple effects. *J. Steroid Biochem. Mol. Biol.* **2011**, *127*, 27–34. [CrossRef]
3. Corrales, J.; Kristofco, L.A.; Steele, W.B.; Yates, B.S.; Breed, C.S.; Williams, E.S.; Brooks, B.W. Global Assessment of Bisphenol A in the Environment: Review and Analysis of Its Occurrence and Bioaccumulation. *Dose Response* **2015**, *13*, 1559325815598308. [CrossRef]
4. Michalowicz, J. Bisphenol A—Sources, toxicity and biotransformation. *Environ. Toxicol. Pharmacol.* **2014**, *37*, 738–758. [CrossRef]
5. Burgos-Aceves, M.A.; Abo-Al-Ela, H.G.; Faggio, C. Impact of phthalates and bisphenols plasticizers on haemocyte immune function of aquatic invertebrates: A review on physiological, biochemical, and genomic aspects. *J. Hazard. Mater.* **2021**, *419*, 126426. [CrossRef]
6. Takeuchi, T.; Tsutsumi, O. Serum bisphenol a concentrations showed gender differences, possibly linked to androgen levels. *Biochem. Biophys. Res. Commun.* **2002**, *291*, 76–78. [CrossRef]
7. Zhang, T.; Sun, H.; Kannan, K. Blood and urinary bisphenol A concentrations in children, adults, and pregnant women from china: Partitioning between blood and urine and maternal and fetal cord blood. *Environ. Sci. Technol.* **2013**, *47*, 4686–4694. [CrossRef]
8. Vandenberg, L.N.; Chahoud, I.; Heindel, J.J.; Padmanabhan, V.; Paumgartten, F.J.; Schoenfelder, G. Urinary, circulating, and tissue biomonitoring studies indicate widespread exposure to bisphenol A. *Ciência Saúde Coletiva* **2012**, *17*, 407–434. [CrossRef]
9. Gounden, V.; Warasally, M.Z.; Magwai, T.; Naidoo, R.; Chuturgoon, A. A pilot study: Bisphenol-A and Bisphenol-A glucuronide levels in mother and child pairs in a South African population. *Reprod. Toxicol.* **2019**, *89*, 93–99. [CrossRef]
10. Lee, J.; Choi, K.; Park, J.; Moon, H.B.; Choi, G.; Lee, J.J.; Suh, E.; Kim, H.J.; Eun, S.H.; Kim, G.H.; et al. Bisphenol A distribution in serum, urine, placenta, breast milk, and umbilical cord serum in a birth panel of mother-neonate pairs. *Sci. Total Environ.* **2018**, *626*, 1494–1501. [CrossRef]
11. Xu, X.; Hong, X.; Xie, L.; Li, T.; Yang, Y.; Zhang, Q.; Zhang, G.; Liu, X. Gestational and lactational exposure to bisphenol-A affects anxiety- and depression-like behaviors in mice. *Horm. Behav.* **2012**, *62*, 480–490. [CrossRef]
12. Jasarevic, E.; Williams, S.A.; Vandas, G.M.; Ellersieck, M.R.; Liao, C.; Kannan, K.; Roberts, R.M.; Geary, D.C.; Rosenfeld, C.S. Sex and dose-dependent effects of developmental exposure to bisphenol A on anxiety and spatial learning in deer mice (*Peromyscus maniculatus* bairdii) offspring. *Horm. Behav.* **2013**, *63*, 180–189. [CrossRef]
13. Lee, B.E.; Park, H.; Hong, Y.C.; Ha, M.; Kim, Y.; Chang, N.; Kim, B.N.; Kim, Y.J.; Yu, S.D.; Ha, E.H. Prenatal bisphenol A and birth outcomes: MOCEH (Mothers and Children's Environmental Health) study. *Int. J. Hyg. Environ. Health* **2014**, *217*, 328–334. [CrossRef]
14. Panzica-Kelly, J.M.; Zhang, C.X.; Augustine-Rauch, K.A. Optimization and Performance Assessment of the Chorion-Off [Dechorinated] Zebrafish Developmental Toxicity Assay. *Toxicol. Sci.* **2015**, *146*, 127–134. [CrossRef]
15. To, K.T.; St Mary, L.; Wooley, A.H.; Wilbanks, M.S.; Bednar, A.J.; Perkins, E.J.; Truong, L.; Tanguay, R.L.; Garcia-Reyero, N. Morphological and Behavioral Effects in Zebrafish Embryos after Exposure to Smoke Dyes. *Toxics* **2021**, *9*, 9. [CrossRef]
16. Tran, C.M.; Do, T.N.; Kim, K.T. Comparative Analysis of Neurotoxicity of Six Phthalates in Zebrafish Embryos. *Toxics* **2021**, *9*, 5. [CrossRef]
17. Parker, M.O.; Brock, A.J.; Walton, R.T.; Brennan, C.H. The role of zebrafish (Danio rerio) in dissecting the genetics and neural circuits of executive function. *Front. Neural Circuits* **2013**, *7*, 63. [CrossRef]
18. Kalueff, A.V.; Stewart, A.M.; Gerlai, R. Zebrafish as an emerging model for studying complex brain disorders. *Trends Pharmacol. Sci.* **2014**, *35*, 63–75. [CrossRef]
19. Itoh, M.; Kim, C.H.; Palardy, G.; Oda, T.; Jiang, Y.J.; Maust, D.; Yeo, S.Y.; Lorick, K.; Wright, G.J.; Ariza-McNaughton, L.; et al. Mind bomb is a ubiquitin ligase that is essential for efficient activation of Notch signaling by Delta. *Dev. Cell* **2003**, *4*, 67–82. [CrossRef]
20. Faustino, A.I.; Tacão-Monteiro, A.; Oliveira, R.F. Mechanisms of social buffering of fear in zebrafish. *Sci. Rep.* **2017**, *7*, 44329. [CrossRef]
21. Golzio, C.; Willer, J.; Talkowski, M.E.; Oh, E.C.; Taniguchi, Y.; Jacquemont, S.; Reymond, A.; Sun, M.; Sawa, A.; Gusella, J.F.; et al. KCTD13 is a major driver of mirrored neuroanatomical phenotypes of the 16p11.2 copy number variant. *Nature* **2012**, *485*, 363–367. [CrossRef]
22. Kimmel, C.B.; Ballard, W.W.; Kimmel, S.R.; Ullmann, B.; Schilling, T.F. Stages of embryonic development of the zebrafish. *Dev. Dyn.* **1995**, *203*, 253–310. [CrossRef]
23. de Esch, C.; Slieker, R.; Wolterbeek, A.; Woutersen, R.; de Groot, D. Zebrafish as potential model for developmental neurotoxicity testing: A mini review. *Neurotoxicol. Teratol.* **2012**, *34*, 545–553. [CrossRef]
24. Buss, R.R.; Drapeau, P. Synaptic drive to motoneurons during fictive swimming in the developing zebrafish. *J. Neurophysiol.* **2001**, *86*, 197–210. [CrossRef]
25. Stehr, C.M.; Linbo, T.L.; Incardona, J.P.; Scholz, N.L. The developmental neurotoxicity of fipronil: Notochord degeneration and locomotor defects in zebrafish embryos and larvae. *Toxicol. Sci.* **2006**, *92*, 270–278. [CrossRef]
26. Costa-Pinto, F.A.; Cohn, D.W.; Sa-Rocha, V.M.; Sa-Rocha, L.C.; Palermo-Neto, J. Behavior: A relevant tool for brain-immune system interaction studies. *Ann. N. Y. Acad. Sci.* **2009**, *1153*, 107–119. [CrossRef]

27. Selderslaghs, I.W.; Hooyberghs, J.; De Coen, W.; Witters, H.E. Locomotor activity in zebrafish embryos: A new method to assess developmental neurotoxicity. *Neurotoxicol. Teratol.* **2010**, *32*, 460–471. [CrossRef]
28. Chen, J.; Liu, N.; Zhang, H.; Zhao, Y.; Cao, X. The effects of Aeromonas hydrophila infection on oxidative stress, nonspecific immunity, autophagy, and apoptosis in the common carp. *Dev. Comp. Immunol.* **2020**, *105*, 103587. [CrossRef]
29. Rotimi, O.A.; Olawole, T.D.; De Campos, O.C.; Adelani, I.B.; Rotimi, S.O. Bisphenol A in Africa: A review of environmental and biological levels. *Sci. Total Environ.* **2021**, *764*, 142854. [CrossRef] [PubMed]
30. Gould, J.C.; Leonard, L.S.; Maness, S.C.; Wagner, B.L.; Conner, K.; Zacharewski, T.; Safe, S.; McDonnell, D.P.; Gaido, K.W. Bisphenol A interacts with the estrogen receptor alpha in a distinct manner from estradiol. *Mol. Cell. Endocrinol.* **1998**, *142*, 203–214. [CrossRef]
31. Burkhardt, F.; Schulz, S.D.; Hellwig, E.; Vach, K.; Tomakidi, P.; Polydorou, O. Low-dose Bisphenol A and its analogues Bisphenol F and S activate estrogen receptor ss and slightly modulate genes in human gingival keratinocytes. *Dent. Mater.* **2021**, *37*, 625–635. [CrossRef]
32. Sang, C.; Song, Y.; Jin, T.W.; Zhang, S.; Fu, L.; Zhao, Y.; Zou, X.; Wang, Z.; Gao, H.; Liu, S. Bisphenol A induces ovarian cancer cell proliferation and metastasis through estrogen receptor-alpha pathways. *Environ. Sci. Pollut. Res. Int.* **2021**, *28*, 36060–36068. [CrossRef]
33. Ejaredar, M.; Lee, Y.; Roberts, D.J.; Sauve, R.; Dewey, D. Bisphenol A exposure and children's behavior: A systematic review. *J. Expo. Sci. Environ. Epidemiol.* **2017**, *27*, 175–183. [CrossRef]
34. Rochester, J.R.; Bolden, A.L.; Kwiatkowski, C.F. Prenatal exposure to bisphenol A and hyperactivity in children: A systematic review and meta-analysis. *Environ. Int.* **2018**, *114*, 343–356. [CrossRef]
35. Kimmel, C.B.; Warga, R.M.; Schilling, T.F. Origin and organization of the zebrafish fate map. *Development* **1990**, *108*, 581–594. [CrossRef] [PubMed]
36. Hanneman, E.; Westerfield, M. Early expression of acetylcholinesterase activity in functionally distinct neurons of the zebrafish. *J. Comp. Neurol.* **1989**, *284*, 350–361. [CrossRef]
37. Wilson, S.W.; Ross, L.S.; Parrett, T.; Easter, S.S., Jr. The development of a simple scaffold of axon tracts in the brain of the embryonic zebrafish, Brachydanio rerio. *Development* **1990**, *108*, 121–145. [CrossRef] [PubMed]
38. Billat, P.A.; Brochot, C.; Brion, F.; Beaudouin, R. A PBPK model to evaluate zebrafish eleutheroembryos' actual exposure: Bisphenol A and analogs' (AF, F, and S) case studies. *Environ. Sci. Pollut. Res. Int.* **2022**, *30*, 7640–7653. [CrossRef]
39. Firestein, B.L.; Firestein, B.L.; Brenman, J.E.; Aoki, C.; Sanchez-Perez, A.M.; El-Husseini, A.E.; Bredt, D.S. Cypin: A cytosolic regulator of PSD-95 postsynaptic targeting. *Neuron* **1999**, *24*, 659–672. [CrossRef]
40. Paletzki, R.F. Cloning and characterization of guanine deaminase from mouse and rat brain. *Neuroscience* **2002**, *109*, 15–26. [CrossRef]
41. Akum, B.F.; Chen, M.; Gunderson, S.I.; Riefler, G.M.; Scerri-Hansen, M.M.; Firestein, B.L. Cypin regulates dendrite patterning in hippocampal neurons by promoting microtubule assembly. *Nat. Neurosci.* **2004**, *7*, 145–152. [CrossRef]
42. Fernandez, J.R.; Welsh, W.J.; Firestein, B.L. Structural characterization of the zinc binding domain in cytosolic PSD-95 interactor (cypin): Role of zinc binding in guanine deamination and dendrite branching. *Proteins* **2008**, *70*, 873–881. [CrossRef]
43. Patel, M.V.; Swiatkowski, P.; Kwon, M.; Rodriguez, A.R.; Campagno, K.; Firestein, B.L. A Novel Short Isoform of Cytosolic PSD-95 Interactor (Cypin) Regulates Neuronal Development. *Mol. Neurobiol.* **2018**, *55*, 6269–6281. [CrossRef]
44. Braunschweig, D.; Krakowiak, P.; Duncanson, P.; Boyce, R.; Hansen, R.L.; Ashwood, P.; Hertz-Picciotto, I.; Pessah, I.N.; Van de Water, J. Autism-specific maternal autoantibodies recognize critical proteins in developing brain. *Transl. Psychiatry* **2013**, *3*, e277. [CrossRef] [PubMed]
45. Schretlen, D.J.; Harris, J.C.; Park, K.S.; Jinnah, H.A.; del Pozo, N.O. Neurocognitive functioning in Lesch-Nyhan disease and partial hypoxanthine-guanine phosphoribosyltransferase deficiency. *J. Int. Neuropsychol. Soc.* **2001**, *7*, 805–812. [CrossRef] [PubMed]
46. Ogungbemi, A.O.; Teixido, E.; Massei, R.; Scholz, S.; Kuster, E. Automated measurement of the spontaneous tail coiling of zebrafish embryos as a sensitive behavior endpoint using a workflow in KNIME. *MethodsX* **2021**, *8*, 101330. [CrossRef]
47. Yu, H.; Ma, L.; Liu, D.; Wang, Y.; Pei, X.; Duan, Z.; Ma, M.; Zhang, Y. Involvement of NMDAR/PSD-95/nNOS-NO-cGMP pathway in embryonic exposure to BPA induced learning and memory dysfunction of rats. *Environ. Pollut.* **2020**, *266*, 115055. [CrossRef]
48. Charych, E.I.; Akum, B.F.; Goldberg, J.S.; Jornsten, R.J.; Rongo, C.; Zheng, J.Q.; Firestein, B.L. Activity-independent regulation of dendrite patterning by postsynaptic density protein PSD-95. *J. Neurosci.* **2006**, *26*, 10164–10176. [CrossRef]
49. Wong, W.T.; Wong, R.O. Rapid dendritic movements during synapse formation and rearrangement. *Curr. Opin. Neurobiol.* **2000**, *10*, 118–124. [CrossRef]
50. Chen, H.; Firestein, B.L. RhoA regulates dendrite branching in hippocampal neurons by decreasing cypin protein levels. *J. Neurosci.* **2007**, *27*, 8378–8386. [CrossRef] [PubMed]

Disclaimer/Publisher's Note: The statements, opinions and data contained in all publications are solely those of the individual author(s) and contributor(s) and not of MDPI and/or the editor(s). MDPI and/or the editor(s) disclaim responsibility for any injury to people or property resulting from any ideas, methods, instructions or products referred to in the content.

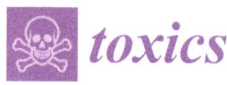

Article

A Metabolome and Microbiome Analysis of Acute Myeloid Leukemia: Insights into the Carnosine–Histidine Metabolic Pathway

Binxiong Wu [1,†], Yuntian Xu [2,3,†], Miaomiao Tang [2,3,†], Yingtong Jiang [2,3,†], Ting Zhang [4], Lei Huang [2,3], Shuyang Wang [2,3], Yanhui Hu [5], Kun Zhou [2,6], Xiaoling Zhang [1,*] and Minjian Chen [2,3,*]

1. Department of Hygienic Analysis and Detection, School of Public Health, Nanjing Medical University, Nanjing 211166, China; wubinxiong@stu.njmu.edu.cn
2. State Key Laboratory of Reproductive Medicine and Offspring Health, Center for Global Health, School of Public Health, Nanjing Medical University, Nanjing 211166, China; uu11ut@163.com (Y.X.); tmm_2023@163.com (M.T.); ytjiang61@163.com (Y.J.); 18756555623@163.com (L.H.); wsy8032@163.com (S.W.); zk@njmu.edu.cn (K.Z.)
3. Key Laboratory of Modern Toxicology of Ministry of Education, School of Public Health, Nanjing Medical University, Nanjing 211166, China
4. Women's Hospital of Jiangnan University, Wuxi 214002, China; zhangting@njmu.edu.cn
5. Sir Run Run Hospital of Nanjing Medical University, Nanjing 211166, China; njjshyh@126.com
6. Department of Epidemiology, Center for Global Health, School of Public Health, Nanjing Medical University, Nanjing 211166, China
* Correspondence: zhangxl3@njmu.edu.cn (X.Z.); minjianchen@njmu.edu.cn (M.C.)
† These authors contributed equally to this work.

Abstract: Metabolism underlies the pathogenesis of acute myeloid leukemia (AML) and can be influenced by gut microbiota. However, the specific metabolic changes in different tissues and the role of gut microbiota in AML remain unclear. In this study, we analyzed the metabolome differences in blood samples from patients with AML and healthy controls using UPLC-Q-Exactive. Additionally, we examined the serum, liver, and fecal metabolome of AML model mice and control mice using UPLC-Q-Exactive. The gut microbiota of the mice were analyzed using 16S rRNA sequencing. Our UPLC-MS analysis revealed significant differences in metabolites between the AML and control groups in multiple tissue samples. Through cross-species validation in humans and animals, as well as reverse validation of Celastrol, we discovered that the Carnosine–Histidine metabolic pathway may play a potential role in the occurrence and progression of AML. Furthermore, our analysis of gut microbiota showed no significant diversity changes, but we observed a significant negative correlation between the key metabolite Carnosine and *Peptococcaceae* and *Campylobacteraceae*. In conclusion, the Carnosine–Histidine metabolic pathway influences the occurrence and progression of AML, while the gut microbiota might play a role in this process.

Keywords: acute myeloid leukemia; gut microbiota; metabolomics; metabolic pathway

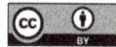

1. Introduction

Acute myeloid leukemia (AML) is a malignant tumor characterized by abnormal proliferation, differentiation disorders, and blocked apoptosis of myeloid stem cells. The accumulation of leukemia cells causes damage by inhibiting normal hematopoiesis and infiltrating other tissues and organs. The prognosis of the disease is poor, with an average survival period of only about 3 months without specific treatment, and the 5-year survival rate after treatment is only about 10–35% [1]. For decades, chemotherapy has remained the main treatment for AML [2], with the goal of inducing remission. However, elderly patients, who are the main population affected by the disease, often have difficulty tolerating chemotherapy [3]. In addition, relapse is difficult to avoid, and the survival rate drops sharply after relapse. AML is highly heterogeneous, and there has been little progress in treatment methods for a long time. Therefore, a better understanding of the development and progression mechanisms of AML is required in order to effectively prevent the disease and mitigate its incidence.

Metabolomics is the scientific study of the metabolite profile of an organism under specific physiological or pathological conditions. By analyzing the types and quantities of metabolites in an organism, it can reveal the metabolic pathways, regulatory mechanisms, and associations with disease development. Metabolic changes may play an important role in the occurrence and development of AML. In AML research, metabolomics techniques have been widely used to analyze the blood metabolism of groups of patients with AML and controls, in order to discover metabolic pathways and molecular biomarkers associated with AML [4], and to aid in disease diagnoses and outcome prediction [5,6]. However, organismal metabolism is a complex system involving multiple metabolic pathways and molecular interactions. Single-type samples may not fully reflect the overall changes in organismal metabolism. Studies have found that plasma has better reproducibility, while serum has higher sensitivity [7,8]. Using different sample types can lead to more comprehensive results. Therefore, in this study, we analyzed the metabolic changes in serum, liver, and fecal samples of mice, as well as serum and plasma samples from human subjects to complement each other and to enhance population metabolic information, for validation and replication. Additionally, in the mouse experiments, we used a natural compound, Celastrol, which has been shown to possess anti-leukemia activity, as a reversing agent [9], to further validate key metabolites.

The gut microbiota, a crucial microbial component residing in the gastrointestinal tract, have been found to play a significant role in metabolism and immunity due to their large numbers and diverse genomes. *Helicobacter pylori*, through chronic inflammation and specific virulence factors, has emerged as a major risk factor for gastric cancer [10]. Similarly, *Fusobacterium nucleatum* has been implicated in inducing colorectal cancer metastasis by downregulating m6A gene modification [11]. It has been reported that the gut microbiota can regulate and maintain normal hematopoiesis [12]. In the research of AML, researchers have discovered that the composition of the gut microbiota is related to the treatment [13]. Currently, fecal microbiota transplantation (FMT) is being used in clinical practice to correct gut dysbiosis and eradicate multidrug-resistant bacteria, thereby treating diseases. These findings suggest that the gut microbiota may also play a role in the occurrence and development of AML. Therefore, it is necessary to explore the complex relationship between the gut microbiota and the development of AML.

The gut microbiota can influence the human body by producing metabolites, with short-chain fatty acids (SCFAs) [14] and tryptophan [15] being among the most extensively studied. These metabolites help maintain gut barrier integrity and reduce disease-related effects. Feces consist of undigested food residues, bacterial metabolites, and other waste materials from the intestines, making changes in fecal metabolites reflective of the metabolic activities of the gut microbiota. By analyzing 16S rRNA in feces, we can gain insights into the composition and function of the gut microbiota, and further investigate the relationship between the gut microbiota and human health. The regulation of organismal metabolism by the gut microbiota genome plays a crucial role in normal physiological functions and disease responses. However, there is still a lack of research on microbiota-dependent metabolites in AML. Additionally, the gut microbiota are susceptible to influences from the diet [16], medications [17], and the environment, making it challenging to conduct population studies with limited confounding variables. Therefore, we aimed to elucidate the alterations in the gut microbiota in the context of AML using a mouse model, which provides a relatively stable and controlled environment. Additionally, we sought to investigate the relationship between changes in the gut microbiota and metabolic alterations.

This study aimed to investigate the non-targeted metabolic changes in multiple samples of AML using a mouse model and blood samples from patients with AML, employing UPLC-MS technology. Additionally, a reversal experiment was conducted using an AML inhibitor, Celastrol, to elucidate key metabolic processes. Furthermore, changes in the gut microbiota were revealed through 16S rRNA amplicon sequencing, and the potential mechanisms of gut microbiota in AML metabolic changes were inferred through statistical and biological correlations. The significance of this study lies in the establishment of a mouse model and the utilization of various techniques to uncover the overall metabolic changes in multiple samples and across species in AML, as well as exploring the potential connections between these changes and the gut microbiota. This research is important for a deeper understanding of the pathogenesis of AML, and identification of new prevention and treatment targets.

2. Materials and Methods

2.1. AML Mouse Model

SPF-grade BALB/c nude mice (male, 5 weeks old, weighing 18–20 g) were purchased from Shanghai Lingchang Biotechnology Co., Ltd. (Shanghai, China). and housed at the Animal Experimental Center of Nanjing Medical University. The mice were kept under constant environmental conditions with a humidity of $55 \pm 10\%$ and a temperature of $22 \pm 2\,°C$, with a 12 h light/dark cycle. They had unrestricted access to water and food. The principles of the 3Rs were followed to ensure the welfare of the experimental animals. After one week of adaptation, the mice were randomly divided into a control group ($n = 8$) and a treatment group ($n = 25$). There was no statistically significant difference of weight between groups (Figure S1). HL-60 cells in the logarithmic growth phase were resuspended in PBS at a density of 5×10^7 cells/mL and subcutaneously injected into the right dorsal axillary region of the treatment group mice, with an injection volume of 100 µL. The control group mice were injected with an equal volume of physiological saline. When the tumor volume reached 200–250 mm^3, the mice were randomly divided into the AML group ($n = 8$), low-dose Celastrol treatment group ($n = 8$), and high-dose Celastrol treatment group ($n = 9$). The Celastrol treatment groups were intraperitoneally injected with 200 µL of a solution containing Celastrol at concentrations of 0.1 mg/mL and 0.2 mg/mL, respectively, once daily. Previous research has demonstrated the inhibitory efficacy of Celastrol against AML at these specific concentrations [18,19]. The control group and AML group were given an equal volume of physiological saline daily. When the tumor volume of the AML group mice reached 2500–3000 mm^3, samples were collected. Adequate fecal samples were collected from the intestines of the dissected mice and stored in clean containers for 16S rRNA gene sequencing. Various organs were also collected and stored in liquid nitrogen for the subsequent analysis.

2.2. Study Population

This section describes a cross-sectional study that included two groups: an AML group ($n = 19$) diagnosed between October 2020 and December 2020 and a recruited healthy control group ($n = 35$) at Jiangsu Provincial Hospital and Nanyang First People's Hospital. The inclusion criteria for the AML group were as follows: diagnosed with AML based on blood cell examination with no liver or kidney diseases, and no recent use of medications that could affect metabolism. The inclusion criteria for the healthy control group were the exclusion of individuals with common endocrine disorders, acute or chronic gastroenteritis, severe impairment of cardiac, hepatic, pulmonary, or renal structure and function, and individuals with tumors. Basic information, including age, gender, and medical history, was recorded for all participants for the subsequent analysis. Fasting blood samples were collected in the morning after an 8–12 h fast (plasma group: $n = 30$, serum group: $n = 24$) and stored at $-80\,°C$ for the subsequent UPLC-MS analysis. This study was conducted in accordance with the ethical standards of Jiangsu Provincial Hospital and Nanyang First People's Hospital. All participants involved in this study provided informed consent.

2.3. Metabolomic Analysis

The metabolomic analysis of plasma, serum, liver, and feces was performed using the UPLC-Q-Exactive platform (UPLC Ultimate 3000 system, Dionex, Germering, GER; Q-Exactive Orbitrap, Thermo Fisher Scientific, Bremen, GER) according to our previous report [20]. Briefly, protein precipitation was conducted with a methanol–water mixture containing isotope-labeled internal standards. The fecal samples were homogenized using vortexing and ultrasonic wave treatment as described in our previous study [21]. The supernatant was concentrated to dryness using a centrifugal concentrator (Labconco, Kansas, MO, USA). The dried sample was reconstituted and ready for the analysis. A Hypersil GOLD C18 column (100 mm × 2.1 mm, 1.9 µm, Thermo Fisher Scientific, Vilnius, Lithuania) was used for a chromatography system. Acetonitrile containing 0.1% formic acid was used as mobile phase A and ultrapure water containing 0.1% formic acid was used as mobile phase B. The flow rate was set at 0.40 mL/min (column temperature at 40 °C). The ionization mode for mass spectrometry was heated electrospray ionization (HESI). The spray voltage was set at 3.5 kV for positive ion mode and 2.5 kV for negative ion mode. Full scan mode was used with a scan range of 70 to 1050 m/z and a resolution of 70,000. The accurate mass and retention time of metabolites were compared with those of metabolite standards using a self-built standard library using TraceFinder 3.1 software for metabolite identification. All samples were analyzed in a randomized fashion to avoid bias of the injection order. The data were further analyzed after integral normalization [22]. An equivalent volume from each sample under investigation was combined to create quality control (QC) samples, and a blank solvent was utilized as the reference blank. The same procedural steps applied to the test samples were followed for the QC and blank samples. The QC samples were injected after every fifth sample injection during the analysis of the test samples. The ropls package (v1.30.0) was used to perform a partial least squares discriminant analysis (PLS-DA) and extract important features based on variable importance in projection (VIP).

2.4. The 16S rRNA Gene Sequencing and Amplicon Analysis

The 16S rRNA gene sequencing was performed by Shanghai Meiji Biomedical Technology Co., Ltd. (Shanghai, China). The specific steps are as follows: After extracting the microbial community genomic DNA from the samples using the E.Z.N.A.® soil DNA kit (Omega Bio-tek, Atlanta, GA, USA) according to the manufacturer's instructions, the quality of the DNA was checked using 1% agarose gel electrophoresis, and the DNA concentration and purity were measured using NanoDrop2000 (Thermo Fisher Scientific, Waltham, MA, USA). Specific primers with barcodes were synthesized for the conserved sequences of the V3-V4 region of the 16S rRNA gene (338F: 5′-ACTCCTACGGGAGGCAGCAG-3′ and 806R: 5′-GGACTACHVGGGTWTCTAAT-3′), and PCR amplification was performed using TransStart Fastpfu DNA Polymerase (TransGen Biotech, Beijing, China). This step was carried out on an ABI GeneAmp® 9700 (ABI, Foster City, CA, USA) thermal cycler. Each sample was amplified in triplicate, and the mixed products were checked using 2% agarose gel electrophoresis. The PCR products were then gel-extracted using the AxyPrep DNA Gel Extraction Kit (Axygen Biosciences, Union City, CA, USA) and eluted with Tris-HCl. After constructing the Miseq library using the NEXTFLEX Rapid DNA-Seq Kit (Bioo Scientific, Austin, TX, USA), sequencing was performed on the Miseq PE300 platform (Illumina, San Diego, CA, USA). The paired-end (PE) reads from sequencing data, which were split based on barcodes and primers, were merged and quality-controlled using FLASH (v1.2.11), fastp (v0.20.1), and vsearch (v2.15.0). The analysis of amplicons includes the concatenation and quality control of raw data, operational taxonomic unit (OTU) clustering and annotation, a diversity analysis, and functional prediction. The specific steps are as follows:

QIIME1 (v1.9.1) was used for OTU clustering, annotation, and phylogenetic tree construction. (1) The merged and quality-controlled sequences were clustered into OTUs at a 97% similarity threshold using the usearch61 algorithm. Representative sequences were selected for each OTU. (2) The rdp algorithm was then used to annotate the representative sequences at a confidence threshold of 0.7, based on the Silva 16S rRNA database (v132), resulting in a table of annotated OTUs. (3) The PyNAST algorithm was used to align the representative sequences, and gaps were filtered out to construct a phylogenetic tree for a downstream analysis. Rare OTUs (<0.005%) and unnecessary taxonomic groups were filtered out, and the OTU table was rarefied based on the minimum sample abundance for the downstream analysis.

A species diversity analysis included an analysis of species abundance and composition. An α-diversity analysis focused on the diversity within individual samples and reflected the richness and evenness of microbial communities. Metrics such as Sobs, Chao, Shannon, Simpson, and PD indices were used to characterize sample diversity. A β-diversity analysis is used to compare the differences in microbial composition between groups and to analyze the similarity between samples. The Weighted UniFrac distance algorithm is used to construct a hierarchical clustering tree based on the similarity of samples between groups. A DESeq2 analysis was used to identify significantly different taxonomic groups. Taxa with $p < 0.05$ and fold change > 2 were considered as significantly altered taxa.

PICRUSt2 software v2.3.0b0 was used to predict the metabolic functional profiles of bacteria corresponding to the 16S rRNA gene sequences. First, an evolutionary tree with gene information (species and quantity) was constructed based on known gene sequences and gene abundances. Then, the 16S rRNA gene sequences obtained from sequencing were matched to their phylogenetic relatives in the tree to predict their gene information. The predicted gene information was then assigned biological significance by identifying the corresponding metabolic pathways using the MetaCyc database. To examine the differences in metabolic pathways between different groups, we employed Welch's t-tests and fold change to compare the abundance of pathways in each group. Pathways with a p-value less than 0.05 and a fold change greater than 2 were considered significantly different between the groups.

2.5. Statistical Analysis

Quantitative data were presented as the mean $\pm$ standard deviation (M $\pm$ SD). Two group comparisons were performed using t-tests or Wilcoxon rank-sum tests. A one-way analysis of variance (ANOVA) was used when the comparison was conducted in three groups followed by Dunnett's test. Rate comparisons were conducted using chi-square tests or Fisher's exact tests. Spearman rank correlation coefficients were used to assess correlation. R software (v4.2.1) was used for all analyses and preparation of figures. To improve the statistical robustness, we used VIP > 1 in combination with the p-value < 0.05 to find significant metabolomic changes [23,24]. Unless otherwise specified, $p < 0.05$ was considered statistically significant.

3. Results

3.1. Multi-Sample Metabolomic Analysis of AML Mice and Human Population

3.1.1. Carnosine and L-Histidine: Key Players in AML Revealed in Mouse Model

In order to investigate the overall metabolic changes in AML, we constructed an AML mouse model and selected mouse serum, liver, and feces as the study objects. These sample sources represent different levels of metabolic reactions, with mouse serum and liver metabolism reflecting the host's metabolic status, and fecal metabolism reflecting the metabolic activity of the gut microbiota. Through the metabolic analysis of these samples, we hope to uncover the changes and correlations between host metabolism and gut microbiota metabolism, and provide new clues for further research.

In the AML group, nude mice developed rice-sized white tumors subcutaneously around 10 days after HL-60 cell inoculation, indicating successful modeling of tumor-bearing nude mice. A total of 160 endogenous metabolites were detected in all mouse samples. PLS-DA models were established for the metabolomic data of serum, liver, and feces. However, the liver sample data failed to establish a successful model, indicating that the metabolic changes were mild between different groups. On the other hand, successful models were established for the feces and serum groups. As shown in Figure 1A,B, the AML group and the control group were clearly separated in the 3D plots, with Q2(cum) values of 0.694 and 0.815, respectively. Permutation tests also indicated the stability of the predictive results.

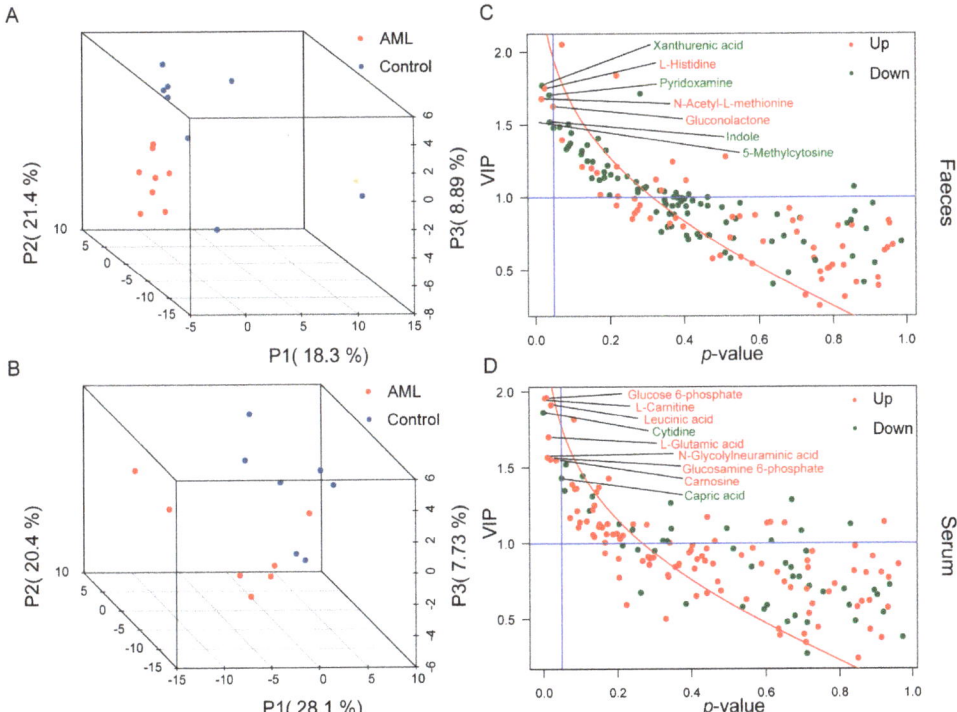

Figure 1. Metabolomic analysis of mouse feces and serum. (**A,B**) PLS-DA score plots of mouse feces and serum, with each point representing a sample and colored by group. Red represents the AML group, while blue represents the control group. (**C,D**) VIP-p plots of mouse feces and serum metabolites, with each point representing a metabolite. The x-axis represents the p-value from the t-test between metabolite groups, while the y-axis represents the VIP value of metabolites after PLS-DA analysis. The blue lines represent the screening thresholds, where VIP > 1 and p-value < 0.05. Red indicates upregulation in the AML group, while green indicates downregulation in the AML group.

After the multivariate statistical analysis, t-tests, the differences and importance distributions of the two groups of metabolites were displayed using VIP-p plots (Figure 1C,D). Using a criterion of VIP > 1 and $p < 0.05$, a total of seven different metabolites were screened in the feces, including Xanthurenic acid, Pyridoxamine, Indole, and 5-Methylcytosine, which decreased in the AML group, and L-Histidine, N-Acetyl-L-methionine, and Gluconolactone, which increased in the AML group (Figure S2A). In the serum, a total of nine different metabolites were screened, including Cytidine and Capric acid, which decreased in the AML group, and Glucosamine 6-phosphate, L-Carnitine, Leucinic acid, L-Glutamic acid, N-Glycolylneuraminic acid, Glucose 6-phosphate, and Carnosine, which increased in the AML group (Figure S2B).

These results indicated that serum and fecal metabolites, as representatives of host and microbial metabolism, represented more sensitive changes in AML compared to liver metabolism.

In order to further understand the role of these metabolites in AML, we conducted administration experiments of Celastrol, which is an agent that can inhibit the proliferation of HL-60 cells. As shown in Figure 2, Celastrol exhibited inhibitory effects on tumor growth. There was a statistically significant difference in tumor volume and weight between the AML group and the treatment group (Figure 2A,B). After analyzing the metabolic changes in feces, we found that the level of 5-Methylcytosine decreased in the feces of the AML group, but it returned to normal after high-dose Celastrol treatment (Figure 2C). On the other hand, the level of L-Histidine in the feces of the AML group increased significantly, but it returned to normal after Celastrol treatment (Figure 2D). Interestingly, L-Histidine serves as a downstream metabolite in the aforementioned Carnosine metabolic pathway, suggesting that the Carnosine–Histidine pathway could potentially play a role in the initiation and advancement of AML.

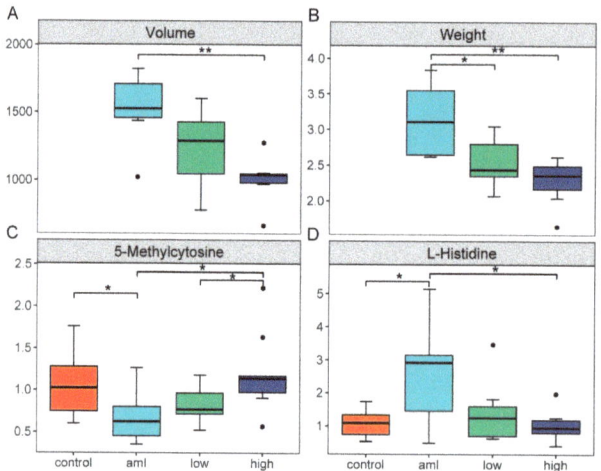

Figure 2. Reversal effect of Celastrol on metabolism in AML mouse model. (**A**,**B**) Box plots showing tumor volume (mm^3) and weight (g) in mice after Celastrol treatment, color-coded by group; The black dots represent outliers; * indicates $p < 0.05$, and ** indicates $p < 0.01$. (**C**,**D**) Box plots showing levels of 5-Methylcytosine and L-Histidine in mice after Celastrol treatment, with the mean of the control group as the reference, color-coded by group; The black dots represent outliers; * indicates $p < 0.05$.

3.1.2. Consistent Metabolic Changes in AML in Humans and Mice: Validation of Carnosine as a Key Metabolite

To further investigate AML-related metabolic changes, we conducted a study on blood metabolism in human populations to compare and validate the findings from the mouse model. We collected both serum and plasma samples to obtain comprehensive metabolic information. The study on human blood metabolism included 35 patients with AML and 19 healthy participants. Table 1 presents the demographic characteristics of the two groups, including gender, age, and blood type. After propensity score matching (PSM), the variables between the case and control groups in serum and plasma were balanced ($p > 0.05$).

Table 1. Study population features.

	AML (N = 19)	HC (N = 35)	Overall (N = 54)	p-Value
Sex				
Female	11 (57.9%)	19 (54.3%)	30 (55.6%)	1
Male	8 (42.1%)	16 (45.7%)	24 (44.4%)	
Age (year)				
Mean (SD)	56.3 (16.9)	52.8 (17.8)	54.0 (17.4)	0.474
Median [Min, Max]	58.0 [14.0, 80.0]	62.0 [22.0, 75.0]	58.5 [14.0, 80.0]	
Type				
Plasma	14 (73.7%)	10 (28.6%)	24 (44.4%)	
Serum	5 (26.3%)	25 (71.4%)	30 (55.6%)	

Using the described metabolomics approach, a total of 186 endogenous metabolites were detected in the human blood samples. The PLS-DA models (Figure 3A,B) showed clear separation between the AML and control groups in both serum and plasma samples, with estimated predictive abilities (Q2(cum)) of 0.867 and 0.687, respectively, and statistically significant permutation test p-values. This indicated that AML could also affect blood metabolism in human populations. These data could be utilized for a subsequent further analysis to investigate in depth the relationship between metabolism and AML.

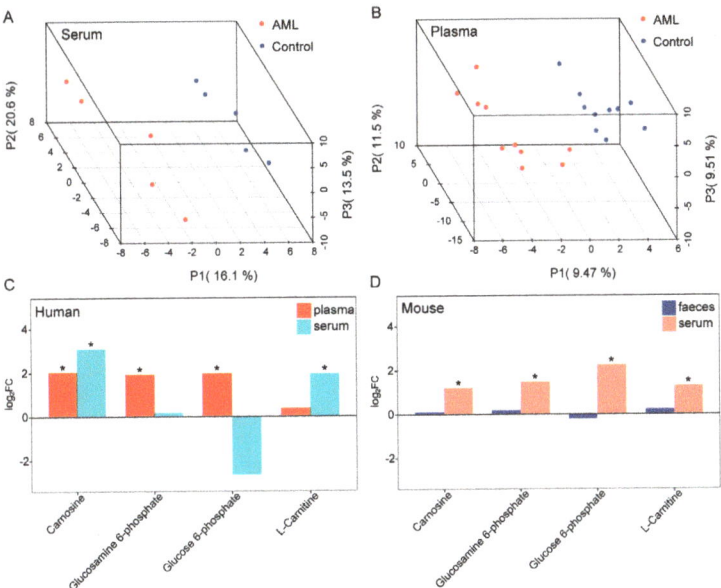

Figure 3. Shared differential metabolites between AML groups and control groups in mice and humans. (A,B) PLS-DA score plots of human population serum and plasma, with each point representing a sample and colored by group. Red represents the AML group, while blue represents the control group. (C,D) Histograms showing the shared differential metabolites in each tissue between groups in humans and mice. Considering the differences in metabolism between species and complexity in human population study, we used a threshold of $p < 0.1$ for human population and a criterion of VIP > 1 and $p < 0.05$ for mice. The x-axis represents the shared differential metabolites, and the y-axis represents the $\log_2$FC values of metabolite levels. * indicates significance, color-coded by group.

Next, we compared the metabolites in the samples of both groups to identify commonalities in AML metabolic changes in humans and mice. As shown in Figure 3C,D, significantly increased levels of Carnosine, Glucosamine 6-phosphate, Glucose 6-phosphate, and L-Carnitine were observed in the differential metabolites of both mice and human populations in the AML group (Figure S3). This suggests that AML has a certain degree of consistency about metabolism in humans and mice. Notably, Carnosine increased in both human serum and plasma, and mice serum. Through validation in humans and animals, we successfully identified Carnosine as the key metabolite.

3.2. Alterations in Diversity, Composition, and Functionality of Gut Microbiota in AML Mice

3.2.1. Satisfactory Sequencing Depth and Coverage in Amplicon Sequencing

After amplicon sequencing of mouse fecal samples, a total of 297,507 and 310,818 raw sequences were obtained for the control and AML groups, respectively, with an average sequence length of 464 bp, which is close to the length of V3–V4 region sequences. After data optimization and removal of noise, a total of 297,465 and 310,773 clean sequences were obtained. The number of sequences, base pairs, and average sequence length before and after optimization for each sample are shown in Table S1. There was no statistically significant difference in the number of sequences between the two groups ($p > 0.05$) (Figure 4A,B). Based on 97% nucleotide sequence similarity, a total of 742 high-abundance operational taxonomic units (OTUs) were identified (control = 711, AML = 738), with 707 shared OTUs between the control and AML groups (Figure 4C).

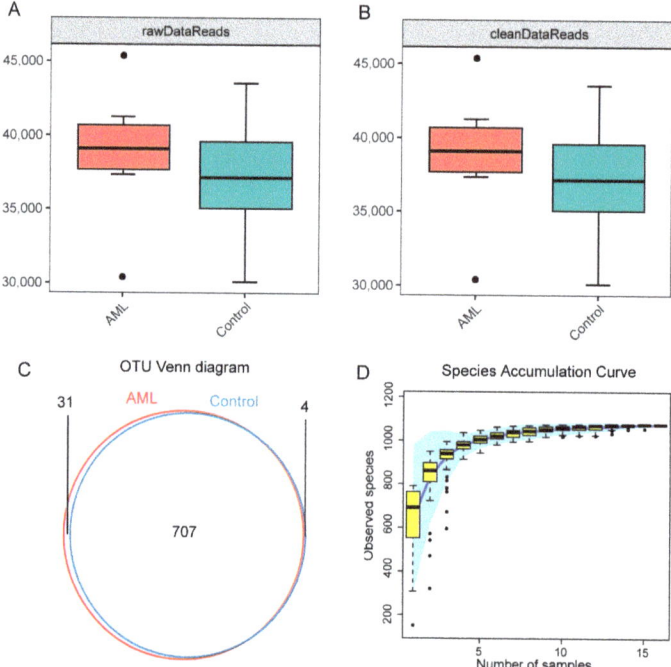

Figure 4. Sequencing depth and coverage of gut microbiota amplicon sequencing. (**A,B**) Box plots of raw and clean sequence reads in AML and control groups. The black dots represent outliers. (**C**) Venn diagram showing the number of OTUs after clustering the sequencing data in AML and control groups. (**D**) Accumulated species abundance curve, with the x-axis representing the number of randomly sampled samples and the y-axis representing the Sobs index at the OTU level after clustering. The black dots represent outliers.

To demonstrate that the sequencing depth and richness of all samples reached a satisfactory level, species accumulation curves were generated by resampling and counting the clustered OTUs. The species accumulation curves showed that the number of discovered species gradually approached a plateau as the number of sampled sequences increased (Figure 4D), indicating that the sequencing sample size was reasonable and that a larger sample size would only yield a small number of new species. Therefore, the sequencing sample size was sufficiently large to reflect the majority of microbial species composition in the gut.

3.2.2. Stable Gut Microbiota Diversity but Decreased Firmicutes Abundance in AML

To further assess the richness and evenness of the gut microbiota community, we calculated multiple indices. The results showed no significant differences in the five diversity indices between the two groups ($p > 0.05$, Figure 5A), indicating that there was no significant difference in α diversity between the two groups. However, the standard deviation and range of diversity indices in the AML group (Table S2) were larger than those in the control group, suggesting that the diversity indices of samples in the AML group were more dispersed and had greater variation. For β diversity, we used the Weighted UniFrac distance algorithm to construct a hierarchical clustering tree to visually display the distance between sample branches (Figure 5B). The samples from both groups clustered well, indicating high within-group similarity and low between-group similarity.

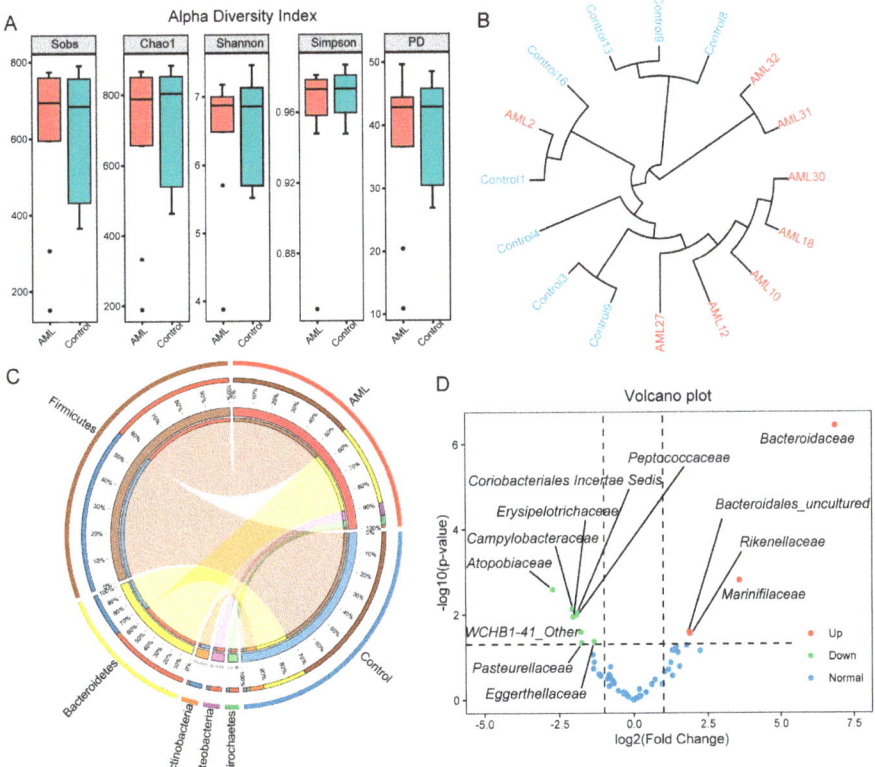

Figure 5. Analysis of gut microbiota diversity, composition, and differences in mice. (**A**) Box plots of α-diversity indices, including Sobs index, Chao1 index, Shannon index, Simpson index, and PD index, comparing AML group and control group. *t*-Test was used to determine the significance of differences between groups, and no significant differences were observed among the indices. The

black dots represent outliers. (**B**) Circular dendrogram of hierarchical clustering of samples, with shorter branches indicating higher similarity in species composition. The red color represents the AML group, while the blue color represents the control group. (**C**) Taxonomic-group-sample circle plot at the phylum level. The left side of the outer circle represents taxonomic groups, while the right side represents sample groups. The length of the arcs represents the relative proportions. The inner circle shows the group proportions of taxonomic groups and the taxonomic group proportions of sample groups, connected by colored ribbons. (**D**) Volcano plot of microbial community at the family level. The y-axis represents the negative logarithm (base 10) of p-values obtained from DESeq2 analysis, while the x-axis represents the logarithm (base 2) of the fold change. Each point represents a specific type of microorganism, with red indicating increased abundance in AML and green indicating decreased abundance in AML.

To investigate the changes in gut microbiota composition under AML conditions, we used a taxon sample circle plot (Figure 5C) and a hierarchical sample circle plot (Figures S4 and S5) to illustrate the gut microbiota composition and its relationship with samples at different taxonomic levels. At the phylum level, the dominant taxa in the AML group were *Firmicutes* (54%) and *Bacteroidetes* (35%), while in the control group, the dominant taxa were *Firmicutes* (71%) and *Bacteroidales* (19%). The proportion of *Firmicutes* and *Bacteroidales* in the AML group decreased compared to the control group. The changes in dominant taxa at different taxonomic levels were mainly characterized by a decrease in the abundance of *Firmicutes* and its corresponding taxonomic levels, as well as an increase in the abundance of *Bacteroidetes* and its corresponding taxonomic levels.

To further analyze the differences in species abundance between the two groups, identify significantly different species, and examine the consistency of these differences, we conducted a DESeq2 analysis on the microbial community at the family level. The analysis revealed significant differences in abundance between the AML group and the control group for certain microbial taxa. Using a significance threshold of $p < 0.05$ and a fold change > 2 or fold change < −2, we identified 12 differentially abundant taxa. Specifically, *Bacteroidaceae*, *Marinifilaceae*, *Bacteroidales_uncultured*, and *Rikenellaceae* showed increased abundance in the AML group, while *Atopobiaceae*, *Campylobacteraceae*, *Coriobacteriales Incertae Sedis*, *Peptococcaceae*, *Erysipelotrichaceae*, *WCHB1-41_Other*, *Eggerthellaceae*, and *Pasteurellaceae* showed decreased abundance in the AML group.

3.2.3. Functional Analysis of Gut Microbiota Suggests Consistent Metabolic Changes with the Host

Using PICRUSt2 based on the IMG microbiome genome database, gene prediction was performed on the 16S sequencing results. The predicted results were then annotated using the MetaCyc database to obtain functional predictions for the 16S rRNA amplicon sequencing. After annotating all metabolic pathways, differences in pathway functionality between groups were analyzed using Welch's t-test and a fold change analysis, as shown in Figure S6. The PCA plot (Figure S6A) demonstrated that when using predicted pathway abundances for dimension reduction, the separation between the first and second principal components of the two groups was more pronounced compared to using OTU abundances. This indicates that there are differences in bacterial genome composition and metabolic functionality among different taxa, and these differences are better manifested at the functional level than at the species level.

The predicted analysis using PICRUSt2 revealed that the 16S rRNA gene sequences of bacteria in the samples corresponded to a total of 330 metabolic pathways. The statistical analysis identified 11 significantly different metabolic pathways (Figure S6B) between the two groups. Overall, these differential metabolisms involve various aspects of metabolism, including amino acid metabolism, vitamin metabolism, and carbohydrate and polysaccharide metabolism. These metabolic changes in the microbial communities are somewhat consistent with the host's metabolism.

3.3. Peptococcaceae and Campylobacteraceae were Key Families Related to Carnosine Metabolism

To further investigate the role of gut microbiota in AML-related metabolic changes, we first utilized the MetOrigin website to identify the sources of detected metabolites in mouse samples. The results revealed that out of all the detected metabolites, 7 were independently metabolized by the host, 14 were independently metabolized by the microbiota, and 102 were co-metabolized by both the host and the microbiota (Figure S7). These findings clearly demonstrated the significant role of gut microbiota in host metabolism, although the underlying correlations require further investigation.

In order to gain a deeper understanding of the association between gut microbiota and metabolites in mice, we conducted a Spearman correlation analysis to determine the correlation coefficients between differentially abundant microbial taxa at the family level and differentially abundant metabolites across various sample types. Based on the pathway associations between metabolites, we constructed a metabolite–microbiota network, as shown in Figure 6. It is worth noting that there was a significant negative correlation between serum Carnosine levels and the abundance of *Peptococcaceae* and *Campylobacteraceae*, and in the AML group, Carnosine levels increased while the abundance of these two gut microbial taxa decreased compared to the control group. In fecal samples, there was a significant positive correlation between Indole levels and the abundance of *Coriobacteriales Incertae Sedis* and *Atopobiaceae*, and in the AML group, both Indole levels and the abundance of these two microbial taxa decreased. These relationships might play an important role in maintaining the homeostasis of the mouse gut microbiota.

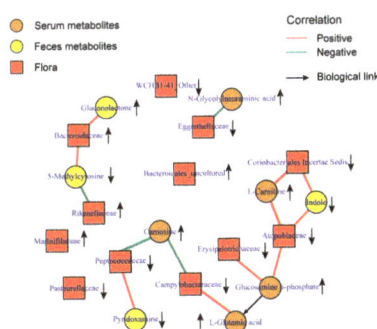

Figure 6. Association between differential metabolites and microbial communities. Network diagram shows the association between differential metabolites and differential microbial communities in mice. Squares represent microbial communities, circles represent metabolites, and the color of the circles represents the source of the differential metabolites. The lines connecting microbial communities and metabolites represent their correlation, with red indicating positive correlation and green indicating negative correlation. Upward arrows indicate an increase in the level of metabolites or microbial communities in the AML group, while downward arrows indicate a decrease.

4. Discussion

The metabolic profile of various tissues in an organism reflects its activity processes and outcomes, providing valuable information. Given the significant impact of the gut microbiota on host health and their ability to produce metabolites through their large genome [25,26], it is crucial to investigate changes in host metabolism and gut microbiota composition, as well as their interrelationships with host diseases. AML is a malignant disease with poor outcomes, and current treatment methods still require significant improvements to encompass a broader range of patients [27]. With the continuous advancement of science, technology, and the field of medicine, there is an increasing focus on the prevention and intervention of such serious diseases. This study utilized metabolomics and microbiome sequencing to uncover key host metabolism and gut microbiota in AML.

The metabolic profiles of serum and feces in mice are indicative of the metabolism of the host and gut microbiota, respectively. Significant differences in the serum and fecal metabolomes were observed between the AML group and control group of mice, and the PLS-DA model successfully distinguished between the two sample groups. These findings suggested a potential link between AML and alterations in both host and gut microbiota metabolism. Furthermore, our cross-species comparisons have revealed that AML also affects human blood metabolism, exhibiting similarities to the metabolic changes observed in mice. Notably, AML-related metabolic changes primarily involved amino acid metabolism and glucose metabolism.

In terms of amino acid metabolism, we observed a significant increase in Carnosine levels in the blood of AML mice and patients with AML. Carnosine is a dipeptide composed of β-alanine and Histidine. A study that constructed a cancer cachexia diagnostic model through metabolomics demonstrated that Carnosine, as a potential biomarker, was increased in cachexia patients [28]. Additionally, elevated levels of fecal L-Histidine, a downstream metabolite of Carnosine, were also observed in AML mice. In the Celastrol reversal model, a decrease in fecal L-Histidine levels with the dose was found. These findings suggested that the Carnosine–Histidine metabolism pathway might have a potential role in the occurrence and development of AML. Furthermore, L-Histidine serves as a donor of one-carbon (1C) units, which cancer cells could utilize for nucleotide synthesis, methylation modifications, and the generation of reducing cofactors. Upregulation of 1C-unit metabolism might provide metabolic flexibility to cancer cells, allowing them to sustain proliferation under stress conditions [29]. However, the levels of L-Histidine returned to control group levels under the reversal effect of Celastrol. Therefore, L-Histidine might play a role as a pro-cancer factor in AML. Moreover, an analysis of AML-related metabolic genes in the population had also shown that amino acid metabolism, including Histidine, was more active in the high-risk subgroup [30]. This is consistent with our study, indicating that changes in amino acid metabolism, represented by the Carnosine–Histidine–1C-unit pathway, might play a crucial role in AML.

Our research findings suggested that the majority of metabolites detected in the mouse samples were produced through the combined metabolism of the host and the microbiota (Figure S7). We specifically focused on metabolites and microbiota associated with the AML disease state, as there is a close relationship between them. Through a correlation analysis, we observed a significant negative correlation between the key metabolite Carnosine mentioned earlier and the families *Peptococcaceae* and *Campylobacteraceae*. The abundance of these two gut microbial taxa decreased compared to the control group. *Peptococcaceae* and *Campylobacteraceae* are also the common bacteria shared by gut microbiota of mice and humans [31,32]. The family *Pedococcaceae* is classified under the phylum *Firmicutes*, which was found to exhibit a decreasing trend in the gut (Figure 5). Consistent with our findings, previous population studies had also reported a decrease in the abundance of *Firmicutes* in the gut of patients with AML [33]. Many bacteria belonging to the phylum *Firmicutes*, which have the potential to act as probiotics [34], and playing a role in alleviating intestinal inflammation and combating specific microorganisms, were significantly reduced in the AML group. Another bacterium, *Campylobacteraceae*, which was related to Carnosine and exhibited decreased abundance, belongs to the phylum *Epsilonbacteraeota* and is derived from the former class ε-*Proteobacteria* [35]. It is a native bacterium in the human gut. The microbiota that reside in the human gut for an extended period and coexist with the host play a role in maintaining the stability of the gut microbiome.

Our analysis also revealed a decrease in *Coriobacteriales Incertae Sedis* and *Atopobiaceae*, which belong to *Actinobacteria*, a Gram-positive bacterium, and its associated amino acid metabolite Indole. Indole, a tryptophan degradation product of bacteria, exhibits various biological activities in the human body, including the regulation of the immune system [36], inhibition of inflammation [37], and modulation of tumor cell growth and apoptosis. We observed a significant decrease in Indole levels in mouse feces. The reduction in indole levels might weaken immune surveillance ability, rendering leukemia cells more susceptible to evading the immune system's attack. Additionally, decreased Indole levels might exacerbate intestinal inflammation, thereby accelerating the development of AML.

In terms of metabolism, we observed an increase in the concentrations of Glucose 6-phosphate and Glucosamine 6-phosphate in both human and mice models. Glucose 6-phosphate is a primary product of glycolysis and antioxidant pathways, and its elevation might reflect enhanced activity of the glycolytic pathway to generate more ATP to meet the energy demands of cancer cells. Additionally, Glucose 6-phosphate could participate in the pentose phosphate pathway to produce NADPH, which is an important component in maintaining the reducing capacity of glutathione and involved in scavenging free radicals and inhibiting lipid peroxidation to counteract the oxidative environment of cancer cells. Glucosamine 6-phosphate is an intermediate product in the metabolism of amino sugars. Its synthesis is the initial step in the hexosamine biosynthetic pathway (HBP). The final product of this pathway is UDP-GlcNAc, which plays a role in the post-translational modification of intracellular proteins involved in regulating nutrient sensing and stress response [38]. UDP-GlcNAc is the donor sugar for O-GlcNAcylation, and studies had shown that increased O-GlcNAcylation could promote the progression of hepatocellular carcinoma [39]. In addition, the synthesis enzyme of Glucosamine 6-phosphate, Glucosamine-6-phosphate synthetase, is also considered a potential carcinofetal marker [40] and a promising target for antimicrobial and antidiabetic drugs [41]. Therefore, the alterations in AML glucose metabolism primarily manifest as enhanced glycolysis, antioxidant activity, and glycosylation modifications. These changes confer protective and promotive effects on cancer cells, enhancing their metastasis and dissemination. These alterations serve as potential preventive and therapeutic targets.

5. Conclusions

This study investigated alterations in the levels of multiple metabolites in human and mouse tissue samples under conditions of AML. Through cross-species validation in mice and humans, as well as reversal validation using Celastrol, we identified the potential involvement of the Carnosine–Histidine metabolic pathway in the development and progression of AML. Importantly, the key metabolite Carnosine might be affected by the gut microbiota including families *Peptococcaceae* and *Campylobacteraceae*. These findings provide a deeper understanding of AML from the perspective of metabolite–gut-microbiota interactions.

Supplementary Materials: The following supporting information can be downloaded at: https://www.mdpi.com/article/10.3390/toxics12010014/s1, Figure S1: Bar graph of mouse body weight during grouping, $p > 0.05$. Figure S2: Differential metabolite heatmap in mouse samples. Figure S3: Differential metabolite heatmap in human samples. Figure S4: Hierarchical sample circle plot of gut microbiota in AML group mice; Figure S5: Hierarchical sample circle plot of gut microbiota in control group mice; Figure S6: Picrust2 analysis results of mouse gut microbiota. (A) PCA score plots of predicted pathway abundance. The top left plot shows the first principal component (PC1) and the second principal component (PC2), the top right plot shows PC2 and the third principal component (PC3), and the bottom left plot shows PC1 and PC3. Each point represents a sample, color-coded by group. (B) Extended error bar plots of pathway, showing only items with p-value < 0.05 and fold change > 2, color-coded by group. Figure S7: Bar chart showing the sources of all detected metabolites in the mouse samples; Table S1: Quality information for amplified sub-sequence raw data and clean data; Table S2: Comparison of five alpha-diversity indices between AML group and control group.

Author Contributions: Conceptualization, X.Z. and M.C.; methodology, X.Z. and M.C.; software, M.C.; validation, Y.X., M.T., and Y.J.; formal analysis, B.W.; investigation, B.W. and S.W.; resources, T.Z., Y.H., K.Z., X.Z., and M.C.; data curation, Y.J. and L.H.; writing—original draft preparation, B.W. and Y.J.; writing—review and editing, X.Z. and M.C.; visualization, B.W. and L.H.; supervision, X.Z. and M.C.; project administration, X.Z. and M.C.; funding acquisition, M.C. All authors have read and agreed to the published version of the manuscript.

Funding: This research was funded by China National Key Research & Development (R&D) Plan (grant number: 2021YFC2700600), Natural Science Foundation of China (grant numbers: 82273668,

81872650), Excellent Young Backbone Teachers of "Qinglan Project" of Colleges and Universities in Jiangsu Province, the Wuxi City Health Committee top-notch talent (grant number: BJ2020077), and the Priority Academic Program Development of Jiangsu Higher Education Institutions (PAPD).

Institutional Review Board Statement: The study was conducted in accordance with the Declaration of Helsinki and approved by the Institutional Review Board of Jiangsu Provincial Hospital and Nanyang First People's Hospital. The animal study protocol was approved by the Institutional Review Board of Nanjing Medical University, 2014-SRFA-130, 4 March 2014.

Informed Consent Statement: Informed consent was obtained from all subjects involved in the study.

Data Availability Statement: Data are contained within the article or Supplementary Material.

Acknowledgments: We would like to thank all the participants that contributed to the human population study.

Conflicts of Interest: The authors declare no conflicts of interest.

References

1. Döhner, H.; Weisdorf, D.J.; Bloomfield, C.D. Acute Myeloid Leukemia. *N. Engl. J. Med.* **2015**, *373*, 1136–1152. [CrossRef] [PubMed]
2. Stein, E.M.; Tallman, M.S. Emerging therapeutic drugs for AML. *Blood* **2016**, *127*, 71–78. [CrossRef] [PubMed]
3. De Kouchkovsky, I.; Abdul-Hay, M. Acute myeloid leukemia: A comprehensive review and 2016 update. *Blood Cancer J.* **2016**, *6*, e441. [CrossRef] [PubMed]
4. Stockard, B.; Garrett, T.; Guingab-Cagmat, J.; Meshinchi, S.; Lamba, J. Distinct Metabolic features differentiating FLT3-ITD AML from FLT3-WT childhood Acute Myeloid Leukemia. *Sci. Rep.* **2018**, *8*, 5534. [CrossRef]
5. Wang, Y.; Zhang, L.; Chen, W.-L.; Wang, J.-H.; Li, N.; Li, J.-M.; Mi, J.-Q.; Zhang, W.-N.; Li, Y.; Wu, S.-F.; et al. Rapid diagnosis and prognosis of de novo acute myeloid leukemia by serum metabonomic analysis. *J. Proteome Res.* **2013**, *12*, 4393–4401. [CrossRef] [PubMed]
6. Musharraf, S.G.; Siddiqui, A.J.; Shamsi, T.; Choudhary, M.I.; Rahman, A.-U. Serum metabonomics of acute leukemia using nuclear magnetic resonance spectroscopy. *Sci. Rep.* **2016**, *6*, 30693. [CrossRef] [PubMed]
7. Yu, Z.; Kastenmüller, G.; He, Y.; Belcredi, P.; Möller, G.; Prehn, C.; Mendes, J.; Wahl, S.; Roemisch-Margl, W.; Ceglarek, U.; et al. Differences between human plasma and serum metabolite profiles. *PLoS ONE* **2011**, *6*, e21230. [CrossRef]
8. Paglia, G.; Del Greco, F.M.; Sigurdsson, B.B.; Rainer, J.; Volani, C.; Hicks, A.A.; Pramstaller, P.P.; Smarason, S.V. Influence of collection tubes during quantitative targeted metabolomics studies in human blood samples. *Clin. Chim. Acta* **2018**, *486*, 320–328. [CrossRef]
9. Uttarkar, S.; Dassé, E.; Coulibaly, A.; Steinmann, S.; Jakobs, A.; Schomburg, C.; Trentmann, A.; Jose, J.; Schlenke, P.; Berdel, W.E.; et al. Targeting acute myeloid leukemia with a small molecule inhibitor of the Myb/p300 interaction. *Blood* **2016**, *127*, 1173–1182. [CrossRef]
10. Salvatori, S.; Marafini, I.; Laudisi, F.; Monteleone, G.; Stolfi, C. Helicobacter pylori and Gastric Cancer: Pathogenetic Mechanisms. *Int. J. Mol. Sci.* **2023**, *24*, 2895. [CrossRef]
11. Chen, S.; Zhang, L.; Li, M.; Zhang, Y.; Sun, M.; Wang, L.; Lin, J.; Cui, Y.; Chen, Q.; Jin, C.; et al. Fusobacterium nucleatum reduces METTL3-mediated m6A modification and contributes to colorectal cancer metastasis. *Nat. Commun.* **2022**, *13*, 1248. [CrossRef]
12. Theilgaard-Mönch, K. Gut microbiota sustains hematopoiesis. *Blood* **2017**, *129*, 662–663. [CrossRef] [PubMed]
13. Hakim, H.; Dallas, R.; Wolf, J.; Tang, L.; Schultz-Cherry, S.; Darling, V.; Johnson, C.; Karlsson, E.A.; Chang, T.-C.; Jeha, S.; et al. Gut Microbiome Composition Predicts Infection Risk During Chemotherapy in Children With Acute Lymphoblastic Leukemia. *Clin. Infect. Dis.* **2018**, *67*, 541–548. [CrossRef] [PubMed]
14. Wu, Z.; Huang, S.; Li, T.; Li, N.; Han, D.; Zhang, B.; Xu, Z.Z.; Zhang, S.; Pang, J.; Wang, S.; et al. Gut microbiota from green tea polyphenol-dosed mice improves intestinal epithelial homeostasis and ameliorates experimental colitis. *Microbiome* **2021**, *9*, 184. [CrossRef] [PubMed]
15. Su, X.; Gao, Y.; Yang, R. Gut Microbiota-Derived Tryptophan Metabolites Maintain Gut and Systemic Homeostasis. *Cells* **2022**, *11*, 2296. [CrossRef]
16. Gentile, C.L.; Weir, T.L. The gut microbiota at the intersection of diet and human health. *Science* **2018**, *362*, 776–780. [CrossRef]
17. Weersma, R.K.; Zhernakova, A.; Fu, J. Interaction between drugs and the gut microbiome. *Gut* **2020**, *69*, 1510–1519. [CrossRef]
18. Li, H.Y.; Zhang, J.; Sun, L.L.; Li, B.H.; Gao, H.L.; Xie, T.; Zhang, N.; Ye, Z.M. Celastrol induces apoptosis and autophagy via the ROS/JNK signaling pathway in human osteosarcoma cells: An in vitro and in vivo study. *Cell Death Dis.* **2015**, *6*, e1604. [CrossRef]
19. Yang, H.; Chen, D.; Cui, Q.C.; Yuan, X.; Dou, Q.P. Celastrol, a triterpene extracted from the Chinese "Thunder of God Vine", is a potent proteasome inhibitor and suppresses human prostate cancer growth in nude mice. *Cancer Res.* **2006**, *66*, 4758–4765. [CrossRef]

20. Zhang, H.; Lu, T.; Feng, Y.; Sun, X.; Yang, X.; Zhou, K.; Sun, R.; Wang, Y.; Wang, X.; Chen, M. A metabolomic study on the gender-dependent effects of maternal exposure to fenvalerate on neurodevelopment in offspring mice. *Sci. Total Environ.* **2020**, *707*, 136130. [CrossRef]
21. Schnizlein, M.K.; Vendrov, K.C.; Edwards, S.J.; Martens, E.C.; Young, V.B. Dietary Xanthan Gum Alters Antibiotic Efficacy against the Murine Gut Microbiota and Attenuates Clostridioides difficile Colonization. *mSphere* **2020**, *5*, e00708-19. [CrossRef] [PubMed]
22. Kohl, S.M.; Klein, M.S.; Hochrein, J.; Oefner, P.J.; Spang, R.; Gronwald, W. State-of-the art data normalization methods improve NMR-based metabolomic analysis. *Metabolomics* **2012**, *8*, 146–160. [CrossRef] [PubMed]
23. Fu, M.; Zhang, X.; Liang, Y.; Lin, S.; Qian, W.; Fan, S. Alterations in Vaginal Microbiota and Associated Metabolome in Women with Recurrent Implantation Failure. *mBio* **2020**, *11*, e03242-19. [CrossRef]
24. Li, Y.; Zhao, H.; Sun, G.; Duan, Y.; Guo, Y.; Xie, L.; Ding, X. Alterations in the gut microbiome and metabolome profiles of septic rats treated with aminophylline. *J. Transl. Med.* **2022**, *20*, 69. [CrossRef] [PubMed]
25. Visconti, A.; Le Roy, C.I.; Rosa, F.; Rossi, N.; Martin, T.C.; Mohney, R.P.; Li, W.; de Rinaldis, E.; Bell, J.T.; Venter, J.C.; et al. Interplay between the human gut microbiome and host metabolism. *Nat. Commun.* **2019**, *10*, 4505. [CrossRef] [PubMed]
26. Ma, J.; Piao, X.; Mahfuz, S.; Long, S.; Wang, J. The interaction among gut microbes, the intestinal barrier and short chain fatty acids. *Anim. Nutr.* **2022**, *9*, 159–174. [CrossRef]
27. Nair, R.; Salinas-Illarena, A.; Baldauf, H.-M. New strategies to treat AML: Novel insights into AML survival pathways and combination therapies. *Leukemia* **2021**, *35*, 299–311. [CrossRef]
28. Yang, Q.-J.; Zhao, J.-R.; Hao, J.; Li, B.; Huo, Y.; Han, Y.-L.; Wan, L.-L.; Li, J.; Huang, J.; Lu, J.; et al. Serum and urine metabolomics study reveals a distinct diagnostic model for cancer cachexia. *J. Cachexia Sarcopenia Muscle* **2018**, *9*, 71–85. [CrossRef]
29. Li, A.M.; Ducker, G.S.; Li, Y.; Seoane, J.A.; Xiao, Y.; Melemenidis, S.; Zhou, Y.; Liu, L.; Vanharanta, S.; Graves, E.E.; et al. Metabolic Profiling Reveals a Dependency of Human Metastatic Breast Cancer on Mitochondrial Serine and One-Carbon Unit Metabolism. *Mol. Cancer Res.* **2020**, *18*, 599–611. [CrossRef]
30. Zhou, H.; Wang, F.; Niu, T. Prediction of prognosis and immunotherapy response of amino acid metabolism genes in acute myeloid leukemia. *Front. Nutr.* **2022**, *9*, 1056648. [CrossRef]
31. Moon, J.M.; Finnegan, P.; Stecker, R.A.; Lee, H.; Ratliff, K.M.; Jäger, R.; Purpura, M.; Slupsky, C.M.; Marco, M.L.; Wissent, C.J.; et al. Impact of Glucosamine Supplementation on Gut Health. *Nutrients* **2021**, *13*, 2180. [CrossRef] [PubMed]
32. Liu, F.; Ma, R.; Wang, Y.; Zhang, L. The Clinical Importance of Campylobacter concisus and Other Human Hosted Campylobacter Species. *Front. Cell Infect. Microbiol.* **2018**, *8*, 243. [CrossRef] [PubMed]
33. Wang, R.; Yang, X.; Liu, J.; Zhong, F.; Zhang, C.; Chen, Y.; Sun, T.; Ji, C.; Ma, D. Gut microbiota regulates acute myeloid leukaemia via alteration of intestinal barrier function mediated by butyrate. *Nat. Commun.* **2022**, *13*, 2522. [CrossRef] [PubMed]
34. Markowiak-Kopeć, P.; Śliżewska, K. The Effect of Probiotics on the Production of Short-Chain Fatty Acids by Human Intestinal Microbiome. *Nutrients* **2020**, *12*, 1107. [CrossRef] [PubMed]
35. Waite, D.W.; Vanwonterghem, I.; Rinke, C.; Parks, D.H.; Zhang, Y.; Takai, K.; Sievert, S.M.; Simon, J.; Campbell, B.J.; Hanson, T.E.; et al. Comparative Genomic Analysis of the Class Epsilonproteobacteria and Proposed Reclassification to Epsilonbacteraeota (phyl. nov.). *Front. Microbiol.* **2017**, *8*, 682. [CrossRef]
36. Fiore, A.; Murray, P.J. Tryptophan and indole metabolism in immune regulation. *Curr. Opin. Immunol.* **2021**, *70*, 7–14. [CrossRef]
37. Rothhammer, V.; Mascanfroni, I.D.; Bunse, L.; Takenaka, M.C.; Kenison, J.E.; Mayo, L.; Chao, C.-C.; Patel, B.; Yan, R.; Blain, M.; et al. Type I interferons and microbial metabolites of tryptophan modulate astrocyte activity and central nervous system inflammation via the aryl hydrocarbon receptor. *Nat. Med.* **2016**, *22*, 586–597. [CrossRef]
38. Lam, C.; Low, J.-Y.; Tran, P.T.; Wang, H. The hexosamine biosynthetic pathway and cancer: Current knowledge and future therapeutic strategies. *Cancer Lett.* **2021**, *503*, 11–18. [CrossRef]
39. Zhou, P.; Chang, W.-Y.; Gong, D.-A.; Xia, J.; Chen, W.; Huang, L.-Y.; Liu, R.; Liu, Y.; Chen, C.; Wang, K.; et al. High dietary fructose promotes hepatocellular carcinoma progression by enhancing O-GlcNAcylation via microbiota-derived acetate. *Cell Metab.* **2023**, *35*, 1961–1975.e6. [CrossRef]
40. Tsuiki, S.; Miyagi, T. Carcinofetal alterations in glucosamine-6-phosphate synthetase. *Ann. N. Y. Acad. Sci.* **1975**, *259*, 298–306. [CrossRef]
41. Stefaniak, J.; Nowak, M.G.; Wojciechowski, M.; Milewski, S.; Skwarecki, A.S. Inhibitors of glucosamine-6-phosphate synthase as potential antimicrobials or antidiabetics—Synthesis and properties. *J. Enzyme Inhib. Med. Chem.* **2022**, *37*, 1928–1956. [CrossRef] [PubMed]

Disclaimer/Publisher's Note: The statements, opinions and data contained in all publications are solely those of the individual author(s) and contributor(s) and not of MDPI and/or the editor(s). MDPI and/or the editor(s) disclaim responsibility for any injury to people or property resulting from any ideas, methods, instructions or products referred to in the content.

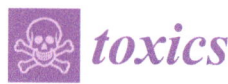

Review

Progress in Research on the Role of the Thioredoxin System in Chemical Nerve Injury

Xinwei Xu [1], Lan Zhang [1], Yuyun He [1], Cong Qi [2] and Fang Li [1,*]

[1] School of Medicine, Jiangsu University, Zhenjiang 212013, China; 2212213084@stmail.ujs.edu.cn (X.X.); 19805662010@163.com (L.Z.); 19802596761@163.com (Y.H.)
[2] Department of Pharmacy, Jurong People's Hospital, Jurong 212400, China; wsqca@163.com
* Correspondence: lfsjy@ujs.edu.cn

Abstract: (1) Background: Various factors, such as oxidative stress, mitochondrial dysfunction, tumors, inflammation, trauma, immune disorders, and neuronal toxicity, can cause nerve damage. Chemical nerve injury, which results from exposure to toxic chemicals, has garnered increasing research attention. The thioredoxin (Trx) system, comprising Trx, Trx reductase, nicotinamide adenine dinucleotide phosphate, and Trx-interacting protein (TXNIP; endogenous Trx inhibitor), helps maintain redox homeostasis in the central nervous system. The dysregulation of this system can cause dementia, cognitive impairment, nerve conduction disorders, movement disorders, and other neurological disorders. Thus, maintaining Trx system homeostasis is crucial for preventing or treating nerve damage. (2) Objective: In this review study, we explored factors influencing the homeostasis of the Trx system and the involvement of its homeostatic imbalance in chemical nerve injury. In addition, we investigated the therapeutic potential of the Trx system-targeting active substances against chemical nerve injury. (3) Conclusions: Chemicals such as morphine, metals, and methylglyoxal interfere with the activity of TXNIP, Trx, and Trx reductase, disrupting Trx system homeostasis by affecting the phosphatidylinositol-3-kinase/protein kinase B, extracellular signal-regulated kinase, and apoptotic signaling-regulated kinase 1/p38 mitogen-activated protein kinase pathways, thereby leading to neurological disorders. Active substances such as resveratrol and lysergic acid sulfide mitigate the symptoms of chemical nerve injury by regulating the Ras/Raf1/extracellular signal-regulated kinase pathway and the miR-146a-5p/TXNIP axis. This study may guide the development of Trx-targeting modulators for treating neurological disorders and chemical nerve injuries.

Keywords: chemical nerve injury; Trx system; Trx reductase; Trx-interacting protein

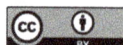

Citation: Xu, X.; Zhang, L.; He, Y.; Qi, C.; Li, F. Progress in Research on the Role of the Thioredoxin System in Chemical Nerve Injury. *Toxics* **2024**, *12*, 510. https://doi.org/10.3390/toxics12070510

Academic Editors: Michael Caudle and Robyn L. Tanguay

Received: 15 May 2024
Revised: 30 June 2024
Accepted: 4 July 2024
Published: 15 July 2024

Copyright: © 2024 by the authors. Licensee MDPI, Basel, Switzerland. This article is an open access article distributed under the terms and conditions of the Creative Commons Attribution (CC BY) license (https://creativecommons.org/licenses/by/4.0/).

1. Introduction

Nerve damage results from the disruption of nerve structure integrity and the subsequent impairment of nerve function. Tumors, inflammation, trauma, and immune disorders can damage the nervous system, leading to dementia, cognitive impairment, nerve conduction disorder, movement disorder, and nutritional disorder in the damaged area. In addition, nerve damage—central or peripheral—can lead to various disorders such as Parkinson's disease (PD), diabetic peripheral neuropathy (DPN), Alzheimer's disease (AD), and autism spectrum disorder [1]. This shows that nerve damage is widespread. As per the 2015 Global Disease Study, neurological disorders are the second leading cause of mortality, accounting for 16.8% of all deaths worldwide. Over the past 25 years, a 36% increase has been noted in the rate of mortality from neurological disorders [2].

Chemical nerve injury refers to toxic chemical-induced nerve damage. Exposure—through contact, inhalation, accidental ingestion, or environmental exposure to severe pollution—to these chemicals (e.g., metals) damages the nervous system (in both humans and animals) by disrupting normal nerve conduction. Owing to the ubiquity of chemical substances, particularly neurotoxic chemicals, increasing research attention has been paid to chemical nerve injury.

Recent evidence implicates the Trx system in the maintenance of redox homeostasis in the central and peripheral nervous systems, while its results are altered in PD [3], DPN [4], and AD [5]. Genetic and environmental factors (nutrition, metals, and toxins) are known to impact the function of the Trx system, thereby contributing to neuropsychiatric disease [6]. Chemicals such as morphine, metals, and methylglyoxal can disrupt the homeostasis of the Trx system, resulting in nerve damage. Timely regulation of the Trx system can prevent chemical nerve injury. Therefore, the concept of targeting this system for treating nerve damage has gained increased attention in the research community. Thus, we conducted this review to identify the factors influencing the homeostasis of the Trx system, assess the involvement of its homeostatic imbalance in chemical nerve injury, and investigate the therapeutic potential of Trx system-targeting active substances against chemical nerve injury.

2. Trx System

The Trx system primarily comprises different isoforms of Trx and Trx-like proteins, isoforms of Trx reductase (TrxR), nicotinamide adenine dinucleotide phosphate (NADPH; reduced coenzyme II or triphosphopyridine nucleotide), and several Trx-interacting proteins, including TXNIP and apoptotic signaling-regulated kinase 1 (ASK1). This system is a widely distributed in vivo NADPH-dependent disulfide reductase system. It is a major defense mechanism against oxidative stress and apoptosis. Enhanced TrxR activity alleviates intracellular oxidative stress and protects cellular functions [7], thereby maintaining redox homeostasis in the central nervous system. Under oxidative stress and in inflammatory conditions, nerve cells release Trx into the extracellular compartment, where Trx exerts cytoprotective effects [8]. TXNIP binds Trx within the cell. Notably, elevated levels of TXNIP result in the direct inhibition of Trx expression.

2.1. Trx

Trx is an oxidoreductase essential for oxidized proteins to recover to their reduced active form. It possesses antioxidative, pro-cell growth, protein-binding, and antiapoptotic properties. To date, Trx has been described as a cytokine for which many cell-activating effects have been observed in the micromolar range and whose cellular effects require adjuvants for activation [9]. Trx was first isolated from *Escherichia coli* in 1964 by Laurent et al. [10]. With technological advancements, Trx has been detected in many prokaryotic and eukaryotic organisms. In mammalian cells, it is categorized into Trx1, Trx2, and Trx3 (specific to spermatogonial cells). Trx1 is found in the cytoplasm and nucleus, whereas Trx2 is found exclusively in the mitochondria. Trx1 and Trx2 are the predominant isoforms of Trx in humans. Both isoforms feature two cysteines in their active sites. However, only Trx1 has three additional cysteine residues at the carboxyl terminus; these residues (-Cys62-Cys69-Cys73-) are involved in protein nitrosylation. By contrast, Trx2 has an additional 60-amino acid sequence at the amino terminus; this signal guides the transfer of Trx2 to the mitochondria (Figure 1) [11]. The active center of Trx (-Cys32-Gly-Pro-Cys35-) is responsible for its antioxidative properties. Any alteration in this sequence leads to conformational changes in Trx, destabilizes this biomolecule, and interferes with its reducing ability [12].

Trx dysfunction has been implicated in various diseases, including cancer, neurodegenerative disorders, and cardiovascular disease. Intravenous injection or overexpression of Trx protects against ischemic stroke injury and extends lifespan [13]. Mice overexpressing Trx exhibit reduced susceptibility to ischemia-induced brain injury. Trx regulates nerve growth factor-mediated signaling and PC12 cell growth. Consistent with this observation, Trx protects neurons (SH-SY5Y and PC12 cells) against the severe oxidative stress and injury induced by the PD-associated neurotoxin 1-methyl-4-phenylpyridinium ion (MPP$^+$) [14]. Tumors exhibit elevated expression levels of Trx1. Trx1 expression is upregulated in the intestines of patients with bowel cancer. Notably, a higher expression level of Trx1 is associated with a poorer prognosis [15]. In mice lacking Trx1, a reduction was noted in the level of the Trx1–ASK1 complex in the cytoplasm, but an increase was observed in the level of ASK1 phosphorylation. These findings suggest that Trx1 knockout promotes apoptosis. Mice lacking mitochondrial Trx2 exhibit markedly reduced mitochondrial adenosine triphosphate (ATP) production, diminished electron transfer chain activity, enhanced mitochondrial apoptosis, increased reactive oxygen species (ROS) production and oxidative damage, and elevated sensitivity to apoptosis [16]. Trx is essential for mammalian development; the absence of Trx1 or Trx2 proves lethal to mouse embryos [17].

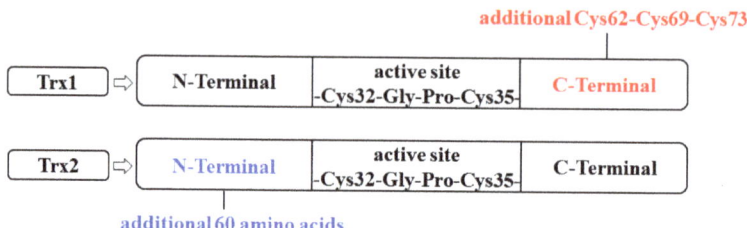

Figure 1. Structure of Trx. The active center of Trx is "-Cys32-Gly-Pro-Cys35-". Trx1 has 3 additional cysteine residues at the carboxyl terminus; Trx2 has an additional 60-amino acid sequence at the amino terminus, this signal guides the transfer of Trx2 to the mitochondria. Trx: thioredoxin; Cys: cysteine residues.

2.2. TrxR

TrxR, a major functional component of the Trx system, converts the conversion of oxidized Trx or Trx-S_2 to reduced Trx or Trx-$(SH)_2$ by using electrons from NADPH (Figure 2) [18]. Mammalian TrxR contains a selenocysteine residue in the C-terminal active site; however, low-molecular-weight prokaryotic TrxR lacks this residue. Owing to this specific nature of selenocysteine, mammalian TrxR has a distinct catalytic mechanism and a broad substrate spectrum, unlike prokaryotic TrxR. Selenocysteine is susceptible to attacks by electrophilic compounds such as 1-chloro-2,4-dinitrobenzene. In an electrophilic attack, the selenocysteine residue of mammalian TrxR alkylates with neighboring cysteine residues, which inhibits TrxR activity, and TrxR is subsequently converted into NADPH oxidase [19]. Three isoforms of TrxR can be found in the human body: TrxR1 in the cytoplasm and nucleus, TrxR2 in the mitochondria, and TrxR3 in the testicular tissue [20]. In a relevant animal study, TrxR activity persisted in the rat brain under severe selenium deficiency conditions; this observation highlights the importance of TrxR in brain function [21].

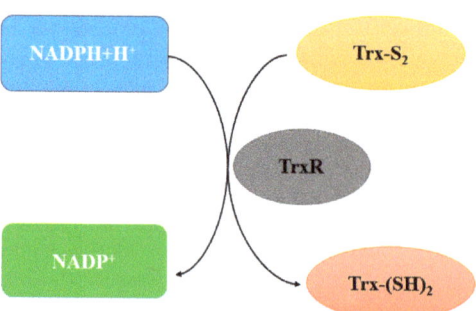

Figure 2. Trx system. TrxR converts the conversion of oxidized Trx or Trx-S_2 to reduced Trx or Trx-$(SH)_2$ by using electrons from NADPH. Trx: thioredoxin; TrxR: Trx reductase; NADPH: nicotinamide adenine dinucleotide phosphate.

TrxR is integral to various cellular functions. It participates in all signaling pathways where Trx serves as a reducing agent. Mutations or deletions in the TrxR gene have been implicated in many neurological disorders. The expression of Trx and TrxR was found to be downregulated in the substantia nigra of a mouse model of PD and the brain tissues of deceased patients with PD. Neuronal expression of this selenoprotein is essential for the development of interneurons, which prevent seizures in addition to playing other roles [22]. TrxR is also essential for growth and development; mouse embryos lacking TrxR1 and TrxR2 exhibit abnormal growth and embryonic death on gestational days 8 and 13 [23]. TrxR reduces ribonucleotides to deoxyribonucleotides and contributes to DNA repair [24]. Furthermore, TrxR-dependent pathways maintain redox homeostasis in human-induced pluripotent stem cells and their differentiated progeny cells under varying levels of oxidative stress. Inhibition of TrxR under a low oxidative load strongly affects oxidative stress resistance [25].

2.3. NADPH

NADPH has been described as the universal currency for anabolic reduction reactions [26]. Through electron transfer, NADPH facilitates the TrxR-mediated reduction of Trx-S_2 into Trx-$(SH)_2$ (Figure 2). In some cases, NADPH contributes to oxidative stress by transferring electrons to molecular oxygen via the NADPH enzyme. Overstimulation of NADPH may lead to the overproduction of ROS [27].

2.4. TXNIP

TXNIP, a regulator of oxidative stress, is involved in cell proliferation, differentiation, and apoptosis. This protein is expressed in both the cytoplasm and mitochondria. It is the sole endogenous Trx-binding protein inhibiting Trx activity, thereby inducing oxidative stress and causing neurological disorders (e.g., dementia and cognitive deficit) [28]. TXNIP expression is upregulated in neurodegenerative disorders (e.g., AD) and cerebrovascular diseases (e.g., stroke) [5]. TXNIP overexpression has been observed in the hippocampus of transgenic mice with familial AD. The inhibition of TXNIP expression reduces the hippocampal levels of inflammatory factors such as interleukin-1β [29]. Under oxidative stress conditions, TXNIP dissociates from the TXNIP–Trx complex and binds to the nucleotide-binding domain, leucine-rich-containing family, and pyrin domain-containing-3 (NLRP3) inflammasome. This binding activates the NLRP3 inflammasome, activating caspase-1, which contributes to oxidative stress and leads to apoptosis and inflammation (Figure 3) [30].

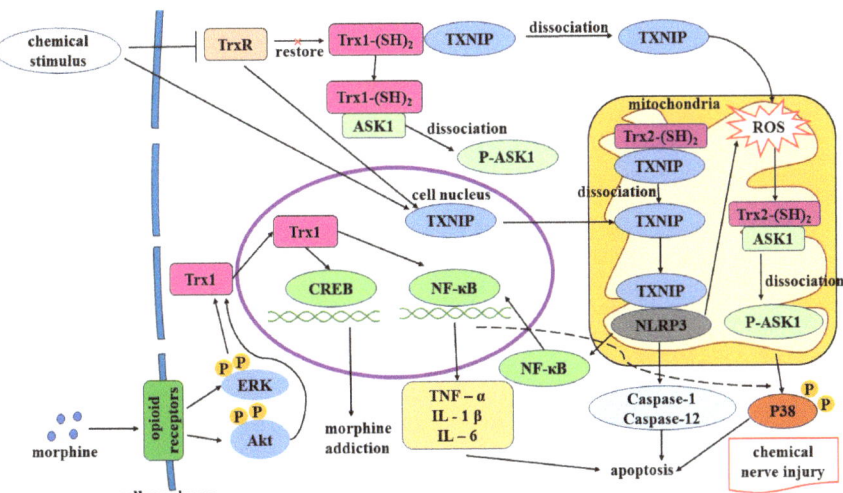

Figure 3. Hypothetical diagram of the mechanisms of neurological damage due to homeostatic derangements of the Trx system caused by chemical toxins. Chemical stimuli (like methylglyoxal and

nitrous oxide) inhibit TrxR, inhibit Trx reduction, or directly cause TXNIP to enter mitochondria. In the cytoplasm, TrxR cannot reduce Trx1, and TXNIP dissociates from the Trx1-TXNIP complex, causing cellular oxidative stress. Moreover, ASK1 separates from the Trx-ASK1 complex, resulting in apoptosis. In mitochondria, TXNIP dissociates from the Trx2-TXNIP complex and binds to NLRP3, releasing caspase-1 and -12 to cause apoptosis. At the same time, NF-κB undergoes nuclear translocation, releases inflammatory factors (TNF-α, IL-1 β, IL-6), activates p38, and ultimately causes apoptosis. The TXNIP-NLRP3 complex in mitochondria induces oxidative stress. ASK1 then separates from the Trx2-ASK1 complex, activating p38 and triggering apoptosis. Morphine phosphorylates ERK and Akt, activating the Trx1/CREB pathway, causing morphine addiction. Trx: thioredoxin; TrxR: Trx reductase; TXNIP: Trx-interacting protein; NLRP3: pyrin domain-containing-3; NF-κB: nuclear transcription factor-κB; ASK1: apoptotic signaling-regulated kinase 1; ERK: extracellular signal-regulated kinase; Akt: protein kinase B; CREB: cyclic adenosine monophosphate-responsive element-binding protein; TNF-α: tumor necrosis factor-α; IL-6: interleukin-6; IL-1β: interleukin-1β; ROS: reactive oxygen species.

3. Chemicals Damaging Nerves by Disrupting Trx System Homeostasis

3.1. Chemicals Damaging Nerves through Abnormal Trx Expression

3.1.1. Morphine-Induced Overexpression of Trx Causes Nerve Damage

Opioids, such as morphine, are the most effective analgesics for the clinical treatment of chronic pain. However, their clinical use induces various side effects, including increased susceptibility to respiratory depression, withdrawal syndrome, and reward effects inherent to opioid use. Moreover, opioids do not eliminate the risk of relapse. Dopaminergic neurons in brain regions such as the ventral tegmental area (VTA), nucleus accumbens (NAc), and hippocampus have been implicated in morphine addiction, which interferes with the long-term plasticity of the brain [31]. Luo et al. [32] demonstrated that after treatment of SH-SY5Y cells with 10 μM of morphine for 24 h, Western blot showed elevated levels of Trx1. Morphine induced the expression of Trx1 in SH-SY5Y cells by activating opioid receptors; this induction resulted in hypermotility, reward effects, and withdrawal syndrome. The nerve growth factor triggers the binding of cyclic adenosine monophosphate (cAMP)-responsive element-binding protein (CREB) to the cAMP-responsive element of the Trx promoter and subsequently mediates the nuclear translocation of Trx. The nerve growth factor induces the expression of Trx1 through the extracellular signal-regulated kinase (ERK) and cyclic adenosine monophosphate-responsive element (CRE)/CREB pathways. Trx1, an essential element of the Trx promoter, is a downstream target of the phosphatidylinositol-3-kinase (PI3K)/protein kinase B (Akt) and ERK pathways. Morphine treatment increases the levels of Akt and ERK phosphorylation by inducing the translocation of Trx1 from the cytoplasm to the nucleus; consequently, the nuclear level of Trx1 is increased. By contrast, PI3K and ERK inhibitors reduce the level of Trx1. When SH-SY5Y cells were treated with a PI3K inhibitor (LY294002) or an ERK inhibitor (PD98059) for 30 min and then co-cultured with 10 μM morphine for 24 h, a morphine-induced increase in Trx1 expression was inhibited. In the nucleus, Trx1 promotes gene transcription by enhancing the interactions of nuclear transcription factor-κB (NF-κB) and CREB with DNA or coactivators (Figure 3). Evidence suggests that NF-κB and CREB play key roles in morphine addiction [33]. Therefore, Trx1 overexpression mediates morphine addiction. Long-term morphine addiction can directly inhibit the respiratory center and affect the central nervous system, causing cerebral ischemia and hypoxia [34]. Morphine addiction can induce compulsive drug-taking behavior and high rates of relapse. When withdrawing from morphine, there are withdrawal reactions such as severe anxiety and depression. Opioid receptor antagonists are commonly used to induce morphine withdrawal [35,36].

3.1.2. Methamphetamine-Induced Inhibition of Trx Expression Causes Nerve Damage

Methamphetamine, a common psychostimulant, belongs to the family of phenylisopropylamine drugs. The misuse of methamphetamine can lead to oxidative stress, dopamine neuron toxicity, and neurological impairment. Prolonged methamphetamine abuse increases the risk of PD [37]. Yang et al. [38] revealed that methamphetamine induces apoptosis and autophagy in dopaminergic neurons through the endoplasmic reticulum stress pathway mediated by CCAAT/enhancer-binding protein homologous protein (CHOP). Methamphetamine exposure increases glutamatergic transmission (N-methyl-D-aspartate receptor subunit 2B and glutamate) and autophagy in mice, induces endoplasmic reticulum stress, upregulates the expression of CHOP, glucose-regulated protein 78 antigen, and B-cell lymphoma-2 (Bcl-2)-associated X protein (Bax; proapoptotic factor) in the VTA and NAc, and downregulates the expression of Bcl-2 (antiapoptotic factor) and caspase-12. Furthermore, methamphetamine exposure leads to a marked reduction in the expression level of Trx1 in the VTA and NAc of mice after intraperitoneal injection of methamphetamine (2.5 mg/kg) for 8 days. Similarly, this is caused by increased glutamatergic transmission in VTA and NAc by methamphetamine exposure, through activation of the CHOP-mediated endoplasmic reticulum stress signaling pathway and mitochondrial apoptosis, resulting in brain damage, rewarding effects, and central nervous system injury. Overexpression of Trx1 using transgenic technology can inhibit the methamphetamine-induced increase in glutamatergic transmission and can reduce endoplasmic reticulum stress, thereby mitigating methamphetamine-induced nerve damage.

3.2. Chemicals Damaging Nerves through the Inhibition of TrxR Activity

3.2.1. Methylglyoxal Inhibits TrxR-Induced Nerve Damage

Methylglyoxal, a metabolite found in many organisms, spontaneously reacts with biopolymers, which are rearranged to form stable advanced glycosylation end products. These end products are involved in the development of aging-related diseases such as neurodegenerative disorders, cancer, and diabetes mellitus (DM) [39].

The neuronal cell line HT22 serves as an excellent model for studying neurodegenerative disorders. Dafre et al. [40] observed increased glycosylation, inactivation of TrxR1 in the nucleus and cytoplasm, and inhibition of Trx1 expression in methylglyoxal-treated HT22 cells. The content of Trx1 in HT22 cells was decreased after treatment with 0.75 mM methylglyoxal for 24 h. Treated with the same concentration for 30 min, the content of TrxR1 decreased; however, no TrxR1 glycosylation was observed in untreated cells. There is a direct effect of methylglyoxal on TrxR1, resulting in inactivation. It was also observed that TrxR2, which is expressed in mitochondria, was reduced by 25% when HT22 cells were treated with 0.75 mM methylglyoxal for 8 h. These findings suggest that Trx and TrxR are key targets for the toxic effects of methylglyoxal. Schmitz et al. [41] demonstrated that the toxic effects of methylglyoxal on hippocampal brain slices and HT22 cells were exacerbated when TrxR activity was suppressed using 2-acetylamino-3-[4-(2-acetylamino-2-carboxyethylsulfanylthiocarbonylamino)phenylthiocarbamoylsulfanyl]propionic acid (2-AAPA) and auranofin. Treatment of SH-SY5Y cells with 625 µM methylglyoxal alone for 24 h did not cause cell death, whereas pretreatment of SH-SY5Y cells with either 10 µM 2-AAPA or 0.5 µM auranofin for 30 min, followed by treatment with 625 µM methylglyoxal for 24 h, resulted in a decrease in cell viability by about 20%. As a result, TrxR inhibition increases the toxicity of methylglyoxal, exacerbating oxidative stress in nerve cells and acting in concert with each other. Furthermore, elevated levels of methylglyoxal have been detected in the plasma of patients with DM; thus, methylglyoxal may be involved in the onset and progression of DPN [42]. The increased intracellular accumulation of methylglyoxal reduces the activity and expression of Trx2 in the mitochondria, leading to the dissociation of Trx2 and ASK1 and the activation of the ASK1/p38 mitogen-activated protein kinase (MAPK) pathway (Figure 3). These events increase the levels of mitochondrial ROS, leading to mitochondrial dysfunction, impaired insulin synthesis and secretion, and β-cell apoptosis [43].

3.2.2. Metals and Metalloids Inhibit Trx and TrxR, Inducing Nerve Damage

Metal or metal-like ions, such as gold, silver, platinum, mercury, and arsenic, are typically soft acids. The deprotonated forms of the selenol of Sec in TrxR can function as a soft base, exhibiting a high affinity for soft acids. Partial deprotonation of thiols in the N-terminal Cys-Val-Asn-Val-Gly-Cys (CVNVGC) active site transforms the active site into a site targeting soft acids. The interactions between soft bases and acids inhibit TrxR activity and convert Trx-(SH)$_2$ to Trx-S$_2$ (Figure 2), leading to DNA damage, elevated ROS levels, cell cycle changes, enzyme activity loss, and apoptosis. Compounds of gold—both Au(I) and Au(III) states—exhibit cytotoxicity. These compounds can selectively inhibit mammalian TrxR activity, block Trx reduction, oxidize Trx, and generate ROS [44]. Wang et al. [45] observed that treatment of SH-SY5Y cells with 10 µM cadmium chloride for 12 or 24 h resulted in a decrease in TrxR1 levels. Cadmium markedly suppresses endogenous TrxR1 expression and enzyme activity in neurons, reduces cell viability, and increases intracellular ROS levels and apoptosis, thereby impairing the differentiation of adult hippocampal neurons. These findings suggest that TrxR1 is a key target for cadmium [46]. A recent study claims that the expression of the TXNIP and NLRP3 proteins was upregulated after SH-SY5Y cells were treated with 10 µM cadmium chloride for 24 h. Cadmium can also induce endoplasmic reticulum stress and excess ROS, leading to neuroinflammation [47].

Auranofin, a gold-containing compound, serves as a mitochondrial toxicant. It substantially increases the severity of mechanical anomalous pain and the level of mechanical nociceptive sensitization in painful peripheral neuropathy [48]. Yumnamcha et al. [49] demonstrated that auranofin specifically inhibits TrxR1 and TrxR2, leading to mitochondrial dysfunction in retinal pigment epithelial cells, mitochondrial autophagy, and inflammatory pyroptosis. The aforementioned findings suggest that auranofin's interference with the Trx/TrxR pathway contributes to cellular oxidative stress, mitochondrial dysfunction, altered mitochondrial autophagy, lysosomal damage, and proinflammatory cell death in retinal neurodegenerative disorders. Therefore, maintaining the homeostasis of the Trx/TrxR redox system may prevent the progression of various neurodegenerative disorders.

3.3. Chemicals Damaging Nerves through the Activation of TXNIP

3.3.1. Streptozotocin-Induced Activation of TXNIP Causes Nerve Damage

Streptozotocin is a classical compound that induces DM and DPN [50]. Gao et al. [51] found that the expression of TXNIP is upregulated in the dorsal root ganglion of rats with streptozotocin-induced DM (55 mg/kg for 3 days). The researchers indicated that TXNIP binds to Trx and inhibits its function and expression, enhancing NLRP3 inflammasome activation and inducing caspase-1 activation and inflammatory factor (tumor necrosis factor-α (TNF-α)) release. These events lead to apoptosis in pancreatic β-cells and abnormal nerve conduction through the induction of oxidative stress and the inflammatory response, resulting in DPN [4].

3.3.2. Nitrous Oxide-Induced Activation of TXNIP Causes Nerve Damage

Nitrous oxide (laughing gas) is a colorless, nonirritating compound [52]. Its abuse has become a global problem. This gas is commonly used to induce anesthesia during outpatient dental procedures. However, recently, nitrous oxide has become popular among teenagers, who use it for recreational purposes [53]. Prolonged nitrous oxide abuse causes neurological damage, leading to myeloneuropathy [54] and motor axonal neuropathy [55]. cAMP is a secondary messenger essential for maintaining neuronal growth and orchestrating successful axonal regeneration. This compound phosphorylates CREB, which subsequently upregulates arginase 1 expression, increases polyamine production, and stimulates axon development. CREB regulates the body's responses to neurotrophic factors, such as brain-derived growth factors [56]. Liu et al. [57] demonstrated that nitrous oxide (70% nitrous oxide, 5% carbon dioxide, and 25% oxygen for 6 h) promotes the release of inflammatory factors by activating the TXNIP/NLRP3 pathway. This activation results in the abnormal localization of NF-κB in the nucleus, which leads to the excessive release of inflammatory factors (TNF-α, interleukin-6 (IL-6), and interleukin-1β (IL-1β)). This cascade activates p38 MAPK, thereby causing hippocampal neuronal damage (Figure 3).

4. Regulation of Trx System Homeostasis Mitigates Nerve Damage

4.1. Upregulation of Trx Transcription and Expression Mitigates Nerve Damage

4.1.1. Sulforaphane-Induced Expression of Trx Mitigates Nerve Damage

Sulforaphane, an aliphatic isothiocyanate, exhibits diverse biological activities, including antioxidative, anti-inflammatory, antitumor, antiangiogenic, and brain health-protective activities. Long-term diabetes increases the risk of diabetic retinopathy, in which Trx plays a key role [58]. Tang et al. [59] found that sulforaphane (0.5 µM for 24 h) upregulates the expression of Trx1 in the primary hippocampal neuron cells of Tubby mutant mice. In contrast to treatment with lysergic sulfanilamide alone, 4-week combination treatment with sulforaphane and PX12—an exogenous inhibitor of Trx1—markedly increases the rate of apoptosis and upregulates the expression of CHOP, Bax, phosphorylated c-Jun N-terminal kinase (JNK), and caspase-12. This is accompanied by the downregulation of Bcl-2 expression. Both the endoplasmic reticulum and mitochondria have damage similar to that observed in diabetic mice. These findings implicate Trx1 in the sulforaphane-mediated prevention of neuronal apoptosis in diabetic mice.

The Ras/Raf/ERK (MAPK) pathway, which is essential for intra- and extracellular communication, serves as a central effector in signaling cell differentiation during the normal growth and development of various tissues. This pathway regulates basic cellular functions such as cell survival, growth, and differentiation. It is necessary for the survival and maintenance of many neuronal cell populations [60]. Kong et al. [61] found that the intracardiac injection of sulforaphane (25 mg/kg for 1 day) had effects on the retinal levels of Trx in mice after 72 h of light exposure. Sulforaphane decelerates retinal degeneration by upregulating the expression of nuclear factor erythroid 2-related factor 2 and Trx in retinal nerves through the activation of the Ras/Raf1/ERK pathway, suppressing the release of cytochrome C and the activity of calpain I, regulating the rate of apoptosis, and protecting photoreceptor cells against photodamage. Sulforaphane activates ERK, which, in turn, induces the transactivation of the Ras and MAPK cascades and upregulates the expression of Trx, thereby preventing the downregulation of tubule-associated antioxidants and the death of cells.

4.1.2. N-Acetylcysteine-Induced Expression of Trx Mitigates Nerve Damage

N-acetylcysteine, a synthetic derivative of endogenous L-cysteine, has been used for the management of neurodegenerative disorders, including spinal cerebellar ataxia, PD, delayed dyskinesia, and Unverricht–Lundborg-type myoclonic epilepsy. It is also used as adjunctive therapy for various diseases, such as multiple sclerosis, amyotrophic lateral sclerosis, and AD [62]. In starved neuronal cells (SH-SY5Y), treatment with 2.5 mM N-acetylcysteine for 24 h prevents TrxR1 knockout-mediated protein hydrolysis dysfunction, reduces protein aggregation, and enhances cell survival [63]. Li et al. [64] found that in neurodegenerative disorders caused by type 1 DM, a combination of N-acetylcysteine and insulin considerably increases Trx1 and Trx2 levels compared with insulin alone. This combination enhances the body's antioxidative activity, mitigating oxidative damage in the brain. This discovery offers new insights for managing type 1 DM and its complications.

4.2. Selenium Supplementation-Induced Enhancement of TrxR1 Activity Mitigates Nerve Damage

Selenocysteine is present in at least 25 human selenoproteins that are involved in a wide range of biological functions. The active site of TrxR, a selenoprotein, contains selenocysteine residues [65]. Selenium is a key element that exhibits antioxidative and neuroprotective activities in various models of toxicity. It plays a central role in preventing and regulating a diverse range of diseases, such as cancer, diabetes, AD, psychiatric disorders, cardiovascular disease, fertility impairment, inflammation, and infections [66]. Wang et al. [46] found that selenium supplementation substantially reduces cadmium cytotoxicity in neuronal cells (SH-SY5Y) by enhancing TrxR1 activity and increasing TrxR1 levels in these cells. These changes exert antioxidative effects, reducing ROS production and apoptosis and mitigating cadmium-induced apoptosis. The researchers also found that, compared with 20 µM selenium selenite, 5 µM selenium selenite markedly enhanced TrxR1 activity in neuronal cells. This finding suggests that exposure to low concentrations of selenium can protect the nervous system. Thus, selenium may be applied in the prevention and treatment of neurodegenerative disorders, such as AD and PD, by enhancing TrxR1 activity and strengthening antioxidative effects.

4.3. Inhibition of TXNIP Mitigates Nerve Damage

4.3.1. Vitamin D_3-Induced Inhibition of TXNIP Mitigates Nerve Damage

Vitamin D_3 (cholecalciferol) serves as a pleiotropic neurosteroid in the brain. Its active form, $1,25(OH)_2D_3$, also serves as a neurosteroid, acting as both a hormone and a paracrine/autocrine agent in the brain [67]. Epidemiologic and clinical evidence suggests that a higher level of vitamin D in serum is associated with higher cognitive performance; by contrast, a low level of vitamin D is associated with AD development [68]. Lu et al. [69] reported that vitamin D_3 (233.3 U/kg body weight/week for 6 months) alleviates retinal inflammation by reducing ROS production (in the retinal vascular endothelium of rats), the activity of the TXNIP/NLRP3 pathway, the Bax/Bcl-2 ratio, retinal apoptosis, and retinal tissue damage, thereby ameliorating DM-related retinal damage. Gao et al. [51] revealed that peripheral nerve conduction velocity in patients with DM is associated with TXNIP. Vitamin D_3 can inhibit inflammation and reduce neuronal apoptosis, thereby preserving peripheral nerve function in patients with DM. The downregulation of TXNIP expression mitigates oxidative stress in patients with DPN.

4.3.2. Resveratrol-Induced Inhibition of TXNIP Expression Mitigates Nerve Damage

Resveratrol, which is derived from grape seeds, is a polyphenolic organic compound. It is easily absorbed by the gastrointestinal tract, metabolized, and excreted through the urine and feces. Han et al. [70] established an animal model of DM by feeding SD rats a high-fat, high-sugar diet and by injecting (laparoscopically) the animals with 1% streptozotocin. Then, these animals were treated with resveratrol (10 mg/kg intraperitoneally for 6 weeks). As a TXNIP inhibitor, resveratrol decreased the synthesis of NLRP3 and suppressed TXNIP expression. This increased sciatic nerve conduction velocity, mitigated pathological changes in sciatic nerve myelin, and lessened symptoms associated with sciatic nerve conduction injury. Notably, miR-146a-5p, the most abundant miRNA in exosomes [71], is involved in cell proliferation [72]. Fan et al. [73] implicated microglia-specific miR-146a-5p in the development of depression, revealing a new therapeutic target for this condition. Hu et al. [74] indicated that resveratrol ameliorates DM-induced cognitive impairment through the miR-146a-5p/TXNIP axis. In patients with DPN, miR-146a-5p increases nerve conduction velocity, mitigates morphological damage, and reduces sciatic nerve demyelination. TXNIP may be a target of miR-146a-5p because miR-146a-5p overexpression considerably downregulates the expression of TXNIP. Resveratrol upregulates the expression of miR-146a-5p, thereby inhibiting TXNIP expression and alleviating the cognitive impairment associated with diabetic encephalopathy. Together, these findings highlight the potential of resveratrol as an inhibitor of TXNIP expression.

5. Summary and Outlook

Several studies have revealed the crucial role of the Trx system in the regulation of nerve injury. Trx and TrxR serve as key targets in chemical nerve injury. In addition to these targets, TXNIP—an endogenous Trx-binding inhibitory protein—was explored in this review. We mentioned that the Trx system plays a role in the maintenance of redox homeostasis in the central and peripheral nervous systems, which is altered in neurodegenerative disorders. Studies on postmortem brains from different neurodegenerative disorders have revealed a differential modulating pattern in these disorders by the Trx system. Reduced levels of selenium and Trx1 in the brains of patients with AD are linked to the oxidation of Trx1 caused by Aβ peptides, which separates Trx1 from ASK1 and initiates apoptosis. In the brains of individuals after death, TrxR1 levels may rise compensatorily. In the brains of patients with Parkinson's disease, the neurotoxic MPP$^+$ is generated, which results in lowered levels of both Trx1 and TrxR2. The brains of patients with Parkinson's disease lack the antioxidant protein DJ-1, which prevents it from co-immunoprecipitating with free ASK1, which ultimately triggers apoptosis through the caspase-12 pathway. Patients with Huntington's disease have diminished TrxR1 and Trx1 levels due to dysregulated glutathione (GSH) redox. TXNIP is high in brain stroke patients, and the ASK1/p38 pathway is activated. TXNIP inhibitors cause thromboembolic stroke prevention [6].

We found that chemicals such as morphine, metals, and methylglyoxal induce nerve injury by inhibiting Trx and TrxR expression and upregulating TXNIP expression. Of course, the chemicals that target the Trx system to cause chemical nerve damage go far beyond what we have discussed. The anti-cancer drug paclitaxel causes peripheral neuropathy with neuropathic pain. Research says it induces sciatic nerve pain in rats by inhibiting TrxR2 [48]. Botulinum neurotoxins inhibit Trx/TrxR, leading to peripheral nerve paralysis [75]. A highglucose environment may also induce TXNIP, which causes oxidative stress in microglia and diabetic neuroinflammation [76]. Homeostatic imbalances in the Trx system caused by chemical nerve injury are mediated primarily through the PI3K/Akt, ERK, ASK1/p38 MAPK, TXNIP/NLRP3, or cAMP/CREB pathways. The results of earlier research that were referenced in this study were combined by us. We proposed the hypothesis that, when chemically stimulated, in the cytoplasm, TrxR cannot reduce Trx1, and TXNIP dissociates from the Trx1-TXNIP complex, causing cellular oxidative stress. Moreover, ASK1 separates from the Trx-ASK1 complex, resulting in apoptosis. When cells are stimulated by nitrous oxide, TXNIP in mitochondria dissociates from the Trx2-TXNIP complex and binds to NLRP3, releasing caspase-1 and -12 to cause apoptosis. At the same time, NF-κB undergoes nuclear translocation, releases inflammatory factors (TNF-α, IL-1 β, IL-6), activates p38, and ultimately causes apoptosis. When stimulated by methylglyoxal, the TXNIP-NLRP3 complex in mitochondria induces oxidative stress. ASK1 then separates from the Trx2-ASK1 complex, activating p38 and triggering apoptosis. Chemical nerve damage is the result of this (Figure 3). Researchers have identified multiple therapeutic agents for regulating these pathways—for example, sulforaphane, resveratrol, vitamin D$_3$, and selenium. Research has claimed that docosahexaenoic acid, as an indirect antioxidant, enhances the antioxidant capacity of the Trx system in nerve cells and may have a big breakthrough in neuroprotective research on AD [77]. The upregulation of endogenous Trx1 and Trx2 expression and the administration of exogenous Trx1 inducers can confer neuroprotective effects against AD through the activation of prosurvival pathways (PI3K/Akt and ERK pathways) and the suppression of oxidative stress, inflammation (TXNIP, NLRP3, and NF-κB), and apoptosis (ASK1/JNK/p38 MAPK and the caspase-1 and -12 pathways) [78]. Therefore, maintaining the homeostasis of the Trx system by upregulating Trx1 and Trx2 expression, enhancing TrxR activity, and inhibiting TXNIP may protect against chemical nerve injury. Evidence suggests that both Trx1 suppression and overexpression can lead to nerve damage, and the benefits of Trx1 are not absolute. Morphine phosphorylates ERK and Akt, activating the Trx1/CREB pathway, causing morphine addiction (Figure 3). These findings highlight the need for a practical orientation in targeting Trx1 and Trx2 for the treatment of chemical nerve injury. In conclusion, the precise molecular mechanisms underlying the homeostatic imbalance of the Trx system in chemical nerve injury remain unclear. Strategies for regulating the Trx system to treat nerve damage are in the experimental stage. In the clinical practice of the therapy of chemical nerve injury, Trx1,2 agonists, TrxR agonists, and TXNIP inhibitors may be developed. Researchers can also consider sulforaphane, resveratrol, selenium supplementation, and other substances mentioned that can modulate the homeostasis of the Trx system. Future studies should focus on the clinical applications of these strategies, facilitating the development of Trx system-targeting drugs for the treatment of chemical nerve injury.

Author Contributions: Conceptualization, investigation, writing—original draft preparation, and visualization, X.X.; validation and writing—review and editing, X.X., L.Z., Y.H., C.Q. and F.L.; supervision, L.Z. and Y.H.; project administration, F.L.; funding acquisition, C.Q. All authors have read and agreed to the published version of the manuscript.

Funding: This review was funded by the Science and Technology project of Jurong People's Hospital (FZ2022026).

Institutional Review Board Statement: Not applicable.

Informed Consent Statement: Not applicable.

Data Availability Statement: Not applicable.

Acknowledgments: The authors are grateful to Jiangsu University for providing the necessary support for this research work.

Conflicts of Interest: The authors declare no conflicts of interest.

Abbreviations

2-AAPA	2-acetylamino-3-[4-(2-acetylamino-2-carboxyethylsulfanylthiocarbonylamino)phenylthiocarbamoylsulfanyl]propionic acid
AD	Alzheimer's disease
Akt	Protein kinase B
ASK1	Apoptotic signaling-regulated kinase 1
ATP	Adenosine triphosphate
Bax	B-cell lymphoma-2-associated X protein
Bcl-2	B-cell lymphoma-2
cAMP	Cyclic adenosine monophosphate
CHOP	CCAAT/enhancer-binding protein homologous protein
CRE	Cyclic adenosine monophosphate-responsive element
CREB	Cyclic adenosine monophosphate-responsive element-binding protein
CVNVGC	-Cys-Val-Asn-Val-Gly-Cys-
DM	Diabetes mellitus
DPN	Diabetic peripheral neuropathy
ERK	Extracellular signal-regulated kinase
GSH	Glutathione
IL-1β	Interleukin-1β
IL-6	Interleukin-6
JNK	Phosphorylated c-Jun N-terminal kinase
MAPK	Mitogen-activated protein kinase
MPP+	1-methyl-4-phenylpyridinium ion
NAc	Nucleus accumbens
NADPH	Nicotinamide adenine dinucleotide phosphate
NF-κB	Nuclear transcription factor-κB
NLRP3	Pyrin domain-containing-3
PD	Parkinson's disease
PI3K	Phosphatidylinositol-3-kinase
ROS	Reactive oxygen species
TNF-α	Tumor necrosis factor-α
Trx	Thioredoxin
TrxR	Trx reductase
TXNIP	Trx-interacting protein
VTA	Ventral tegmental area

References

1. Pena, S.A.; Iyengar, R.; Eshraghi, R.S.; Bencie, N.; Mittal, J.; Aljohani, A.; Mittal, R.; Eshraghi, A.A. Gene Therapy for Neurological Disorders: Challenges and Recent Advancements. *J. Drug Target.* **2020**, *28*, 111–128. [CrossRef]
2. Gunata, M.; Parlakpinar, H.; Acet, H.A. Melatonin: A Review of Its Potential Functions and Effects on Neurological Diseases. *Rev. Neurol.* **2020**, *176*, 148–165. [CrossRef]

3. Yang, H.; Li, L.; Jiao, Y.; Zhang, Y.; Wang, Y.; Zhu, K.; Sun, C. Thioredoxin-1 Mediates Neuroprotection of Schisanhenol against MPP+-Induced Apoptosis via Suppression of ASK1-P38-NF-κB Pathway in SH-SY5Y Cells. *Sci. Rep.* **2021**, *11*, 21604. [CrossRef]
4. Vincent, A.M.; Edwards, J.L.; McLean, L.L.; Hong, Y.; Cerri, F.; Lopez, I.; Quattrini, A.; Feldman, E.L. Mitochondrial Biogenesis and Fission in Axons in Cell Culture and Animal Models of Diabetic Neuropathy. *Acta Neuropathol.* **2010**, *120*, 477–489. [CrossRef]
5. Ishrat, T.; Mohamed, I.N.; Pillai, B.; Soliman, S.; Fouda, A.Y.; Ergul, A.; El-Remessy, A.B.; Fagan, S.C. Thioredoxin-Interacting Protein: A Novel Target for Neuroprotection in Experimental Thromboembolic Stroke in Mice. *Mol. Neurobiol.* **2015**, *51*, 766–778. [CrossRef]
6. Bjørklund, G.; Zou, L.; Peana, M.; Chasapis, C.T.; Hangan, T.; Lu, J.; Maes, M. The Role of the Thioredoxin System in Brain Diseases. *Antioxidants* **2022**, *11*, 2161. [CrossRef] [PubMed]
7. Mohamed, I.N.; Hafez, S.S.; Fairaq, A.; Ergul, A.; Imig, J.D.; El-Remessy, A.B. Thioredoxin-Interacting Protein Is Required for Endothelial NLRP3 Inflammasome Activation and Cell Death in a Rat Model of High-Fat Diet. *Diabetologia* **2014**, *57*, 413–423. [CrossRef] [PubMed]
8. Mahmood, D.F.D.; Abderrazak, A.; El Hadri, K.; Simmet, T.; Rouis, M. The Thioredoxin System as a Therapeutic Target in Human Health and Disease. *Antioxid. Redox Signal.* **2013**, *19*, 1266–1303. [CrossRef] [PubMed]
9. Pekkari, K.; Holmgren, A. Truncated Thioredoxin: Physiological Functions and Mechanism. *Antioxid. Redox Signal.* **2004**, *6*, 53–61. [CrossRef]
10. Laurent, T.C.; Moore, E.C.; Reichard, P. Enzymatic Synthesis of Deoxyribonucleotides. IV. Isolation and Characterization of Thioredoxin, the Hydrogen Donor from *Escherichia coli* B. *J. Biol. Chem.* **1964**, *239*, 3436–3444. [CrossRef]
11. Xinastle-Castillo, L.O.; Landa, A. Physiological and Modulatory Role of Thioredoxins in the Cellular Function. *Open Med.* **2022**, *17*, 2021–2035. [CrossRef] [PubMed]
12. Jastrząb, A.; Skrzydlewska, E. Thioredoxin-Dependent System. Application of Inhibitors. *J. Enzym. Inhib. Med. Chem.* **2021**, *36*, 362–371. [CrossRef] [PubMed]
13. Nasoohi, S.; Ismael, S.; Ishrat, T. Thioredoxin-Interacting Protein (TXNIP) in Cerebrovascular and Neurodegenerative Diseases: Regulation and Implication. *Mol. Neurobiol.* **2018**, *55*, 7900–7920. [CrossRef] [PubMed]
14. Chiueh, C.; Lee, S.; Andoh, T.; Murphy, D. Induction of Antioxidative and Antiapoptotic Thioredoxin Supports Neuroprotective Hypothesis of Estrogen. *Endocrine* **2003**, *21*, 27–31. [CrossRef] [PubMed]
15. Noike, T.; Miwa, S.; Soeda, J.; Kobayashi, A.; Miyagawa, S. Increased Expression of Thioredoxin-1, Vascular Endothelial Growth Factor, and Redox Factor-1 Is Associated with Poor Prognosis in Patients with Liver Metastasis from Colorectal Cancer. *Hum. Pathol.* **2008**, *39*, 201–208. [CrossRef] [PubMed]
16. Roman, M.G.; Flores, L.C.; Cunningham, G.M.; Cheng, C.; Allen, C.; Hubbard, G.B.; Bai, Y.; Saunders, T.L.; Ikeno, Y. Thioredoxin and Aging: What Have We Learned from the Survival Studies? *Aging Pathobiol. Ther.* **2020**, *2*, 126–133. [CrossRef] [PubMed]
17. Oberacker, T.; Kraft, L.; Schanz, M.; Latus, J.; Schricker, S. The Importance of Thioredoxin-1 in Health and Disease. *Antioxidants* **2023**, *12*, 1078. [CrossRef]
18. Arnér, E.S.J.; Holmgren, A. Physiological Functions of Thioredoxin and Thioredoxin Reductase. *Eur. J. Biochem.* **2000**, *267*, 6102–6109. [CrossRef] [PubMed]
19. Ren, X.; Zou, L.; Lu, J.; Holmgren, A. Selenocysteine in Mammalian Thioredoxin Reductase and Application of Ebselen as a Therapeutic. *Free. Radic. Biol. Med.* **2018**, *127*, 238–247. [CrossRef]
20. Zhang, J.; Li, X.; Han, X.; Liu, R.; Fang, J. Targeting the Thioredoxin System for Cancer Therapy. *Trends Pharmacol. Sci.* **2017**, *38*, 794–808. [CrossRef]
21. Ren, X.; Zou, L.; Zhang, X.; Branco, V.; Wang, J.; Carvalho, C.; Holmgren, A.; Lu, J. Redox Signaling Mediated by Thioredoxin and Glutathione Systems in the Central Nervous System. *Antioxid. Redox Signal.* **2017**, *27*, 989–1010. [CrossRef] [PubMed]
22. Wirth, E.K.; Conrad, M.; Winterer, J.; Wozny, C.; Carlson, B.A.; Roth, S.; Schmitz, D.; Bornkamm, G.W.; Coppola, V.; Tessarollo, L.; et al. Neuronal Selenoprotein Expression Is Required for Interneuron Development and Prevents Seizures and Neurodegeneration. *FASEB J.* **2010**, *24*, 844–852. [CrossRef] [PubMed]
23. Leonardi, A.; Evke, S.; Lee, M.; Melendez, J.A.; Begley, T.J. Epitranscriptomic Systems Regulate the Translation of Reactive Oxygen Species Detoxifying and Disease Linked Selenoproteins. *Free. Radic. Biol. Med.* **2019**, *143*, 573–593. [CrossRef] [PubMed]
24. Maqbool, I.; Ponniresan, V.K.; Govindasamy, K.; Prasad, N.R. Understanding the Survival Mechanisms of Deinococcus Radiodurans against Oxidative Stress by Targeting Thioredoxin Reductase Redox System. *Arch. Microbiol.* **2020**, *202*, 2355–2366. [CrossRef] [PubMed]
25. Ivanova, J.; Guriev, N.; Pugovkina, N.; Lyublinskaya, O. Inhibition of Thioredoxin Reductase Activity Reduces the Antioxidant Defense Capacity of Human Pluripotent Stem Cells under Conditions of Mild but Not Severe Oxidative Stress. *Biochem. Biophys. Res. Commun.* **2023**, *642*, 137–144. [CrossRef] [PubMed]
26. Miller, C.G.; Holmgren, A.; Arnér, E.S.J.; Schmidt, E.E. NADPH-Dependent and -Independent Disulfide Reductase Systems. *Free. Radic. Biol. Med.* **2018**, *127*, 248–261. [CrossRef] [PubMed]
27. Yang, F.; Gao, W.; Fan, C.; Yuan, Y.; Ma, Q.; Li, Y.; Tang, M. NAD/NADP and the Role in Neurodegenerative Diseases by Mediating Oxidative Stress Molecular neurobiology. *Prog. Mod. Biomed.* **2018**, *18*, 4382–4385+4381. [CrossRef]
28. Zhang, J.; Liu, L.; Zhang, Y.; Yuan, Y.; Miao, Z.; Lu, K.; Zhang, X.; Ni, R.; Zhang, H.; Zhao, Y.; et al. ChemR23 Signaling Ameliorates Cognitive Impairments in Diabetic Mice via Dampening Oxidative Stress and NLRP3 Inflammasome Activation. *Redox Biol.* **2022**, *58*, 102554. [CrossRef]

29. Sbai, O.; Djelloul, M.; Auletta, A.; Ieraci, A.; Vascotto, C.; Perrone, L. AGE-TXNIP Axis Drives Inflammation in Alzheimer's by Targeting Aβ to Mitochondria in Microglia. *Cell Death Dis.* **2022**, *13*, 302. [CrossRef]
30. Sun, X.; Jiao, X.; Ma, Y.; Liu, Y.; Zhang, L.; He, Y.; Chen, Y. Trimethylamine N-Oxide Induces Inflammation and Endothelial Dysfunction in Human Umbilical Vein Endothelial Cells via Activating ROS-TXNIP-NLRP3 Inflammasome. *Biochem. Biophys. Res. Commun.* **2016**, *481*, 63–70. [CrossRef]
31. Jiang, C.; Wang, X.; Le, Q.; Liu, P.; Liu, C.; Wang, Z.; He, G.; Zheng, P.; Wang, F.; Ma, L. Morphine Coordinates SST and PV Interneurons in the Prelimbic Cortex to Disinhibit Pyramidal Neurons and Enhance Reward. *Mol. Psychiatry* **2021**, *26*, 1178–1193. [CrossRef] [PubMed]
32. Luo, F.-C.; Feng, Y.-M.; Zhao, L.; Li, K.; Wang, S.-D.; Song, J.-Y.; Bai, J. Thioredoxin-1 Expression Regulated by Morphine in SH-SY5Y Cells. *Neurosci. Lett.* **2012**, *523*, 50–55. [CrossRef] [PubMed]
33. Yang, J.; Yu, J.; Jia, X.; Zhu, W.; Zhao, L.; Li, S.; Xu, C.; Yang, C.; Wu, P.; Lu, L. Inhibition of Nuclear Factor-κB Impairs Reconsolidation of Morphine Reward Memory in Rats. *Behav. Brain Res.* **2011**, *216*, 592–596. [CrossRef] [PubMed]
34. Liu, J.; Yi, S.; Shi, W.; Zhang, G.; Wang, S.; Qi, Q.; Cong, B.; Li, Y. The Pathology of Morphine-Inhibited Nerve Repair and Morphine-Induced Nerve Damage Is Mediated via Endoplasmic Reticulum Stress. *Front. Neurosci.* **2021**, *15*, 618190. [CrossRef]
35. Listos, J.; Łupina, M.; Talarek, S.; Mazur, A.; Orzelska-Górka, J.; Kotlińska, J. The Mechanisms Involved in Morphine Addiction: An Overview. *Int. J. Mol. Sci.* **2019**, *20*, 4302. [CrossRef] [PubMed]
36. Ye, J.; Yang, Z.; Li, C.; Cai, M.; Zhou, D.; Zhang, Q.; Wei, Y.; Wang, T.; Liu, Y. NF-κB Signaling and Vesicle Transport Are Correlated with the Reactivation of the Memory Trace of Morphine Dependence. *Diagn. Pathol.* **2014**, *9*, 142. [CrossRef] [PubMed]
37. Qiao, H.-H.; Zhu, L.-N.; Wang, Y.; Hui, J.-L.; Xie, W.-B.; Liu, C.; Chen, L.; Qiu, P.-M. Implications of Alpha-Synuclein Nitration at Tyrosine 39 in Methamphetamine-Induced Neurotoxicity in Vitro and in Vivo. *Neural Regen. Res.* **2019**, *14*, 319–327. [CrossRef] [PubMed]
38. Yang, L.; Guo, N.; Fan, W.; Ni, C.; Huang, M.; Bai, L.; Zhang, L.; Zhang, X.; Wen, Y.; Li, Y.; et al. Thioredoxin-1 Blocks Methamphetamine-Induced Injury in Brain through Inhibiting Endoplasmic Reticulum and Mitochondria-Mediated Apoptosis in Mice. *NeuroToxicology* **2020**, *78*, 163–169. [CrossRef]
39. Kold-Christensen, R.; Johannsen, M. Methylglyoxal Metabolism and Aging-Related Disease: Moving from Correlation toward Causation. *Trends Endocrinol. Metab.* **2020**, *31*, 81–92. [CrossRef]
40. Dafre, A.L.; Goldberg, J.; Wang, T.; Spiegel, D.A.; Maher, P. Methylglyoxal, the Foe and Friend of Glyoxalase and Trx/TrxR Systems in HT22 Nerve Cells. *Free. Radic. Biol. Med.* **2015**, *89*, 8–19. [CrossRef]
41. Schmitz, A.E.; de Souza, L.F.; dos Santos, B.; Maher, P.; Lopes, F.M.; Londero, G.F.; Klamt, F.; Dafre, A.L. Methylglyoxal-Induced Protection Response and Toxicity: Role of Glutathione Reductase and Thioredoxin Systems. *Neurotox. Res.* **2017**, *32*, 340–350. [CrossRef]
42. Lu, J.; Randell, E.; Han, Y.; Adeli, K.; Krahn, J.; Meng, Q.H. Increased Plasma Methylglyoxal Level, Inflammation, and Vascular Endothelial Dysfunction in Diabetic Nephropathy. *Clin. Biochem.* **2011**, *44*, 307–311. [CrossRef]
43. Liu, C.; Cao, B.; Zhang, Q.; Zhang, Y.; Chen, X.; Kong, X.; Dong, Y. Inhibition of Thioredoxin 2 by Intracellular Methylglyoxal Accumulation Leads to Mitochondrial Dysfunction and Apoptosis in INS-1 Cells. *Endocrine* **2020**, *68*, 103–115. [CrossRef] [PubMed]
44. Ouyang, Y.; Peng, Y.; Li, J.; Holmgren, A.; Lu, J. Modulation of Thiol-Dependent Redox System by Metal Ions via Thioredoxin and Glutaredoxin Systems. *Metallomics* **2018**, *10*, 218–228. [CrossRef]
45. Wang, H.; Abel, G.M.; Storm, D.R.; Xia, Z. Cadmium Exposure Impairs Adult Hippocampal Neurogenesis. *Toxicol. Sci.* **2019**, *171*, 501–514. [CrossRef]
46. Wang, H.; Sun, S.; Ren, Y.; Yang, R.; Guo, J.; Zong, Y.; Zhang, Q.; Zhao, J.; Zhang, W.; Xu, W.; et al. Selenite Ameliorates Cadmium-Induced Cytotoxicity Through Downregulation of ROS Levels and Upregulation of Selenoprotein Thioredoxin Reductase 1 in SH-SY5Y Cells. *Biol. Trace Elem. Res.* **2023**, *201*, 139–148. [CrossRef] [PubMed]
47. Li, Z.; Shi, Y.; Wang, Y.; Qi, H.; Chen, H.; Li, J.; Li, L. Cadmium-Induced Pyroptosis Is Mediated by PERK/TXNIP/NLRP3 Signaling in SH-SY5Y Cells. *Environ. Toxicol.* **2023**, *38*, 2219–2227. [CrossRef] [PubMed]
48. Xiao, W.H.; Bennett, G.J. Effects of Mitochondrial Poisons on the Neuropathic Pain Produced by the Chemotherapeutic Agents, Paclitaxel and Oxaliplatin. *Pain* **2012**, *153*, 704–709. [CrossRef] [PubMed]
49. Yumnamcha, T.; Devi, T.S.; Singh, L.P. Auranofin Mediates Mitochondrial Dysregulation and Inflammatory Cell Death in Human Retinal Pigment Epithelial Cells: Implications of Retinal Neurodegenerative Diseases. *Front. Neurosci.* **2019**, *13*, 1065. [CrossRef]
50. Sun, Q.; Wang, C.; Yan, B.; Shi, H.X.; Shi, Y.; Qu, L.; Liang, C.X. Expressions of Thioredoxin Interacting Protein/Nucleotide-binding Oligomerization Domain-like Receptor Protein 3 Inflammasome in the Sciatic Nerve of Streptozotocin-induced Diabetic Rats. *J. Chin. Acad. Med. Sci.* **2019**, *41*, 799–805. [CrossRef]
51. Gao, Y.; Chen, S.; Peng, M.; Wang, Z.; Ren, L.; Mu, S.; Zheng, M. Correlation Between Thioredoxin-Interacting Protein and Nerve Conduction Velocity in Patients With Type 2 Diabetes Mellitus. *Front. Neurol.* **2020**, *11*, 733. [CrossRef]
52. Xiang, Y.; Li, L.; Ma, X.; Li, S.; Xue, Y.; Yan, P.; Chen, M.; Wu, J. Recreational Nitrous Oxide Abuse: Prevalence, Neurotoxicity, and Treatment. *Neurotox. Res.* **2021**, *39*, 975–985. [CrossRef] [PubMed]
53. Lan, S.-Y.; Kuo, C.-Y.; Chou, C.-C.; Kong, S.-S.; Hung, P.-C.; Tsai, H.-Y.; Chen, Y.-C.; Lin, J.-J.; Chou, I.-J.; Lin, K.-L.; et al. Recreational Nitrous Oxide Abuse Related Subacute Combined Degeneration of the Spinal Cord in Adolescents—A Case Series and Literature Review. *Brain Dev.* **2019**, *41*, 428–435. [CrossRef] [PubMed]

54. Swart, G.; Blair, C.; Lu, Z.; Yogendran, S.; Offord, J.; Sutherland, E.; Barnes, S.; Palavra, N.; Cremer, P.; Bolitho, S.; et al. Nitrous Oxide-Induced Myeloneuropathy. *Eur. J. Neurol.* **2021**, *28*, 3938–3944. [CrossRef]
55. Berling, E.; Fargeot, G.; Aure, K.; Tran, T.H.; Kubis, N.; Lozeron, P.; Zanin, A. Nitrous Oxide-Induced Predominantly Motor Neuropathies: A Follow-up Study. *J. Neurol.* **2022**, *269*, 2720–2726. [CrossRef]
56. Akram, R.; Anwar, H.; Javed, M.S.; Rasul, A.; Imran, A.; Malik, S.A.; Raza, C.; Khan, I.U.; Sajid, F.; Iman, T.; et al. Axonal Regeneration: Underlying Molecular Mechanisms and Potential Therapeutic Targets. *Biomedicines* **2022**, *10*, 3186. [CrossRef] [PubMed]
57. Liu, W.; Zhang, G.; Sun, B.; Wang, S.; Lu, Y.; Xie, H. Activation of NLR Family, Domain of Pyrin Containing 3 Inflammasome by Nitrous Oxide through Thioredoxin-Interacting Protein to Induce Nerve Cell Injury. *Bioengineered* **2021**, *12*, 4768–4779. [CrossRef]
58. Ren, X.; Li, C.; Liu, J.; Zhang, C.; Fu, Y.; Wang, N.; Ma, H.; Lu, H.; Kong, H.; Kong, L. Thioredoxin Plays a Key Role in Retinal Neuropathy Prior to Endothelial Damage in Diabetic Mice. *Oncotarget* **2017**, *8*, 61350–61364. [CrossRef]
59. Tang, L.; Ren, X.; Han, Y.; Chen, L.; Meng, X.; Zhang, C.; Chu, H.; Kong, L.; Ma, H. Sulforaphane Attenuates Apoptosis of Hippocampal Neurons Induced by High Glucose via Regulating Endoplasmic Reticulum. *Neurochem. Int.* **2020**, *136*, 104728. [CrossRef]
60. Degirmenci, U.; Wang, M.; Hu, J. Targeting Aberrant RAS/RAF/MEK/ERK Signaling for Cancer Therapy. *Cells* **2020**, *9*, 198. [CrossRef]
61. Kong, L.; Liu, B.; Zhang, C.; Wang, B.; Wang, H.; Song, X.; Yang, Y.; Ren, X.; Yin, L.; Kong, H.; et al. The Therapeutic Potential of Sulforaphane on Light-Induced Photoreceptor Degeneration through Antiapoptosis and Antioxidant Protection. *Neurochem. Int.* **2016**, *100*, 52–61. [CrossRef]
62. Bavarsad Shahripour, R.; Harrigan, M.R.; Alexandrov, A.V. N-Acetylcysteine (NAC) in Neurological Disorders: Mechanisms of Action and Therapeutic Opportunities. *Brain Behav.* **2014**, *4*, 108–122. [CrossRef] [PubMed]
63. Nagakannan, P.; Iqbal, M.A.; Yeung, A.; Thliveris, J.A.; Rastegar, M.; Ghavami, S.; Eftekharpour, E. Perturbation of Redox Balance after Thioredoxin Reductase Deficiency Interrupts Autophagy-Lysosomal Degradation Pathway and Enhances Cell Death in Nutritionally Stressed SH-SY5Y Cells. *Free Radic. Biol. Med.* **2016**, *101*, 53–70. [CrossRef] [PubMed]
64. Li, X.; Wu, H.; Huo, H.; Ma, F.; Zhao, M.; Han, Q.; Hu, L.; Li, Y.; Zhang, H.; Pan, J.; et al. N-Acetylcysteine Combined with Insulin Alleviates the Oxidative Damage of Cerebrum via Regulating Redox Homeostasis in Type 1 Diabetic Mellitus Canine. *Life Sci.* **2022**, *308*, 120958. [CrossRef]
65. Steinbrenner, H.; Sies, H. Selenium Homeostasis and Antioxidant Selenoproteins in Brain: Implications for Disorders in the Central Nervous System. *Arch. Biochem. Biophys.* **2013**, *536*, 152–157. [CrossRef] [PubMed]
66. Barchielli, G.; Capperucci, A.; Tanini, D. The Role of Selenium in Pathologies: An Updated Review. *Antioxidants* **2022**, *11*, 251. [CrossRef]
67. Landel, V.; Stephan, D.; Cui, X.; Eyles, D.; Feron, F. Differential Expression of Vitamin D-Associated Enzymes and Receptors in Brain Cell Subtypes. *J. Steroid Biochem. Mol. Biol.* **2018**, *177*, 129–134. [CrossRef]
68. Lin, F.-Y.; Lin, Y.-F.; Lin, Y.-S.; Yang, C.-M.; Wang, C.-C.; Hsiao, Y.-H. Relative D3 Vitamin Deficiency and Consequent Cognitive Impairment in an Animal Model of Alzheimer's Disease: Potential Involvement of Collapsin Response Mediator Protein-2. *Neuropharmacology* **2020**, *164*, 107910. [CrossRef] [PubMed]
69. Lu, L.; Lu, Q.; Chen, W.; Li, J.; Li, C.; Zheng, Z. Vitamin D3 Protects against Diabetic Retinopathy by Inhibiting High-Glucose-Induced Activation of the ROS/TXNIP/NLRP3 Inflammasome Pathway. *J. Diabetes Res.* **2018**, *2018*, 8193523. [CrossRef]
70. Han, L.; Xi, G.; Guo, N.; Guo, J.; Rong, Q. Expression and Mechanism of TXNIP/NLRP3 Inflammasome in Sciatic Nerve of Type 2 Diabetic Rats. *Dis. Markers* **2022**, *2022*, 9696303. [CrossRef]
71. Li, X.; Liao, J.; Su, X.; Li, W.; Bi, Z.; Wang, J.; Su, Q.; Huang, H.; Wei, Y.; Gao, Y.; et al. Human Urine-Derived Stem Cells Protect against Renal Ischemia/Reperfusion Injury in a Rat Model via Exosomal miR-146a-5p Which Targets IRAK1. *Theranostics* **2020**, *10*, 9561–9578. [CrossRef] [PubMed]
72. Chen, X.; Li, W.; Chen, T.; Ren, X.; Zhu, J.; Hu, F.; Luo, J.; Xing, L.; Zhou, H.; Sun, J.; et al. miR-146a-5p Promotes Epithelium Regeneration against LPS-Induced Inflammatory Injury via Targeting TAB1/TAK1/NF-κB Signaling Pathway. *Int. J. Biol. Macromol.* **2022**, *221*, 1031–1040. [CrossRef] [PubMed]
73. Fan, C.; Li, Y.; Lan, T.; Wang, W.; Long, Y.; Yu, S.Y. Microglia Secrete miR-146a-5p-Containing Exosomes to Regulate Neurogenesis in Depression. *Mol. Ther.* **2022**, *30*, 1300–1314. [CrossRef] [PubMed]
74. Hu, Y.; Zhang, Q.; Wang, J.-C.; Wang, J.; Liu, Y.; Zhu, L.-Y.; Xu, J.-X. Resveratrol Improves Diabetes-Induced Cognitive Dysfunction in Part through the miR-146a-5p/TXNIP Axis. *Kaohsiung J. Med. Sci.* **2023**, *39*, 404–415. [CrossRef] [PubMed]
75. Pirazzini, M.; Azarnia Tehran, D.; Zanetti, G.; Megighian, A.; Scorzeto, M.; Fillo, S.; Shone, C.C.; Binz, T.; Rossetto, O.; Lista, F.; et al. Thioredoxin and Its Reductase Are Present on Synaptic Vesicles, and Their Inhibition Prevents the Paralysis Induced by Botulinum Neurotoxins. *Cell Rep.* **2014**, *8*, 1870–1878. [CrossRef] [PubMed]
76. Iwasa, M.; Kato, H.; Iwashita, K.; Yamakage, H.; Kato, S.; Saito, S.; Ihara, M.; Nishimura, H.; Kawamoto, A.; Suganami, T.; et al. Taxifolin Suppresses Inflammatory Responses of High-Glucose-Stimulated Mouse Microglia by Attenuating the TXNIP-NLRP3 Axis. *Nutrients* **2023**, *15*, 2738. [CrossRef] [PubMed]

77. Díaz, M.; Mesa-Herrera, F.; Marín, R. DHA and Its Elaborated Modulation of Antioxidant Defenses of the Brain: Implications in Aging and AD Neurodegeneration. *Antioxidants* **2021**, *10*, 907. [CrossRef]
78. Jia, J.; Zeng, X.; Xu, G.; Wang, Z. The Potential Roles of Redox Enzymes in Alzheimer's Disease: Focus on Thioredoxin. *ASN Neuro* **2021**, *13*, 1759091421994351. [CrossRef]

Disclaimer/Publisher's Note: The statements, opinions and data contained in all publications are solely those of the individual author(s) and contributor(s) and not of MDPI and/or the editor(s). MDPI and/or the editor(s) disclaim responsibility for any injury to people or property resulting from any ideas, methods, instructions or products referred to in the content.

MDPI AG
Grosspeteranlage 5
4052 Basel
Switzerland
Tel.: +41 61 683 77 34

Toxics Editorial Office
E-mail: toxics@mdpi.com
www.mdpi.com/journal/toxics

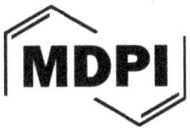

Disclaimer/Publisher's Note: The statements, opinions and data contained in all publications are solely those of the individual author(s) and contributor(s) and not of MDPI and/or the editor(s). MDPI and/or the editor(s) disclaim responsibility for any injury to people or property resulting from any ideas, methods, instructions or products referred to in the content.